DATE OF RETURN
UNLESS RECALLED BY LIBRARY

3 0 NOV 1999	
- 1 FEB 2000	- 8 APR 2002
	1 5 AUG 2002
- 4 MAY 2000	- 8 OCT 2002
3 0 MAY 2000	
2 6 JUN 2000	- 6 JAN 2003
2 2 NOV 2000	1 6 APR 2003
	1 4 JUN 03
2 2 JAN 2001	
	1 9 NOV 2003
3 1 JAN 2001	2 7 APR 2005
1 4 DEC 2001	3 0 OCT 2007
	2 8 JAN 2008

PLEASE TAKE GOOD CARE OF THIS BOOK

Physiotherapy in Stroke Management

For Churchill Livingstone:

Editorial director: Mary Law
Project editor: Dinah Thom
Copy editor: Nicky Haig
Indexer: Jill Halliday
Project Manager: Valerie Burgess
Project Controller: Pat Miller
Design Direction: Judith Wright

Physiotherapy in Stroke Management

Edited by

Marilyn A. Harrison FCSP
Physiotherapy Management Consultant,
East Bridgford, Nottinghamshire, UK

*On behalf of the World Confederation of Physical Therapy-Europe
and the Danish Physiotherapy Association*

Foreword by

Robert A. Rustad MNFF PT MPH
Chairman of the European Region of the
World Confederation for Physical Therapy-Europe

CHURCHILL LIVINGSTONE
EDINBURGH HONG KONG LONDON MADRID MELBOURNE NEW YORK AND
TOKYO 1995

CHURCHILL LIVINGSTONE
Medical Division of Pearson Professional Limited

Distributed in the United States of America by Churchill
Livingstone Inc., 650 Avenue of the Americas, New York,
N. Y. 10011, and by associated companies, branches and
representatives throughout the world.

First published 1995

ISBN 0-443-05228-X

British Library Cataloguing in Publication Data
A catalogue record for this book is available from the British
Library.

Library of Congress Cataloging in Publication Data
A catalog record for this book is available from the Library of
Congress.

The
publisher's
policy is to use
paper manufactured
from sustainable forests

Produced by Longman Singapore Publishers (Pte) Ltd.
Printed in Singapore

Contents

Foreword

The first Congress of WCPT-Europe was a result of several years of planning and preparation by many people. As early as 1990, when the European region of WCPT was established, the concept of staging European congresses within the area of physiotherapy was decided upon as a major task for the regional organization. In reviewing the first Congress I had the pleasure of stating that the event went well, that it fully answered the region's plans and expectations, and that the participants, as far as we know from their evaluations, were more than pleased with what they had had the opportunity to participate in.

The Congress gathered more than 450 participants from nearly 40 different countries. All five regions of the WCPT world organization were represented. A number of different groups of health professionals were present – medical doctors, nurses, occupational therapists and others – though most were physiotherapists and clinicians as well as teachers and researchers. For me it was a very satisfactory feeling to meet and speak with many of the participants. Their obvious devotion to their field of professional interest, and their eagerness to participate and learn more, made me proud and optimistic for the future of our profession. The World Health Organization was also represented at the congress and was, as myself, impressed by the standards of professionalism shown.

There are many people to thank for this: all the workers at the Danish Association who put their efforts into making it a good and friendly event; the Congress organizers who did a fine job; and the staff at the SAS Falconer who welcomed us all to the Congress Centre. However some people were more responsible than others for the success: Elisabeth Haase, the Secretary General of the Danish Association and the Chair of the Organizing Committee; Nina Holten, the Educational officer of the Danish Association and the Vice-chair of the Organizing Committee; and Susanne Testrup, the Chair of the Scientific Committee. All worked hard and deserve warm thanks for their contributions. Also, the then present Vice-chairman of WCPT-Europe, Elizabeth Condie, deserves honours for her major contributions to the making of the congress as a member of the Scientific

Committee. Without her persistence over many years the event would not have turned out as it did.

The Executive Committee of WCPT-Europe and the Organizing Committee decided early on that the lectures from the congress should be documented and published for the benefit of all participants and all those colleagues and others who were not able to participate at the event. It was also considered that a book would give students and others insight into the current trends in physiotherapy stroke management. Lastly, it was considered that a book from the congress was important as a way of documenting treatment procedures within such an important field of physiotherapy and as a way of 'marketing' the profession. I sincerely hope that you will agree that we have accomplished some of this in this book and that you will feel that it has been worth your time reading the chapters. The editor, Marilyn Harrison, has done a thorough job and I thank her, also, warmly for her great contribution.

Good luck with your own professional development in health care and within the field of stroke management.

R.A.R.

Contributors

Sally Ann Adams MSc MCSP SRP
Senior Physiotherapist, Elderly Care Unit, Southampton University
Hospital NHS Trust, Southampton, UK

Ann Ashburn MPhil MCSP
Course Coordinator of MSc in Rehabilitation Studies, University
Rehabilitation Research Unit, University of Southampton, UK

Frøydis Bakke
Physiotherapist, Stroke Unit, Department of Medicine, University
Hospital of Trondheim, Trondheim, Norway

Joseph C. Barbenel BDS BSc MSc PhD
Professor (Head of Unit), Bioengineering Unit, University of Strathclyde,
Glasgow, UK

Birgitta Bergman PhD RPT
Director of Research and Development, LSR, Stockholm, Sweden

Jean-Pierre Bleton
Head of the Rehabilitation Centre, Neurology Department of Professor
Jean de Recondo, Raymond Garcin Centre, Sainte-Anne Hospital, Paris,
France

Gudrun Boysen MD
Department of Neurology, Hvidovre Hospital, University of
Copenhagen, Denmark

Toril Bergerud Buene
President, The Norwegian Physiotherapist Association, Oslo, Norway

Doris Christensen RN
Nurse Consultant, Rønde, Denmark

Elizabeth Condie
Lecturer, National Centre for Training and Education in Prosthetics and
Orthotics, University of Strathclyde, Glasgow, UK

David N. Condie
Technical Director, Tayside Rehabilitation Engineering Services, Dundee
Limb Fitting Centre, Dundee, UK

Bengt Engström
Physiotherapist, Posturalis, Hasselby, Sweden

Peter Fentem
Stroke Association Professor of Stroke Medicine, Division of Stroke
Medicine (University of Nottingham), Stroke Research Unit, Nottingham
City Hospital (NHS) Trust, Nottingham, UK

Amanda C. B. Ferguson DipCOT MCSP MSc PhD
Research Physiotherapist, Bioengineering Unit, University of Strathclyde,
Glasgow, UK

Kjeld Fredens
Assistant Professor, Risskov, Denmark

Michele Gerber PT
Advanced Course Instructor BOBATH, IBITAH, Impasse Aurore,
Sierre, Switzerland

Olav Gjelsvik
Senior Physiotherapist, Department of Neurology, Haukeland University
Hospital, Bergen, Norway

Thomas Glott MD
Sunnaas Rehabilitation Centre, Nesoddtangen, Norway

Malcolm H. Granat BSc PhD
Lecturer, Bioengineering Unit, University of Strathclyde, Glasgow, UK

Esther Greve MD
Neurologist, Holstebro, Denmark

Jos Halfens PT
National Institute for Research and Postgraduate Education in Physical
Therapy/SWSF, Amersfoort, The Netherlands; Hoensbroeck
Rehabilitation Centre, Hoensbroek, The Netherlands; NDT Instructor

Marianne Heidman
Physiotherapist, Lehrkraft fur Krankengymnastik, Neu-Isenberg, Germany

Sverker Johansson RPT
Department of Physiotherapy, Erstagårdskliniken, Nacka, Sweden

Markku Kaste MD PhD
Associate Professor, Chairman, Department of Neurology, University of
Helsinki, Finland

David G. Kerwin MA BEd
Senior Lecturer, Department of Sports Sciences, Loughborough
University, Loughborough, UK

Kennedy R. Lees BSc MB ChB MD FRCP (Glasgow)
Senior Lecturer/Consultant Physician, Bioengineering Unit, University of
Strathclyde, Glasgow, UK

Ivar Lie PhD
Professor in Psychology, Institute of Psychology, University of Oslo,
Oslo, Norway

Nadina B. Lincoln BSc MSc PhD
Consultant Clinical Psychologist/Director, Stroke Research Unit,
Nottingham City Hospital (NHS) Trust, Nottingham, UK

Signe Lind RPT
Lecturer, Department of Physiotherapy, Uppsala College of Health and
Caring Sciences, University Hospital, Uppsala, Sweden

Birgitta Lindmark RPT PhD
Senior Lecturer, Department of Physiotherapy, Uppsala College of
Health and Caring Sciences, University Hospital, Uppsala, Sweden

Marianne Loid
Occupational Therapist, Bagarmossen, Sweden

Michele J. McCreadie MBA MCSP
Clinical Audit Co-ordinator, Disablement Services, Sheffield DSC,
Northern General Hospital, Sheffield, UK

Heather McKibbin MSc MCSP MMACP
Independent Physiotherapist in Clinical Practice, Lecturing and Research,
London, UK

Kenth Malmström RPT
Department of Physiotherapy, Erstagårdskliniken, Nacka, Sweden

Susan Mawson BSc (Hon) MCSP
Senior Lecturer in Physiotherapy, School of Health and Community
Studies, Sheffield Hallam University, Sheffield, UK

Douglas J. Maxwell BSc
Research Fellow, Bioengineering Unit, University of Strathclyde,
Glasgow, UK

Cheryl Mogensen DipPT BHSc(PT) MCPA
President of Mogensen Long Term Care Consulting, Burlington,
Ontario, Canada

Theo Mulder
Sint Maartenskliniek, Head of Department of Research and
Development, Nijmegen, The Netherlands; Professor of Rehabilitation
Research, University of Nijmegen, Neurological Institute, Nijmegen, The
Netherlands

Karen Nielsen
Physiotherapist, Therapiezentrum, Burgau, Germany

Bart Nienhuis
Sint Maartenskliniek, Biomedical Engineer, Department of Research and
Development, Nijmegen, The Netherlands

Francoise Odier PhD
Neuropsychologist, Neurology Department of Professor Jean de
Recondo, Raymond Garcin Centre, Sainte-Anne Hospital, Paris, France

Rob A.B. Oostendorp PhD PT MT
National Institute for Research and Postgraduate Education in Physical
Therapy/SWSF, Amersfoort, The Netherlands

Anne Parry PhD MCSP Dip TP
Reader in Physiotherapy, School of Health and Community
Studies/Health Research Centre, Sheffield Hallam University, Sheffield,
UK

John Pauwels
Sint Maartenskliniek, Experimental Psychologist, Department of Research
and Development, Nijmegen, The Netherlands

Jesus de Pedro-Cuesta MD PhD
Division of Neurology, Department of Clinical Neuroscience and Family
Medicine, Karolinska Institute, Huddinge University Hospital, Sweden

Gitte Rasmussen RPT
Centre for Rehabilitation of Brain Injury, University of Copenhagen,
Copenhagen, Denmark

C. Dorine van Ravensberg PhD PT
National Institute for Research and Postgraduate Education in Physical
Therapy/SWSF, Amersfoort, The Netherlands

Helena Sallnäs RPT
Department of Physiotherapy, Erstagårdskliniken, Nacka, Sweden

Marie-Luise Seisenbacher
Rehabilitationszentrum, Grossgmain, Austria

Martin Sheridan BSc PhD
University Lecturer, Human Performance Laboratory, Department of
Psychology, University of Hull, UK

Karen Margrethe Sødring RPT
Specialist in Physiotherapy, Neurological Rehabilitation MNFF, Clinic
for Geriatric and Rehabilitation Medicine, Ulleval University Hospital,
Oslo, Norway

Maria Thorsteinsdottir PTDip BPT MASc
Associate Professor, Department of Physiotherapy, University of Iceland,
Reykjavik, Iceland

Eric Viel PT PhD
Director of the Graduate Studies Programme, Bois-Larris BP 12
(affiliated to the University of Amiens), France

Paulette van Vliet BAppSc Msc
Research Physiotherapist, Stroke Research Unit, Nottingham City
Hospital (NHS) Trust, Nottingham, UK

Derick Wade FRCP MD
Rivermead Rehabilitation Centre, Oxford, UK

Lotta Widén Holmqvist RPT
Lecturer, Division of Neurology, Department of Clinical Neuroscience
and Family Medicine, Karolinska Institute, Huddinge University
Hospital, Sweden

Introduction

It was appropriate that the first congress held by the European Region of the World Confederation of Physical Therapy (WCPT-Europe) in 1994 should be in Copenhagen, Denmark. It was in Copenhagen, in 1951, that the inaugural meeting of WCPT took place, when representatives of 11 countries came together to discuss the merits of establishing an organization which would enable physiotherapists to promote the interchange of professional and scientific knowledge and to forge closer links between countries. Six of those 'founder' 11 countries were within Europe.

Membership of WCPT now stands at 54 countries with 11 more members elect hoping to have their full membership ratified at the 13th General Meeting in Washington DC, USA in 1995. This represents well over 200 000 physiotherapists worldwide (O'Hare 1994).

At the special meeting of WCPT held in London, UK, in 1988, the idea of regionalization was put forward by the membership and the executive committee. This was later ratified at the 12th General Meeting in London in 1991. Since that date, the structure of WCPT has been that of an international organization operating out of five regions – Africa, Asia–Western Pacific, Europe, North America–Caribbean and South America (O'Hare 1994).

Article 3.4 from the WCPT Regions' Constitution (1991) states that the aims of WCPT are:

To initiate professional activities within the region that will assist in
accomplishing the WCPT objectives to:
• encourage high standards of physical therapy education and practice
• encourage communication and exchange of information
• encourage scientific research
• encourage the development of associations of physical therapists and support
  the efforts of appropriate national organizations to improve the situation of
  physical therapists.

The countries making up WCPT-Europe had already come together between 1988 and 1991, so once ratification of the regions had occurred they were in a good position to start their regional programme of work, one aspect of which was to mount regional congresses. Danske Fysioterapeuter,

The Danish Physiotherapy Association, offered to host the inaugural congress on behalf of WCPT-Europe and thus the 1994 Congress – Physiotherapy in Stroke Management – came into being.

One of the early decisions made by the WCPT-Europe Congress Organizing Committee was that there should be a book based on papers presented by keynote and supplementary speakers at the Congress. This would give the opportunity for those present at the Congress to be reminded of those papers which they had heard and to have copies of those papers which they had been unable to hear due to the programme of concurrent sessions. The book would also provide information for those who were unable to attend the Congress. It would provide a record or bench-mark for a period in time as to 'the state of the art' of those practitioners invited to be either keynote or supplementary speakers.

The Scientific Committee selected and invited all those who subsequently presented papers. The Congress Programme was divided into sections which provided a focus on the current state of stroke management, aspects of clinical practice, measurement and research, and finally psychological aspects and management of change.

The programme is published so that it may act as an index to the chapters which follow. Almost all the speakers in Copenhagen have presented their papers for publication, and their help and co-operation is gratefully acknowledged as without their assistance there would be no book.

Most conferences which professionals, of any discipline, attend in order to keep up to date with current treatment and management, totally omit to consider the patient or client viewpoint. Usually physiotherapy conferences are no different. However, the scientific committee of this WCPT-Europe Congress recognized that the patient's viewpoint is central to any programme devised for stroke management.

So important is the requirement for physiotherapists to understand what the 'patient view' reveals, that immediately following the opening keynote paper which addressed 'A Review of Current Physiotherapy in Stroke Management', and before any subsequent speakers, 'The Patient's point of View' was presented by a speaker from Denmark, Ms Birgit Falner Jensen. This was a very personal presentation by someone with the experience of two major strokes, 12 months apart, some 10 years previously. The first stroke had resulted at the time in a severe right hemiplegia with speech impairment, the second one with a sense of loss of time and space. It took many months for the speaker to recognize and accept the disability and also the cosmetic effect which can be devastating.

It is important for physiotherapists and other medical care workers to note the immediate problem of possibly being admitted to a small hospital, where there is no stroke unit, where staff are insufficiently trained, in that they have no knowledge of such things as positioning, and where there is no possibility of being referred for physiotherapy. Fortunately in the instance described the patient was moved to the neurological ward of a large hospital 3 weeks after the onset of the stroke.

It is one thing to be ill in hospital, but for the patient who has had a stroke there are the added burdens of not knowing what is wrong and having no idea of what the future might hold. There is a great psychological burden in having a body with decreased function and not being able to communicate due to an expressive dysphasia. There is a sense of great helplessness and an immense feeling of fatigue. It is natural for an adult to react to this set of circumstances by becoming depressed.

It is important for physiotherapists to have a clear understanding of the situation, to get to know the patients and to know their backgrounds. The depression is like being in a deep hole without being able to see the light of where to go. There is a view, held by many, that it would be preferable to fight this crisis without medication as it is a natural reaction to be worked through. The depression may worsen prior to going home. The brain damage itself may cause an organic depression.

In the summing up, five clear points emerged as being of great importance to the patient:

- Physiotherapy has to be commenced early following stroke.
- If at all possible the same physiotherapist should follow the treatment through, from acute care to final rehabilitation. If that is not possible, there should then be a core physiotherapist with responsibility for overall management.
- There should be a co-ordination of physiotherapy with other therapies.
- There needs to be a much better co-ordination of the management of patients in transferring them from hospital to home. Services need to be in place in the community.
- Real rehabilitation begins when the patient arrives home.

The patient is going to want the best possible treatment as soon as possible and for as long as possible.

The observations made in the patient's viewpoint presentation were referred to many times by many speakers throughout the congress, particularly during discussion, thereby emphasizing the importance not only of the content of this contribution but also the timing of the presentation, being at the beginning of the Congress.

The presentations from keynote and supplementary speakers follow in the book as separate chapters which cover a diversity of practice.

No congress is complete without a poster exhibition and the Copenhagen Congress was no exception. A considerable number of posters (including video) were presented, and for completeness, the titles of the abstracts and the names and addresses of the presenters are listed in Appendices 1 and 2. A series of workshops were also held at the Congress and these are listed in Appendix 3.

It is hoped that not only will this book be a record of an important congress and first venture for WCPT-Europe but will also provide contact names for continued networking between therapists and all those with an interest in the management of stroke.

Nottinghamshire, 1995   M.H.

O'Hare M 1994 Information supplied by M. O'Hare, Secretary General of WCPT

Programme

Sunday 5 June 1994

The Current state of stroke management

Registration
Trade exhibition

Official opening

Welcome adresses:

Susanne Testrup, Chairman of the Scientific Committee

Inger Brøndsted, President of the Danish Association of Physiotherapists

Robert Rustad, Norway, Chairman, European Region of the World Confederation for Physical Therapy

'Kropskompagniet'
Dance Performance

Opening keynote address

A Review of current physiotherapy in stroke management
Ann Ashburn, PT, (UK)

The Patient's point of view
Birgit Falkner Jensen, (DK)

Break
Official opening of trade exhibition

Plenary sessions

The epidemiology of stroke
Gudrun Boysen, Professor Phd, (DK)

*The socioeconomics of stroke rehabilitation
Anni Ankjær Jensen, Economist (DK)

Panel discussion

Physiotherapy, stroke and society: the challenges
Ann Ashburn, Birgit Falkner, Gudrun Boysen

Welcome reception

Gala dinner at Tivoli Gardens

Monday 6 June 1994

Aspects of clinical practice

Concurrent sessions

Symptoms in adult Hemiplegia – new approaches and their therapeutic implications in the Bobath Concept
Michèle Gerber, PT, (CH)

The use of a cognitive approach in the rehabilitation of hemiplegic upper extremity
Jean-Pierre Bleton, PT, (F)

Orthotics and F.E.S. in stroke rehabilitation
Elizabeth Condie, PT, and Douglas Maxwell, BSc, (UK)

PNF in stroke rehabilitation
Marianne Heidmann, PT, (D)

Break

Concurrent sessions

'The recollection of my whole body in my brain – physiotherapy based on aspects of the affolter concept'
Karen Nielsen, PT, (D)

The motor relearning programme
Maria Thorsteinsdottir, PT, (Iceland)

Adverse neural tension
Heather Mc Kibbin, PT, (UK)

---

*No paper or abstract available

Plenary. audience participation session

How do physiotherapists view Spasticity?
Olav Gjelsvik, PT, (N)

Lunch

Measurement and research

Keynote plenary session

Research on stroke rehabilitation
Nadina Lincoln, Clin Psych, (UK)

The role of the physiotherapist in research
Birgitta Bergmann, PT, Phd, (S)

Concurrent sessions

Scores and scales

The Sødring scale
K.M. Sødring, PT, (N)

The Rivermead motor assessment for stroke
Sally Ann Adams, PT, (UK)

Testing the FIM scale on stroke patients
Thomas Glott, MD, (N)

Quality assurance

The way forward in stroke outcome audit
Michele McCreadie presents for Susan Mawson, PT, (UK)

A positioning programme for the long term care team
Cheryl Mogensen, PT, (Canada)

A stroke protocol for physical therapy in primary health care
Dorine van Ravensberg, PT, (NL)

Examples of Research

A 5 year study of stroke patient recovery
Birgitta Lindmark, PT, MD, (S)

A study of the reaching movements of stroke patients
Paulette van Vliet, PT, (UK)

Comparison of 2 motor function scales (FIM/ RMA)
Marie-Luise Seisenbacher, PT (A)

Break

Keynote plenary session
The question of scales. Measurement in neurological rehabilitation
Derick T. Wade, MD, (UK)

Plenary session
Quality management in physiotherapy
Toril Bergerud Buene, PT, MSc, (N)

Reception at City Hall

Tuesday 7 June 1994

Psychosocial aspects and management of change

Keynote plenary session
The organization of rehabilitation
Ivar Lie, Phd, (N)

Concurrent sessions
Different types of rehabilitation

The acute treatment of stroke,
Frøydis Bakke, PT, (N)

Rehabilitation of Chronic Stroke Patients – Experiences from Sätra Brunn
Signe Lind, and Marianne Loid, OT, (S)

Rehabilitation at home after stroke. A pilot study
Lotta Widèn Holmqvist, PT, (S)

The stroke patient as a person

Body image and sexuality
Esther Greve. MD (DK)

By whom should stroke patients be treated
Markku Kaste, Phd, (SF)

Social implications

Wheel-chairs and seating in stroke
Bengt Engstrøm, PT, (S)

The health needs of people with stroke.
Preliminary study.
Anne Parry, PT, PhD, (UK)

When the therapist stops and the rest is nursing or less
Doris Christensen, RN, (DK)

Break

Plenary session

*****European Consensus on Stroke**
Aushra Shatchkute, Phd, Regional Advisor, WHO

Lunch

Keynote plenary session

Neuroplasticity and movement science
Kjeld Fredens, MD. (DK)

Concurrent sessions

Theory based approach
Assessment of motor dysfunctions towards a disability oriented
approach
Theo Mulder, PhD, (NL)

Community care management and organization of community care
Eric Viel, Director, PT, (F)

Sports and leisure
a) **Cross country skiing**
  Michèle Gerber, PT, (CH)
b) **Aerobics with hemiplegic patients**
  Gitte Rasmussen, PT, (DK)

Cognitive and perceptual approach
Volleyball, music, archery and riding with stroke patients
Kenth Malmström, PT and Helena Salnäs, PT, (S)

---

*No paper or abstract available

Plenary review of congress

Aushra Shatchkute, WHO
Elizabeth Condie, Vice-chairman,
WCPT-Europe, (UK)

Closing ceremony
Robert Rustad, Chairman WCPT- Europe, Norway

Farewell coffee/tea

The Current State Of Stroke Management

1. A review of current physiotherapy in the management of stroke

A. Ashburn

INTRODUCTION

Stroke is a condition that primarily affects the elderly (Andrews et al 1984). It produces significant disability in approximately 50% of survivors as a result of loss or impairment of body movement, difficulties with speech or decline in intellectual function (Effective Health Care 1992). Those who survive the early period can expect some spontaneous recovery. Researchers agree that most recovery takes place within the first 3 months (Skilbeck et al 1983, Wade et al 1985) although some report a continuation to 6 months (Parker et al 1986), and others suggest that a few of the younger severely impaired may continue to recover over a longer period (Lindmark 1988, Ferrucci et al 1993). However, the final level of function is difficult to predict (Wade et al 1983) as it is influenced by so many variables.

The treatment of patients disabled by stroke forms a major work commitment for many physiotherapists in hospital and community rehabilitation settings and is viewed by them as a specialist area of practice. At present it is requested worldwide by doctors, patients and their relatives, but the increasing demand for cost-effective health care provision and limited evidence of treatment efficacy means these demands may often remain unfulfilled. The impact of morbidity from stroke can be devastating with a patient's premorbid ability and concurrent illness affecting the recovery process (Wade et al 1984). Although physiotherapy is likely to be only one of several components in a rehabilitation programme, physical recovery will probably dominate the expectations of patients, staff and family at the expense of cognitive, emotional and social factors (Forster & Young 1992).

Physical dysfunction and the re-education of motor control and functional ability are the main targets for treatment by physiotherapists who may use a combination of observational, verbal, manual and educational skills. Deficits of motor output and abnormalities of tone and sensation can influence initiation and quality of voluntary movement and postural control (Newton 1991). Disabilities, such as difficulties with mobility, or impairments such as loss of movement are more likely to form the focus of a treatment session than the management of handicaps, although physiotherapy may indirectly influence this through treatment of the disability.

Handicaps are the social consequences of impairment and disability and may involve, for example, such activities as going to the shops or visiting friends.

Current practice throughout the world is based on a number of approaches that were developed independently by several pioneers in the 1950s. Traditionally, there has been an assumption that the different approaches strongly oppose each other, but recent reviewers have identified similarities (Kidd et al 1992, Partridge et al 1993) and in some cases promoted an integration of approaches (Sullivan et al 1982, Kidd et al 1992, Connolly & Montgomery 1991). The most commonly used physiotherapy approaches are outlined in this chapter; early publications and recent articles on physiotherapy have been examined. The review has been structured around the following questions:

- What are the different approaches?
- What evidence is there to distinguish one approach from another?
- Who are the approaches designed for?
- Where to next?

The need for research is a theme common to each of these sections.

WHAT ARE THE DIFFERENT APPROACHES?

Prior to the 1950s the physical treatment of patients following stroke focused on encouraging the patient to use the unaffected side of the body to compensate for the disabilities of the affected side. Treatment aimed for function, accepting safe, but abnormal, modes of activity. The affected limbs were not a prime focus for treatment. During the 1950s a number of new physiotherapy approaches emerged. These were developed by practitioners who were dissatisfied with the results of practice at that time and were interested in treating the paresis resulting from stroke. The work of many of these pioneers e.g. Bobath (1969), Brunnstrom (1961, 1970), Knott & Voss (1968) and Rood (Goff 1969) remains influential today. They developed their programmes primarily from observation and experience. Some of the approaches were associated with neurophysiological concepts current at that time, but others were developed from observation alone and then a suitable theory was adopted to explain the effects (Kidd et al 1992).

Peto introduced a different approach which he called conductive education; he founded the Institute for the Motor Disabled in Budapest in the 1950s (Kinsman et al 1988, Kinsman 1989). His work differed from that of others as it was based on educational principles and emphasised the need for an integrated programme that should be implemented throughout the day.

Since that period most of the approaches have continued to evolve, being extended either by their pioneers (Bobath 1990) or by other practitioners (Davies 1985, Johnstone 1980, 1989, Sawner & LaVigne 1992, Sullivan et al 1982). Further programmes have also been developed; one example is Carr & Shepherd's motor relearning programme (1987, 1989), an approach which utilises principles of motor relearning and biomechanics. In addition techniques or tools have been designed as adjuncts to programmes, e.g. biofeedback and functional electrical stimulation (Partridge et al 1993). Although these approaches differ in some respects they all aim to improve motor control.

Limited associations with scientific theories of practice is a feature common to all the approaches. This lack of a knowledge base has resulted in pioneers promoting programmes by emphasising the delivery and successes at a clinical level rather than providing theoretical explanations and reasoning. Interestingly, most of the approaches have been named after their pioneers rather than the principles behind the treatment (Nillson & Nordholm 1992).

The pioneers and their immediate disciples were the purists in following treatment principles, but in recent years modifications have been made to programmes and greater flexibility has been suggested (Kidd et al 1992, Connolly & Montgomery 1991). It is therefore misleading to believe that most physiotherapists will follow an approach in a uniform or purist manner. Most clinicians are selective and adapt techniques and procedures according to their clinical expertise and knowledge of skills, although they are most likely to favour and support one approach.

Until recently documentation of the treatment approaches has been extremely poor. Some pioneers have been better at publishing than others but publications are more likely to be in the form of books which detail treatment procedures; few refer to scientific theories or evaluative evidence. Capturing and describing the practical skills of physiotherapy in words is extremely difficult, which may explain why there are conflicting interpretations of treatment principles and handling procedures. The problem of communicating a practical skill has also limited therapists' opportunities to keep up-to-date on developments or changes in practical handling and conceptual thinking. Training in all of the approaches is given by means of undergraduate education and practical postgraduate courses.

Bower (1993), in a detailed review of physiotherapy for cerebral palsy, divided the treatment approaches for children into three groups: those with a neurological basis, those with an educational basis and those with a mechanical basis. Using her style of documentation, approaches for treating adult hemiplegia can be grouped under the following headings: neurophysiological, theories of learning, and tools and techniques.

Neurophysiological

Bobath

Background. Berta and Karel Bobath developed their approach to the treatment of hemiplegia from their observations and handling of children with cerebral palsy (Bobath 1963, Bobath 1972); their work began in the late 1940s. Their approach has received popular acceptance on an empirical basis. It has influenced physiotherapy practice worldwide including the work of other leading practitioners such as Davies (1985), Johnstone (1989) and Carr & Shepherd (1987).

Aim.

The aim of treatment is to improve the quality of movement on the affected side, so that ultimately the two sides work together as harmoniously as possible within the scope of the cerebral injury (Bobath 1990).

Direct handling of the body at key points such as the trunk, aim to control afferent input and facilitate normal postural reactions (Bobath 1990). The purpose of this control is to allow patients the experience of normal afferent input and normal movement patterns while inhibiting abnormal afferent input and abnormal movement (Bobath 1976, 1990).

Basis of practice. The approach is based on the assumption that increased tone and increased reflex activity will emerge as a result of lack of inhibition from a damaged postural reflex mechanism, and that movement will be abnormal if it stems from a background of abnormal tone (Bobath 1990). A further assumption is that performing abnormal movements will reinforce more abnormal movements. Berta Bobath observed, however, that tone could be influenced by altering the position or movement of proximal joints of the body (Bobath 1976). Such movements, made in a direction opposing spastic synergies, formed the basis of practice in the 1970s and 1980s and were known first as reflex inhibiting positions and later as patterns of movement. These procedures, particularly when used to treat brain damaged children, made use of the developmental sequences (Bower 1993), and were used to encourage movement to emerge in an order that would be expected to occur in normal children. Therefore, the approach is referred to sometimes as the 'neurodevelopmental approach' (Connolly & Montgomery 1991). This term was not used by the pioneers to describe their approach for adults.

Treatment. Treatment centres around the facilitation of corrected movement by a therapist who handles the body at key points of control such as head and spine, shoulders and pelvic girdle and, distally, the feet and hands (Bobath 1990). Manual handling aims to control postural tone and allow normal movement to emerge. Unfortunately, the published literature does not clarify how normal sensory input and awareness can be achieved when there is a damaged sensory system. Volitional activity by the patient is requested only against a background of automatic postural activity. The choice of treatment position is influenced by the pathological distribution of postural tone and static patterning (Partridge et al 1993).

In recent years treatment has become more active and functionally directed, aiming not only at inhibiting abnormal input but at facilitating the relearning of normal movement (Partridge et al 1993). Strategies for enhancing a 'carry-over' effect are being introduced. Treatment is continuously adapted to individual needs in terms of goal, range, speed or pattern of movement; there are no set 'Bobath' exercises (Partridge et al 1993). The patient's response to handling guides the treatment procedure and Bobath states that 'there is a great deal of experimentation in good treatment' (Bobath 1990).

The type of techniques employed depend on the stage of recovery the patient has reached or the stage at which the process of recovery has arrested. Three stages have been identified: the initial stage of flaccidity, the stage of spasticity and the stage of relative recovery (Bobath 1990). Specific muscle strengthening is not viewed as a necessary part of treatment, and the only movements that are performed against resistance are those that use body weight.

In summary, the approach focuses on and aims to control the responses that result from the damaged postural reflex mechanism. Emphasis is placed on the facilitation of normal afferent inputs and normal movement patterns while minimising the experience of abnormal movement. Movements are not isolated to individual joints but take place in patterns. Therapists are encouraged to view handling techniques as interchangeable and requiring constant adjustment according to the patient's response. Primitive reflexes, patterns and associated reactions are inhibited and are not used to facilitate movement. Muscle strengthening is not viewed as part of treatment. In adults, the selection of activities stems from distribution of pathological reactions and functional needs; developmental sequencing does not determine treatment planning, and thus the term 'neurodevelopmental approach' here is misleading. In common with most of the other approaches, the influence of cognitive factors on motor control is not addressed (Connolly & Montgomery 1991). However, the importance of occupational therapists, speech therapists and physiotherapists working together is acknowledged (Bobath 1990).

Brunnstrom

Background. Signe Brunnstrom, a Swedish physiotherapist, worked in New York and popularised her approach in the United States of America and in parts of Europe. She first publicised her approach in the late 1950s (Brunnstrom 1956, 1961). Over time she carefully documented the movement recovery of large numbers of patients (Brunnstrom 1970).

Aim. The approach aims to encourage the return of voluntary movement in patients with hemiplegia through the use of reflex activity and a range of sensory stimulation. The choice of stimulation varies depending on which stage the patient has reached in the motor recovery process (Brunnstrom 1970, Sawner & LaVigne 1992).

Basis of practice. The approach is based on the assumption that recovery progresses from subcortical to cortical control of muscle function. Brunnstrom (1970) felt that normal selective movement did not recover unless patients first progressed through stages of abnormality. She therefore saw the use of mass flexion and extension synergies as a basis of retraining movement – a belief that contrasts with that of the Bobaths, followers of whom would view primitive responses and mass patterns as pathological and in need of inhibition.

The stages of recovery which were indentified by Brunnstrom (Sawner & LaVigne 1992) are:

1. Flaccidity.
2. Presence of basis synergy on a reflex level.
3. Voluntary control of the movement synergies.
4. Ability to mix components of antagonistic synergies but influence of spasticity still observable.
5. More difficult movement combinations mastered; limb synergies lose their dominance.
6. Individual joint movements become possible.
7. Normal motor function is restored.

It was noted that recovery could cease at any point on this scale.

Treatment. Training sessions are planned so that the only tasks that are demanded are those that a patient can master or almost master. The choice and use of sensory stimulation depends on the stage of recovery or pattern of reflex training. Stimulation from tonic neck, labyrinthine reflexes, use of stroking, tapping or slapping of muscles or resistance to movement of the affected or unaffected side are used to elicit a movement synergy. This process is employed until the primitive synergies are established, then facilitation is used to develop some voluntary control. Conditioning of the reflex is subsequently attempted (Brunnstrom 1970, Sawner & LaVigne 1992), first to establish voluntary control over the synergies, then to break away from the synergies by mixing components of movement patterns and leading to skilled activities and normal function. Interestingly, Brunnstrom advocates that preparation for walking should be emphasised early but that extensive walking should be postponed in order to avoid the development of a poor gait pattern. The preparation for walking includes balance training, modification of motor responses in the legs, use of sensory inputs and feedback of knowledge of results to the patient (Sawner & LaVigne 1992, Connolly & Montgomery 1991).

In summary, the Brunnstrom approach, unlike the Bobath approach, uses primitive reflexes to initiate movement and encourages the use of mass patterns in the early stages of motor recovery. The ultimate aim is for normal function with unwanted activity being controlled at more advanced stages of recovery. Tactile, proprioceptive, visual and auditory stimuli are employed, along with asymmetrical tonic neck reflexes, tonic lumbar and tonic labyrinthine reflexes for facilitating movement. Treatment is planned and assessed in stages and movement is encouraged in patterns. The approach does not aim to normalise tone or inhibit the expression of primitive movement.

Knott and Voss

Background. Knott and Voss, both physiotherapists, worked with Kabat, a neurophysiologist, at the Kaiser Foundation in the United States of America during the 1950s, and developed the approach known as proprioceptive neuromuscular facilitation (PNF) (Knott & Voss 1968). This approach has influenced physiotherapy practice worldwide. It was developed primarily for use with patients suffering from neuromuscular dysfunction, although therapists have been encouraged to use it to treat patients with other conditions where an increase in muscle power is required (Kabat et al 1959).

Aim. The approach aims to promote movement and functional synergies of movement by maximising peripheral input (Knott & Voss 1968, Sullivan et al 1982, Kidd et al 1992). Patterns and techniques of proprioceptive neuromuscular facilitation are designed to hasten motor learning by:

1. providing appropriate sensory stimulus
2. following activities in a developmental sequence.

Basis of practice. The approach is based on the assumption that people who move normally have passed through a developmental sequence, and that after damage it is necessary to return to that developmental sequence before recovery will take place. It also assumes that maximal peripheral stimulation is required to recruit motor responses. The use of total patterns of movement is believed to be a way of encouraging and reinforcing movement. This belief is based on the fact that the cortex is thought to control movement in patterns and not as singular muscular actions (Kidd et al 1992). In addition, it is believed that recruitment can take place from strong muscles to weak muscles. Diagonal and spiral patterns of active and passive movements are encouraged since most muscles act in a spiral direction, and stretch reflexes are superimposed on these patterns in order to increase muscle activity (Knott & Voss 1968, Sullivan et al 1982).

Treatment. Appropriate sensory input for enhancing motor learning is applied through the use of handling techniques and patterns of movement. A developmental plan of activities is followed. Sensory stimuli can include manual contact and pressure, verbal commands, elongation of muscles and stretch reflexes, joint traction and approximation, maximal muscle resistance, reversal of direction of movements and repeated muscular contractions.

Whenever possible the patient's voluntary effort is used to promote volitional control of movement and posture. Techniques for stimulation or relaxation are coupled with the patient's effort to initiate movement or overcome resistance to movement. Manual contact and tone of voice are used to modulate the patient's effort to move and careful placement of the therapist's hands are a key aspect of the approach (Knott & Voss 1968, Sullivan et al 1982, Kidd et al 1992). This approach, unlike Brunnstrom's approach, does not utilise primitive reflexes to initiate movement and, unlike Bobath's approach, it does use resisted activities.

In recent years the developmental sequence has been used less rigidly, the selection of tasks being guided more by age appropriateness. It is of interest to note that as early as 1959 a paper reminded therapists that 'they should approach facilitation with an experimental attitude, as only flexible use of the techniques will produce good results' (Kabat et al 1959).

In summary, PNF uses peripheral input such as stretch and resisted movements to reinforce existing motor responses (Kidd et al 1992). Total patterns of movement are used in treatment and activities are followed in a developmental sequence. The approach does not encourage abnormal movements (Kidd et al 1992) and unwanted activities are inhibited. The approach does not address the problems of abnormal tone.

Rood

Background. Margaret Rood, another American physiotherapist, also developed her approach in the 1950s for treating neurological impairment. Unfortunately, she was poor at documenting her programme and it is difficult therefore to form a true interpretation of her approach. Like PNF, the approach focuses on the developmental sequence of recovery and the use of peripheral input to facilitate movement (Goff 1969).

Aim. The approach aims to obtain as normal a motor reponse as possible and, where appropriate, on an automatic level. Sensory stimuli are used to activate or inhibit movement or postural reactions which are progressed through a developmental sequence (Goff 1969).

Basis of practice. The approach is based on the assumption that postural stability and movement patterns are similar in all individuals and follow a developmental sequence. A return to this developmental framework of motor sequences is fundamental to the approach. Sensory input is used to recruit and enhance motor responses. Rood believed that motor and sensory functions are inseparable. She suggests links between motor responses and somatosensory, autonomic and psychological functions (Connolly & Montgomery 1991). Therefore, the relationship between sensory factors and motor functions assumes a major role. She classifies muscles according to their work and describes the developmental sequence in terms of muscle work.

Treatment. Treatment is aimed at stimulating movement, preferably at an autonomic level. The approach is often known as the 'cutaneous approach', and icing, tapping, bone pounding, stroking or brushing along with resisted movements are used to facilitate activities (Goff 1969). Speed and rate of applying stimulation vary according to the working role of the muscle; e.g. cold is used for relaxation, and pressure and stretches are used for postural muscle activation (Connolly & Montgomery 1991). Muscles are classified according to their workloads and their roles within the developmental sequence. Treatment plans are organised according to the classification of motor disability and these are grouped by Rood as hypokinesia, hyperkinesia or hypertonia (Goff 1969).

In summary, the approach emphasises the use of activities in the developmental sequence, sensory stimulation and the classification of muscle work. Unwanted activity is inhibited, total patterns of movement are utilised and the aim is for a normal motor response. The approach does not emphasise the use of functional tasks or provide an overall approach to patient management.

Johnstone

Background. Margaret Johnstone's approach to the management of patients following stroke has evolved since the 1950s, when she first worked with stroke patients. She acknowledges the influence of Bobath on her work and has published several books describing the approach (Johnstone 1980).

Aim. The main aim of the approach is to control spasticity consistently over time.

Basis of practice. The approach is based on the assumption that the damaged postural reflex mechanism can be controlled through positioning and splinting. The main problems identified are the imbalance of muscle tone and the resultant disabling postures. Treatment is based on a hierarchical model with manipulation and control of sensory and motor functions.

Treatment. During the early stages the patient is positioned in side lying and 'air splints' are used to apply even deep pressure to the limbs. Patients are mobilised by means of a hierarchical sequence of activities during which a continual emphasis is placed on correct positioning and use of air splints (Johnstone 1989).

In summary, the approach emphasises the control of spasticity and the facilitation of movement while tone is being controlled. Treatment focuses on the trunk, with total body movements progressing from rolling through to crawling. Family involvement is encouraged. The approach does not utilise abnormal movements.

Theories of learning

Conductive education (Peto)

Background. In the 1950s Peto, a physician and neuropsychologist, founded the Institute for the Neurologically Motor Disabled in Budapest (Bower 1993). His approach, conductive education, focused on teaching and training children with cerebral palsy by means of specially trained conductors.

Aim. The approach aims to teach individuals strategies for dealing with problems of physical disability in order to encourage the child or adult to learn to live with or overcome disability (Kinsman 1989, Bower 1993) in everyday life. It also aims to provide a totally integrated approach emphasising continuity and consistency through the use of a conductor (Kinsman et al 1988).

Basis of practice. The approach is based on the assumption that feelings of failure resulting from physical disability, passive conditioning and dependence can produce a dysfunctional attitude (Cotton & Kinsman 1983), and that such an attitude can prevent rehabilitation. Peto wanted to teach rather than treat individuals; he wanted to teach them strategies for coping with their physical problems so that they would avoid failure. His belief was that individuals will achieve greater functional independence if taught how to control their physical ability.

Peto considered that, under the normal system, the child or adult was disadvantaged by fragmentation of services and confusion about treatment, often brought about by interprofessional conflicts (Cotton & Kinsman 1983), so he introduced the role of the conductor. The conductor (who undergoes 4 years' specialised training), like a conductor of an orchestra, aims to keep the individuals 'in tune' by directing sessions and daily programmes (Cotton & Kinsman 1983). Active movements start with an intention and end with the goal, and the patient requires help to find his way between the two. The conductor's role is to assist the child or adult to achieve control of movement through task analysis and rhythmical intention or verbal reinforcement, and is responsible for organising the daily programme. Treatment techniques are based on educational theories and Peto's approach places an emphasis on brain damaged children learning rather than being recipients of treatment.

Treatment. Treatment involves the integration of therapy and education so that movement, language and function are combined in a programme. Educational principles and repetition are utilised as a method of rote learning. The conductor controls a highly structured day, and treatment centres around group work, task analysis, repetition and reinforcement of a task through rhythmical intention or verbal chanting. Tasks are chosen carefully and task analysis is a key element of the learning process, with all activities or functions broken down into a number of component parts.

Verbal intention and reinforcement accompany the learning of a new skill (Cotton & Kinsman 1983, Kinsman 1989). A common group activity is identified but the steps to achieving that activity may vary for each member. The steps of a task are planned for each individual and are changed as necessary. Rhythmical intention or verbal reinforcement accompanies the movement; e.g. the person may rhythmically chant, 'I lift my arms up' as he performs or attempts to perform the movement. This procedure is viewed as a fundamental aspect of the approach and of the process of learning. The term 'rhythmical intention', employed by Peto, describes a technique that utilises language to facilitate the planning, intention and performance of a movement (Kinsman et al 1988).

Neither manual guidance nor manual sensory input is used by the conductor to facilitate movement; in this respect the approach differs from the neurophysiological approaches. The individual is encouraged to guide his own movements through bilateral activities. Abnormal unwanted activity is controlled only by means of the level of task chosen. The level of learning required for this programme would exclude some of the cognitively impaired.

In summary, the approach emphasises the use of educational principles and repetition to facilitate the independence of individuals in daily activities. Programmes are highly structured and are controlled by the conductor; patients are encouraged to actively learn rather than to be treated. Group work, repetition and task analysis are used to reinforce learning. Manual facilitation is not used as it is in the other approaches; patients guide their own movements through bilateral activities. The approach does not emphasise individual treatment, manipulative guidance for correcting movement or the use of enhancing somatosensory stimuli.

Carr and Shepherd

Background. Carr and Shepherd, both Australian physiotherapists, developed the approach known as the motor relearning programme and first published their ideas on the management of the neurologically impaired in 1980 (Carr & Shepherd 1980). They acknowledged the influence of Bobath on their work. Since that time the programme has been extended and they have published several books documenting their revised thinking (Carr & Shepherd 1987, 1989, 1990). They expressed their frustration with therapists for still following unproven concepts developed three decades before and emphasised the need to look forward rather than backwards. They looked to the literature on behavioural science and biomechanics when developing their programme. More recently they have referred to their programme as a framework for retraining movement.

Aim. The aim of the framework is to enable the disabled person to learn how to perform or improve performance of actions critical to everyday life.

The emphasis is placed on:

• Utilising theories of learning, in particular the use of practice and knowledge of results to encourage people to learn and self monitor.
• Knowledge of biomechanics for analysing movements and performance of tasks.

(Carr & Shepherd 1987)

Basis of practice. The model is based on the assumption that the impaired learn in the same way as the unimpaired, as the principles that they follow stem from work that has focused primarily on the learning responses of normal subjects (Carr & Shepherd 1989). It is also assumed that motor control of posture and movement are interrelated and that appropriate sensory input will help modulate the motor response to a task. The programme is based on four factors thought to be essential for motor relearning:

• elimination of unnecessary muscle activity
• feedback
• practice
• the link between postural adjustment and movement.

Task analysis and measurement are viewed as essential elements of the framework. In addition they underline the importance for therapists to keep abreast of the movement science literature (Carr & Shepherd 1987).

Treatment. Movement analysis and training form the critical part of the framework (Carr & Shepherd 1990) and four steps can be identified (Carr & Shepherd 1987):

1. analysis of the task
2. practice of the missing components
3. practice of the task
4. transference of training.

Principles of biomechanics are used to analyse both the tasks and the motor performance. Missing component parts to the movement are identified and programmes are planned to train the required activity. Movements of the person with a disability are compared with a normal performance and measurement is viewed as critical for evaluation. Instruction, explanation and feedback are considered to be essential parts of the training process. Motor training involves the practice of specific actions with guidance from the therapist. This guidance principally takes the form of instruction and explanation and feedback about performance. Manual guidance is used as a support or for demonstration and, unlike the first group of approaches, it is not used for providing sensory input. Where an action cannot be practised in its entirety, component parts may be practised separately. Unwanted activities are limited by choosing an appropriate level of activity.

An emphasis is placed on providing a clear explanation of the task, identifiable and specified goals, and verbal feedback by the therapist. Patients are encouraged to use observation for monitoring and correcting the quality of their movement. Some unwanted activity is accepted as part of relearning movements; a principle based on the way normal subjects learn new skills. The focus is placed on cognitive learning and thus it is unclear how the intellectually impaired cope with this programme (Carr & Shepherd 1987).

The effects of abnormal movement are not thought to result entirely from tonal change, contrary to the beliefs of Bobath's followers (Carr & Shepherd 1990). In contrast to PNF and Rood's approach, the developmental sequence of activities is not followed and training focuses on a series of functional tasks. A series of tasks has been chosen because learning by normal subjects has been shown to be task-specific with minimal carry-over from one activity to another.

In summary, the appproach emphasises the practice of functional tasks and the importance of relearning real-life activities that have meaning for patients. Careful biomechanical analysis of movements and tasks are highlighted as key to planning treatment and following context-specific training. Principles of learning are emphasised – in particular the importance of practice. The programme can appear to be more prescriptive than Bobath's as a set number of specified functional tasks are practised. The programme does not utilise manual guidance techniques for manipulating movement or providing normal afferent input, thus some unwanted activity may emerge.

Tools and techniques

Biofeedback will be used as an illustration of one approach in this group. In a standard treatment session the physiotherapist provides feedback to a patient about performance and outcome through the use of verbal, visual and manual cues. Instrumentation can also be used; this procedure is known as biofeedback. It is beyond the scope of this chapter to detail the technique but a brief outline will be provided.

When used in the treatment of hemiplegia, biofeedback utilises instrumentation to enhance signals to a patient. These signals are designed to facilitate learning either to inhibit unwanted activity or to facilitate movement. Visual and auditory signals are most likely to be used and are most commonly linked to electromyographic readings.

Marinacci & Horande (1960) were among the first authors to document this process with subjects suffering from neurological inpairment. More recently, researchers have utilised electronic devices designed to feed back information to subjects about their body movements and distribution of weight (Sackley & Baguley 1993, De Weerdt et al 1989).

Horn (1993) discusses the wide-ranging use of biofeedback. She describes the strengths and weaknesses of different techniques as well as highlighting the mixed results from evaluative studies on the procedures. The positive results, she concludes, come from studies in which biofeedback has been used with precision and subjects' needs have been carefully matched with what biofeedback could offer. She recommends that more work must be done to tease out all the factors contributing to its successful use.

It is interesting to note that Mroczec et al (1978) proposed that biofeedback should not be considered as a therapy but as a modality or tool to be used where sensory loss is inhibiting motor control. They suggested that biofeedback could help with isolated tasks or muscle actions but could not be employed for augmenting and guiding multiple integrated factors in the way that a physiotherapist can. De Weerdt & Harrison in 1985 reported that the use of biofeedback in physiotherapy departments in the National Health Service in Great Britain was very limited and had no major impact on the profession.

Summary

Several different physiotherapy approaches are used in the management of patients who have suffered a stroke but these approaches are not mutually exclusive and are rarely delivered in a uniform or purist manner. The theoretical basis of the individual approaches remains unsubstantiated. All of the approaches aim to improve motor control and all of them demand that the therapist has a specialist training in the individual concepts.

There is a spectrum, one end representing those approaches that maximise sensory input for facilitating motor performance, while at the other end are those that use minimal sensory inputs but follow principles of learning. All approaches, with the exception perhaps of Peto's, are working towards normal skills, although the proposed processes for achieving this aim are different. As a group of approaches, they appear to focus singularly on physical function and do not address ways of managing the patient with incontinence or dysfunction of cognition and mood.

Debate between the different followers continues over issues such as:

• type of sensory input to be used and when and how sensory stimuli should be employed
• resisted or no resisted activities
• independent or guided practice
• treatment aim for quality of movement or a functional outcome.

WHAT EVIDENCE IS THERE TO DISTINGUISH ONE APPROACH FROM ANOTHER?

The inevitable question: 'which physiotherapy approach has been shown to be most effective in the clinical setting?' has been asked by physiotherapists, directors of units and budget holders for many years. In the climate of an increasing need for accountability and cost-effective health provision, great demands are being placed on discovering the most efficacious way to manage patients following stroke. Several reviewers (Ernst 1990, Dombovy et al 1986, Wagenaar & Meijer 1991, Lind 1982) have concluded that, although the evidence is not clear-cut, patients suffering from stroke derive benefit from rehabilitation with physiotherapy. The optimal type of physiotherapy, however, is yet to be identified. Comparative research studies discussed by Ashburn et al (1993) found no differences between approaches, which suggests that either it does not matter which treatment approach is used or, if there is an optimal approach, it has not yet been characterised.

Research in this area and delivery of physiotherapy at a clinical level is complex. The multidisciplinary nature of stroke management inevitably influences the application of approaches and makes it difficult to disentangle the treatment effects. The age of the population and complexity of the condition produce a group of patients with wide-ranging problems. In addition, the range of experience that staff possess and the erroneous assumption that therapy is delivered in a uniform manner makes the comparative exercise a difficult one. Despite this, several researchers have attempted to find the answer. Table 1.1 lists the approaches which are compared in articles included in the review.

All of these studies suffered from methodological flaws which could explain their lack of conclusive evidence. For example, the definitions and contents of the treatment approaches used were not provided in the papers. The experience of the physiotherapists in delivering these approaches also was not documented. The research questions posed in all the studies revolved around independence and did not focus directly on patterns of movement or motor control. In most of the studies the principle outcome measure was an activities of daily living (ADL) index, rather than a measure of motor performance, which is the focus of physiotherapy. These methodological limitations, in addition to fundamental study design problems and the lack of suitable tools for determining the outcome of physiotherapy may have contributed to the lack of differences when comparing physiotherapy approaches.

Table 1.1 Types of physiotherapy approaches compared in research studies (number of subjects given in brackets)

Approaches compared	Reference
Bobath & Rood (42) and Traditional (42)	Logigian et al 1983
PNF (31) and Conventional (31)	Stern et al 1970
Traditional (19) and Facilitation (20)	Lord & Hall 1986
Bobath and PNF and Conventional (131)	Dickstein et al 1986
Neurodevelopmental and Brunnstrom (7)	Wagenaar et al 1990

The recommendations made by Ashburn et al (1993) propose that more research is needed into the physiotherapy management of patients following stroke in the clinical setting. However, they suggest that the value of comparing different physiotherapy approaches in the clinical setting is questionable as it assumed, erroneously, that therapy is delivered in a uniform manner and that outcome measures are sensitive enough to detect differential effects of techniques in the clinical environment. Their proposal was that future studies should concentrate first on the identification of best practice and the evaluation of optimal delivery and goal setting, and secondly on research at a neuromuscular level in order to investigate the responses to different handling techniques. They highlight the importance of sound methodology and the involvement of therapists in identification and development of outcome measures which should match aims of treatment and research questions.

WHO ARE THE APPROACHES DESIGNED FOR?

It may seem strange to ask this question, as 'the patient' may appear to be the obvious answer. If this is truly the case, it is necessary to ask why there is so little knowledge about the type of patients who do or do not respond to particular types of approaches. If patients really are central in this situation, knowledge about the range of responses to the different approaches should be readily available. One explanation for this paucity of information could be that patients tend to be fitted into treatment approaches as a result of the therapist controlling the situation, even at the stage of rehabilitation, when patient choice is supposed to be paramount to a successful outcome (Whalley Hammell 1994a,b).

Papers which describe physiotherapy approaches always place the therapist in the leading position, even though patient and physiotherapist must work together. It would not be surprising to find that people respond differently to different treatment approaches; both patient and physiotherapist should feel comfortable with the style of treatment, but choice and negotiation is rarely available. Contraindications to individual approaches are still unknown, as are the characteristics of people who may or may not react favourably to particular programmes. While it is impressive to watch a skilled therapist handling a patient, such observations on their own are insufficient to justify the effectiveness of treatment. Patients' responses to treatment over time need to be measured; the importance lies in what the patient is able to learn and use in daily life (Scrutton 1984).

More knowledge is required concerning the aspects of the therapist's skill which produce the required motor learning with a carry-over effect while preventing unwanted detrimental effects. Working together with individuals under treatment to define and achieve agreed outcomes may be one of these keys to success (Whalley Hammell 1994a).

Baddeley (1993), when discussing ways to achieve progress in neuropsychological rehabilitation, emphasises the importance of learning from patients who have responded positively to treatment in order to know what helped, while at the same time establishing the problems of those who do not respond or who are critical of treatment. A similar recommendation should be made in physiotherapy. Partridge's (1994) report on patients' views of physiotherapy raises a number of positive and negative comments. It was found that, for example, poor communication skills, particularly the inability of people to listen, was a cause of great frustration; on the other hand, patients recognised immediately the skilled and experienced therapist, who stood out favourably in their approach to care.

WHERE TO NEXT?

It is widely acknowledged that the pratice of physiotherapy should be built on a body of knowledge and not on an empirical basis (Newham 1994). The limited association between the approaches used by physiotherapists for managing stroke and scientific theory and evidence is therefore a cause for criticism. It would be foolish, however, to disregard the approaches for their lack of substantiated theory as they have provided, and do provide, very useful frameworks for guiding practice (Connolly & Montgomery 1991, Bower 1993, Hagedorn 1992).

It could also be argued that it is unrealistic to expect one approach to the retraining of movement to meet the needs of all people. Educationally, people learn best in different ways (Entwistle 1988); therefore, there is no reason to believe that responses to rehabilitaion are any different (McLellan personal communication). A range of approaches with their frameworks spanning individual treatments to group sessions, should therefore be welcomed. It is surprising, however, how much is unknown about the type of person who will respond to a particular style of treatment and what sort of response they will make, as well as about the type of therapist who works best in a given environment and the strategy employed.

Frameworks lose their usefulness if they become fixed and, therefore, if they are to be of value, they need to be changed in response to research findings (Connolly & Montgomery 1991). One problem in the use of named approaches is that the loyalty of followers can encourage them to become fixed because the responsibility of therapists to question and challenge the dogma seems to disappear. There is a need to encourage practitioners to focus on and enquire more about both the damaged neuromuscular system they are treating and the processes they are using to modify that system. One possible way of facilitating that shift is to encourage therapists to stop referring to named individual approaches and to refer more to their preferred theoretical and clinical basis of pratice.

Confusion and contention among health care workers does arise from the different approaches, particularly in relation to the promotion of types of techniques to use and when and how they should be employed. The lack of knowledge about responses to techniques at a neuromuscular level, programme contents and optimal delivery of services contributes to the debates. If this confusion is to be unravelled, further research is essential, in order to build on the evidence available.

Overall, there is a need to understand which aspects of treatment or which combinations of aspects lead to change in some or all sufferers of stroke and how treatment, needs and outcome may differ at different stages of recovery and for different subjects. The stability of change in patients' condition over time needs to be investigated and therefore long-term evaluation is required. Studies should seek information from patients and therapists, and monitor responses to treatment and techniques in clinical environments and at a neuromuscular level. A key to the effectiveness of all of these research studies is the use of appropriate outcome measures, designed to record changes in those factors that the treatment being studied aims to influence.

Acknowledgements

Thanks are extented to Lorraine DeSouza and Cecily Partridge for reading this chapter and for providing valuable comments.

REFERENCES

Andrew K, Brocklehurst J, Richards B, Laycock P 1984 The influence of age on the clinical presentation and outcome of stroke. Int Rehab Med 6: 49–53
Ashburn A, Partridge C, DeSouza L 1993 Physiotherapy in the rehabilitation of stroke: a review. Clin Rehab 7: 337–345
Baddeley A 1993 A theory of rehabilitation without a model of learning is a vehicle without an engine: a comment on Caramazza & Hillis. Neuropsych Rehab 3(3): 235–244
Bobath B 1963 Treatment principles and planning in cerebral palsy. Physiotherapy 49: 122–124
Bobath B 1969 The treatment of neuromuscular disorders by improving patterns of coordination. Physiotherapy 55(1): 18–22
Bobath B 1976 Adult hemiplegia: evaluation and treatment. Heinemann, London
Bobath B 1990 Adult hemiplegia: evaluation and treatment, 3rd edn. Heinemann, London
Bobath K 1972 The motor deficits in patients with cerebral palsy. Clinics Development Medicine 23
Bower E 1993 Physiotherapy for cerebral palsy: a historical review. In: Ward C (ed) Baillière's clinical neurology 2(1): 29–54
Brunnstrom S 1956 Associated reactions of the upper extremity in adult hemiplegia: an approach to training. Physical Therapy Review 36: 225–236
Brunnstrom S 1961 Motor behaviour of adult hemiplegic patients. Amer J Occup Ther 15(1): 6–12
Brunnstrom S 1970 Movement therapy in hemiplegia. Harper & Row, London
Carr J, Shepherd R 1980 Physiotherapy in disorders of the brain. Heinemann, London
Carr J, Shepherd R 1987 A motor relearning programme for stroke. Heinemann, London
Carr J, Shepherd R 1989 A motor learning model for stroke rehabilitation. Physiotherapy 75(7): 372–380
Carr J, Shepherd R 1990 A motor learning model for rehabilitation of the movement-disabled. In: Ada L, Canning C (eds) Key issues in neurological physiotherapy. Butterworth-Heinemann, Oxford
Connolly B, Montgomery P 1991 Framework for assessment and treatment. In: Montgomery P, Connolly B (eds) Motor control and physical therapy: theoretical framework and practical applications. Chattanooga,Tennessee

Cotton E, Kinsman R 1983 Conductive education and adult hemiplegia. Churchill Livingstone, Edinburgh

Davies P 1985 Steps to follow: a guide to the treatment of adult hemiplegia. Springer Verlag, Berlin

De Weerdt W, Harrison M 1985 The use of biofeedback in physiotherapy. Physiotherapy 71(1): 9–12

De Weerdt W, Crossley S, Lincoln N, Harrison M 1989 Restoration of balance in stroke patients. A single case study design. Clin Rehab 3: 139–147

Dickstein R, Hocherman S, Pillar T, Shaham R 1986 Stroke rehabilitation: three exercise therapy approaches. Phys Ther 66: 1233–1238

Dombovy M, Sandok B, Basford J 1986 Rehabilitation for stroke: a review. Stroke 17: 363–369

Effective Health care Series 1992 Stroke rehabilitation. Leeds Evaluation Unit, Leeds

Entwistle N 1988 Styles of learning. David Fulton, London

Ernst E 1990 A review of stroke rehabilitation and physiotherapy. Stroke 21: 1081–1085

Ferrucci L, Bandelli S, Guralnik J, Lamponi M, Bertini C, Falchini M, Baroni A 1993 Recovery of functional status after stroke. Stroke 24: 200–205

Forster A, Young J 1992 Stroke rehabilitation. Can we do better? BMJ 305: 1446–1447

Goff B 1969 Appropriate afferent stimulation. Physiotherapy 55: 9–17

Hagedorn R 1992 Occupational therapy: foundations for practice. Churchill Livingstone, Edinburgh

Horn S 1993 Biofeedback. In: Lewith G, Aldridge D (eds) Clinical research methodology for complementary therapies. Hodder & Stoughton, London

Johnstone M 1980 Home care for the stroke patient: living in a pattern. Churchill Livingstone, Edinburgh

Johnstone M 1989 Current advances in the use of pressure splints in the management of adult hemiplegia. Physiotherapy 75(7): 381–384

Kabat H, McLeod M, Holt C 1959 The practical application of proprioceptive neuromuscular facilitation. Physiotherapy 45: 87–92

Kidd G, Lawes N, Musa I 1992 A critical review of contemporary therapies. Understanding neuromuscular plasticity: a basis for clinical rehabilitation. Edward Arnold, London

Kinsman R 1989 A conductive education approach to stroke patients at Barnet General Hospital. Physiotherapy 75(7): 418–421

Kinsman R, Verity R, Waller J 1988 A conductive education approach for adults with neurological dysfunction. Physiotherapy 74(5): 277–230

Knott M, Voss D 1968 Proprioceptive neuromuscular facilitation, 2nd edn. Harper & Row, London

Lind K 1982 A synthesis of studies on stroke rehabilitation. J Chron Dis 35: 133–149

Lindmark B 1988 The improvement of different motor functions after stroke. Clin Rehab 2: 275–283

Logigian M, Samuels M, Falconer J 1983 Clinical exercise trial for stroke patients. Arch Phys Med Rehab 64: 364–367

Lord J, Hall K 1986 Neuromuscular re-education versus traditional programs for stroke rehabilitation. Arch Phys Med Rehab 67: 88–91

Marinacci A, Horande M 1960 Electromyogram in neuromuscular re-education. Bull Los Angeles Neurol Soc 25: 57–71

Mroczec M, Halpern D, McHugh R 1978 Electromyographic feedback and physical therapy for neuromuscular retraining in hemiplegia. Arch Phys Med Rehab 59: 592–596

Newham D 1994 Practical research. Physiotherapy 90(6): 337–339

Newton R 1991 Neural system underlying motor control. In: Montgomery P, Connolly B (eds) Motor control and physical therapy: theoretical framework and practical applications. Chattanooga, Tennessee

Nillson L, Nordholm L 1992 Physical therapy in stroke rehabilitation: bases for Swedish physiotherapists' choice of treatment. Phys Theory & Practice 8: 49–55

Parker V, Wade D, Langton-Hewer R 1986 Loss of arm function after stroke: measurement, frequency and recovery. Int Rehab Med 8: 69–73

Partridge C 1994 Evaluation of physiotherapy for people with stroke. Kings Fund Centre, London

Partridge C, Cornall C, Lynch M, Greenwood R 1993 Physical therapies. In:

Greenwood R, Barnes M, McMillan T, Ward C (eds) Neurological rehabilitation. Churchill Livingstone, Edinburgh

Sackley C, Baguley B 1993 Visual feedback after stroke with the balance performance monitor. Two single case studies. Clin Rehab 7(3): 189–195

Sawner K, LaVigne J 1992 Brunnstrom's movement therapy in hemiplegia: a neurophysiological approach, 2nd edn. Lippincott, Philadelphia

Scrutton D 1984 Aim orientated management. In: Scrutton D (ed) Management of motor disorders of children with cerebral palsy. Spastic International Medical Publication, London

Skilbeck C, Wade D, Langton-Hewer R, Wood V 1983 Recovery after stroke. J Neurol Neurosurg Psychiatry 46: 5–8

Stern P, McDowell F, Miller J, Robinson M 1970 Effects of facilitation exercise techniques in stroke rehabilitation. Arch Phys Med Rehab 51: 526–531

Sullivan P, Markos P, Minor M 1982 An integrated approach to therapeutic exercise. Reston, Virginia

Wade D, Skilbeck C, Langton-Hewer R 1983 Predicting Barthel ADL scores at 6 months after an acute stroke. Arch Phys Med Rehab 64: 24–28

Wade D, Langton-Hewer R, Wood V 1984 Stroke: the influence of age upon outcome. Age & Ageing 13: 357–362

Wade D, Wood V, Langton-Hewer R 1985 Recovery after stroke – the first three months. J Neurol Neurosurg Psychiatry 48: 7–13

Wagenaar R, Meijer O 1991 Effects of stroke rehabilitation. J Rehab Sci 4: 133–149

Wagenaar R, Meijer O, Van Wieringen P, Kuik D, Hazenberg G, Lindeboom J, Wichers F, Rijswijk H 1990 The functional recovery of stroke: a comparison between neuro-developmental treatment and the Brunnstrom method. Scan J Rehab Med 22: 1–8

Whalley Hammell K 1994a Establishing objectives in occupational therapy practice, part 1. BJOT 57(1): 9–14

Whalley Hammell K 1994b Establishing objectives in occupational therapy practice, part 2. BJOT 57(2): 45–48

2. Epidemiology of stroke

G. Boysen

INTRODUCTION

As a result of increasing life expectancy, the total number of patients with stroke will increase since about half of all strokes occur in people over the age of 75 years. At present, stroke is the third leading cause of death in many western countries, and in some areas of China stroke is the second cause of death (Malmgren et al 1987, Terent 1993, World Health Organization 1982, 1991, Aho et al 1980). Stroke survivors are often left with severe disability and there is a great need for physical rehabilitation in the initial phase after stroke as welll as a need for long-term assistance in the late phase. In this chapter, some measures of stroke frequency, such as incidence rate, stroke mortality and case-fatality rate will be considered.

Incidence rate means the number of first-ever strokes per number of inhabitants in a given location or sample per year. Stroke mortality means the number of people dying of stroke per number of inhabitants per year. Case-fatality rate means the percentage of fatal strokes among all strokes in the sample.

Incidence rates can be given either as age- and sex-specific rates, usually for successive 10-year age groups within a specific population, or as age- and sex-adjusted with reference to the population in the country or to the world population (Terent 1993). Reference to the world population renders the incidence rates comparable among countries, while reference to the population from which the study sample is derived enables estimation of the total number of new strokes in the country. The world population is young compared to most developed countries, and because stroke incidence increases dramatically with age the numerical value of the estimated incidence rate will be reduced if the reference population is changed from one with a high proportion of old people to the world population.

STROKE INCIDENCE

Most incidence studies are based on the World Health Organization's definition of stroke: 'an acute disturbance of focal or global cerebral function with symptoms lasting more than 24 hours or leading to death presumably of vascular origin' (Aho et al 1980). This clinical definition includes ischaemic stroke as well as haemorrhagic stroke and subarachnoid haemorrhage. Many epidemiologic studies, however, exclude subarachnoid haemorrhage and some exclude intracerebral haemorrhage, which means that direct comparison between studies often is not useful.

For incidence studies to give a true estimate of given disease it is required that all cases in a defined population are identified (Malmgren et al 1987). Not only should information from hospital records and death certificates be collected, but also cases treated at home or not requiring medical attention should be identified. The latter requirment is the most difficult to fulfil and is the weak point of most incidence studies.

With reference to the world population, the incidence of first-ever stroke ranges from 84 per 100 000 in Umbria, Italy to 144 per 100 000 in Söderhamn, Sweden (Terent 1993). In terms of the much older Swedish population, these incidence rates would change to 141 per 100 000 in Umbria and to 274 per 100 000 in Söderhamn. This example illustrates the importance of knowing to which population a given incidence rate relates.

Stroke incidence varies with sex and age. In young people of less than 35 years of age, where stroke incidence is very low, the rate is slightly higher in woman than in men (Mettinger et al 1984, Lidegaard et al 1986, Nencini et al 1988), while in people over the age of 35 the incidence is higher in men than in women. Studies in the Scandinavian countries have shown stroke incidence in the age group 35–65 years to be twice as high in men as in women. In people over the age of 65, the sex difference decreases and tends to disappear in the oldest age groups.

In spite of this sex difference, the lifetime risk of dying of stroke is higher in women than in men because, in general, women live longer than men and therefore reach the age of high stroke incidence in greater numbers (Bonita 1992).

Secular changes in stroke incidence

In Rochester, Minnesota, USA, stroke incidence decreased from 1945 to 1980 (Garraway et al 1983a), whereas the incidence increased slightly during the 1980s (Broderick et al 1989). A decrease in stroke incidence has also been demonstrated in Finland (Tuomilehto et al 1991) and in Japan (Ueda et al 1981). In Sweden (Terent 1988), Denmark (Boysen et al 1988, Lindenstrøm et al 1992, Jørgensen et al 1992) and New Zealand (Bonita et al 1993), there have been no major changes in the last 20 years and reliable incidence data are not available prior to this period.

CASE-FATALITY RATE AND SURVIVAL

The case-fatality rate represents the proportion of stroke patients who die early, which is usually defined as within 28 or 30 days of onset. In Rochester, Minnesota, case fatality has decreased from 33% to 17% between the 1940s and the 1980s (Garraway et al 1983a). Long-term survival (7 years) improved from 22% to 40% in the same period. Improved treatment of hypertension has been suggested as an explanation for some of the decrease in stroke fatality. Improved medical care with early mobilisation is another important factor. It has recently been documented that management of patients in stroke units or by stroke teams improves survival compared to treatment in general medical wards (Langhorne et al 1993).

Among Japanese men living in Hawaii, the 30-day case-fatality rate decreased from 30% in the period 1969–1972 to 16% in the period 1985–1988 (Kagan et al 1994). In New Zealand, the 28-day case-fatality rate declined from 27% to 22% in men and from 38% to 26% in women from 1981 to 1991 (Bonita et al 1993). In Shanghai, the case-fatality rate was 46% in men in 1990 and slightly lower in women (Hong et al 1994), which is similar to the rate in Denmark 40 years ago (Marquardsen 1969), where it had declined to 19% by 1988 (Boysen et al 1988). In New Zealand the case-fatality rate one year after stroke is about 42% (Bonita et al 1993).

STROKE MORTALITY

The age-specific stroke mortality rate rises sharply with age from fewer than 10 deaths per 100 000 in people less than 45 years of age to more than 1000 per 100 000 in people aged 75 years or older.

Age-standardized mortality rates for the age group 40–69 years were reported from 27 countries and ranged from 249 per 100 000 population in Bulgarian men to 21 per 100 000 in Swiss women (Bonita et al 1990, Bonita & Beaglehole 1993). Stroke mortality has been decreasing in many countries during the last 50 years, although most studies have been carried out within the last 20 years (Figs 2.1 and 2.2). The cause of this decrease has not been fully explained. It may be a consequence of a decrease in

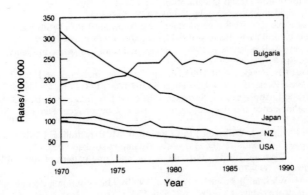

Fig. 2.1   Age-standardized stroke mortality rates (per 100 000 population) in men aged 40–69 years in selected countries from 1970 to 1989. NZ, New Zealand; USA, United States of America. (Reproduced from Bonita & Beaglehole 1993, with permission of Butterworth-Heinemann.)

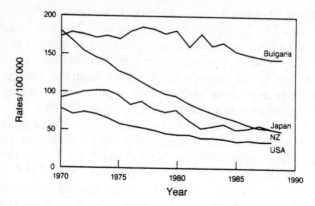

Fig. 2.2 Age-standardized stroke mortality rates (per 100 000 population) in women aged 40–69 years in selected countries from 1970 to 1989. NZ, New Zealand; USA, United States of America. (Reproduced from Bonita & Beaglehole 1993, with permission of Butterworth-Heinemann.)

incidence, in case-fatality rate or in both. From 1970 to 1985 there was a fall in stroke mortality in 25 out of 27 countries; this was most pronounced in Japan. In the eastern part of Europe, where stroke mortality rates are among the highest, the trend was the reverse and the mortality rates have increased in Poland, Hungary, Bulgaria, and in former Yugoslavia. The cause of this increase is unknown but is likely to be multifactorial, probably including poverty, high smoking rate, and unsatisfactory management of hypertension.

REFERENCES

Aho K, Harmsen P, Hatano S, Marquardsen J, Smirnov V E, Strasser T 1980 Cerebrovascular disease in the community: results of a WHO collaborative study. Bulletin of the World Health Organization 58: 113–130
Bonita R 1992 Epidemiology of stroke. Lancet 339: 342–344
Bonita R, Beaglehole R 1993 Stroke mortality. In: Whisnant J P (ed) Stroke: populations, cohorts, and clinical trials. Butterworth-Heinemann, Oxford, pp 59–79
Bonita R, Stewart A, Beaglehole R 1990 International trends in stroke mortality: 1970–1985. Stroke 21: 989–992
Bonita R, Broad J B, Beaglehole R 1993 changes in stroke incidence and case-fatality in Auckland, New Zealand, 1981–91. Lancet 342: 1470–1473
Boysen G, Nyboe J, Appleyard M, Sørensen P S, Boas J, Somnier F, Jensen G, Schnohr P 1988 Stroke incidence and risk factors for stroke in Copenhagen, Denmark. Stroke 19: 1345–1353
Broderick J P, Phillips S J, Whisnant J P, O'Fallon W M, Bergstralh E J 1989 Incidence rates of stroke in the eighties: the end of the decline in stroke? Stroke 20: 577–582
Garraway W M, Whisnant J P, Drury I 1983a The changing pattern of survival following stroke. Stroke 14: 699–703
Garraway W M, Whisnant J P, Furlan A J et al 1983b The continuing decline in the incidence of stroke. Mayo Clin Proc 58: 520–523
Hong Y, Bots M, Pan X, Hofman A, Grobber D E, Chen H 1994 Stroke incidence and mortality in rural and urban Shanghai from 1984 through 1992. Stroke 25: 1165–1169
Jørgensen H S, Plesner A M, Hübbe P, Larsen K 1992 Marked increase of stroke incidence in men between 1972 and 1990, Frederiksberg, Denmark. Stroke 23: 1701–1704

Kagan A, Popper J, Reed D, MacLean C J, Grove J S 1994 Trends in stroke incidence and mortality in Hawaiian Japanese men. Stroke 25: 1170–1175

Langhorne P, Williams B O, Gilchrist W, Howie K 1993 Do stroke units save lives? Lancet 342: 395–398

Lidegaard O, Soe M, Andersen M V N 1986 Cerebral thromboembolism among young women and men in Denmark 1977–1982. Stroke 4: 670–675

Lindenstrøm E, Boysen G, Nyboe J, Appleyard M 1992 Stroke incidence in Copenhagen, 1976–1988 Stroke 23: 28–32

Malmgren R, Warlow C, Bamford J, Sandercock P 1987 Geographical and secular trends in stroke incidence. Lancet 2: 1196–1200

Marquardsen J 1969 The natural history of acute cerebrovascular disease: a retrospective study of 769 patients. Acta Neurol Scandinavica 45 (suppl 38): 9–192

Mettinger K L, Söderström C E, Allander E 1984 Epidemiology of acute cerebrovascular disease before the age of 55 in the Stockholm County 1973–77: I. Incidence and mortality rates. Stroke 15: 795–801

Nencini P, Inzitari D, Baruffi M C et al 1988 Incidence of stroke in young adults in Florence, Italy. Stroke 19: 977–981

Terent A 1988 Increasing incidence of stroke among Swedish women. Stroke 12: 460–466

Terent A 1993 Stroke morbidity. In: Whisnant J P (ed) Stroke : populations, cohorts, and clinical trials. Butterworth-Heinemann, Oxford, pp 37–58

Tuomilehto J, Bonita R, Stewart A, Nissinen A, Salonen J T 1991 Hypertension, cigarette smoking, and the decline in stroke incidence in eastern Finland. Stroke 22: 7–11

Ueda K, Omae T, Hirota Y et al 1981 Decreasing trend in incidence and mortality from stroke in Hisayama residents, Japan. Stroke 12: 154–160

World Health Organization 1982 Cancer incidence in five continents, vol. 4. International Agency for Research on Cancer, Lyon

World Health Organization 1991 World Health Statistics Annual, pp 362–366

Aspects of clinical practice

3. Symptoms in adult hemiparesis – new approaches and their therapeutic implications in the Bobath concept

M. Gerber

INTRODUCTION

The Bobath concept is an *active, functional, re-education process* aimed at improving the quality of life in patients with central nervous system deficits by enabling them to develop new strategies for completing the tasks in their daily lives.

The treatment is a constant interplay between patient and therapist. The concept is in continuous evolution. Several instructors, such as Joan Mohr and Susan Ryerson in the USA, Patricia Davies, Mary Lynch and Louise Rutz-Lapitz in Europe and Elia Panturin in Israel, have joined together to form the International Bobath Instructor's Association (IBITAH).They have taken on the challenge of the work of Berta Bobath and her husband, Dr Karel Bobath and have contributed significantly to the continued development of their theory in the light of new neurophysiological and therapeutic discoveries.

The symptoms of adults with a hemiparesis constitute a source of information which can be compared to a 'puzzle'. Each piece is equally important and influences the whole in a significant way.

Spasticity, inefficient stereotyped synergies, associated reactions, soft tissue changes, or the hyperactivity of the unaffected side are all symptoms to be decoded within the framework of a holistic approach towards the patient.

While the Bobath concept used the hierarchical model to support the belief that the symptoms of hemiparesis could be influenced in treatment, others disagreed. These symptoms, now, can be approached holistically using a systems model which integrates multiple systems such as neurophysiological, biomechanical, psychological and enviromental systems.

If the hierarchical model is abandoned as an explanation of the symptoms of central nervous system (CNS) damage, in favour of a much more global model, as proposed by the 'neurotherapeutic systems model' (Horak 1991) and the 'biomechanical notion of degree of freedom' (Bernstein 1967), there will be a new way to describe the Bobath concept. The CNS can be

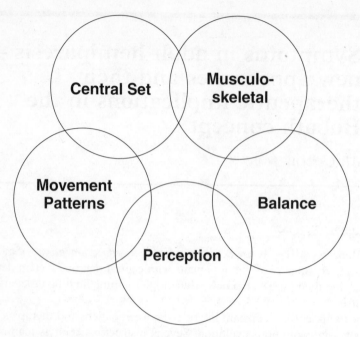

Fig. 3.1 Neurotherapeutic system model (Horak 1990).

compared with a spider's web; if a fly is caught in it, the whole net begins to move. With a stroke, the CNS becomes completely disorganized and the aim of treatment will be to give to the patient the ability of normal function; in order to achieve this, he or she needs normal movement (Panturin, unpublished).

The return to the systems approach of the CNS's functioning fundamentally changes the original explanation of the concept as proposed by Dr Bobath. In surveying the different elements contained in Horak's neurotherapeutic systems model, one can try to relate them to treatment (Horak 1990) (Fig. 3.1).

CENTRAL SET/PREDICTIVE CONTROL

The central set is the ability of the nervous system to prepare the motor system for incoming sensory information and to prepare the sensory system for incoming movement. For example, postural adjustments have been shown to precede self-initiated arm, leg, and trunk movements to minimize postural instability that would otherwise have occurred. It is based on prior experience (Horak 1991). To use this concept in therapy can be very positive if the therapist knows exactly what to expect and uses the set adequately.

Therapists should be encouraged to use the acquired musical experience of patients and to put rhythm into their treatments. A piece of jazz can instil more rhythm into a patient's gait, and allows unsuspected selective movements of the trunk to appear.

The apparent diversion of play in treatment can produce better concentration and may use the concept of predictive control. By using coloured balls, skateboards and musical instruments, therapists can stimulate creativity in the patients and put some 'fun' into long and tedious rehabilitation.

BALANCE PROBLEMS

Normal postural motor behaviour is in the task-orientated approach, the product of the interaction of many components organized around a fundamental behavioural goal to maintain equilibrium and orientation in the environment. These components are the musculoskeletal system, perception and sensory organization, predictive central set and motor coordination (Horak 1991).

Balance reactions are multifactorial as is their training. The emphasis in treatment is on eliciting reactions; this means learning to react to proprioceptive input. This constitutes an important part of the aims for the first stage of recovery, when the flaccid muscle tone.does not allow the accomplishment of function. The training of function in a feedforward or predictive mode will be used, but in the interim stages, the ability of selective movements will be trained through specific activities with an emphasis on the trunk.

Carr & Shepherd (1987) criticize the use of manual contact ('hands on') during balance reactions because it interferes with the patient's reactions. The author does not agree because 'hands on' experience is constructive as long as it prevents an abnormal reaction by providing proprioceptive information, inhibiting abnormal tone or inefficient stereotyped synergies and facilitating normal movement. Cognitive coorperation through visualization of the tasks can be used by some patients. Balance reactions will first be taught in the sitting position. The reactions in standing will be practised as soon as the malalignment in the lower extremities does not produce too many compensatory reactions in the upper extremities. In the next strategy, speed and difficulty will be increased.

MOVEMENT PATTERNS

The associated reactions (per definition on the hemiparetic side) can be interpreted as either a reaction of physiological equilibrium or a result of a pathological perception of the patient's own body in relation to his/her environment. It is a compensatory strategy in which the centre of gravity is overdisplaced and produces 'normal' arm reactions.

Three different shifts of a patient's centre of gravity can be described:

• Category A: dorsal displacement – the patient presents a movement component of flexion/internal rotation at the shoulder, flexion/pronation at the elbow and ulnar abduction at the wrist.

• Category B: ventral displacement – with a component of extension/external rotation at the shoulder, flexion/supination at the elbow and radial abduction at the wrist.

• Category C: lateral displacement – mostly to the unaffected side, with an abduction at the shoulder.

An empirical observation enables the author to describe a geographical distribution of these three categories. The patient in category A is more common in countries with long-term rehabilitation, the so-called 'classical north European hemiparetic'. The second category 'North American hemiparetic' has shorter readaptation and earlier ambulation from the wheelchair. Some European head injury patients present this reaction. The third category (group C) is classically found in groups A and B (Gerber & Vaney 1994). With better trunk and lower extremity control associated reactions will be spontaneously reduced.

PERCEPTION

Is sensation necessary for movement? In the feedforward control, movements are initiated before any sensory stimulus (e.g. in the gastrocnemius-soleus before the heel strike), but it represents only a category of movement. If some movements are possible without sensory feedback, they still need it for regulation and adaptation. The deficits in coordination by well-trained astronauts after a short period of time without gravity demonstrate that the human control system is very precarious.

Affolter (1981) wrote that the unique sensory modality which one can activate directly is the tactile-kinaesthetic system. The understanding of differences between left and right hemiparetic patients allows a better assessment of perception; Davies' description of the 'pusher syndrome' is a well-known example (Davies 1985).

In 1990, the author presented a study on 54 patients comparing the variations in heart rate and modifications of muscle tone during functional activities (e.g. walking up and down stairs or going down to the floor) and found significant differences between left and right hemiparetic patients (Gerber 1990).

Wiard has shown connections between visuospatial neglect and psycho-affective disorders of patients with left hemiparesis (Wiard 1994). All these observations provide new pieces for the puzzle and should influence treatment.

The proprioceptive input will be experienced through weight bearing on the hemiparetic side and will also influence muscle tone. The structured environment will help a patient with perceptual problems by putting him or her in 'a corner'. The surplus of information allows the patient to find the midline and to accept the environment instead of fighting it.

What Paul Beelen, a paediatric Bobath instructor, described as a 'new panorama' is a new interpretation of symptoms by some children with cerebral palsy (Beelen 1990).

The unique possible response of a disturbed perception of the world is an increase of hypertonicity which allows the child to organize himself in the environment. His response is to take refuge in hypertonicity. If the space is felt as bottomless, he may choose immobility. Spasticity or hypertonicity can be seen in these cases as more neurobehaviourally than neurologically influenced.

The strategy used in these cases will be to limit, through fixing, the degrees of freedom, as seen sometimes in ataxia, stroke, multiple sclerosis or head injury. Empirical experience over the years allows the author to notice that with some of those patients, an *aquatic treatment* can be very beneficial; warm water can provide an environment that is an additional source of information about the body and can give astonishing results.

MUSCULOSKELETAL SYSTEM

Some ideas about the inefficient stereotyped synergies and associated reactions have already been described. How will symptoms such as spasticity, soft issue changes and hyperactivity of the unaffected side be explained by the system's approach? The new challenge will consist of looking at the symptoms as 'normal compensations' of an abnormal way. There are always many reasons for a symptom. Intervention by the therapist is easier on compensatory strategies than on the primary result of the neural lesion. This depends more on the plasticity of the brain and the ipsilaterality of some corticospinal tracts.

Malalignment of joints and muscle fibres, neural tension, soft tissue changes (e.g. a deep oedema between muscle fibres) can prevent muscle stretch and stimulate hypertonicity. Change of intrinsic properties in spastic muscles, problems of muscle firing, shortening, weakness or lack of endurance are all pieces of the 'symptoms puzzle'. A correct evaluation will guide the therapist towards specific action.

Bernstein was the first to suggest that the principal problem faced by the CNS is the enormous number of joints and muscles in the human body. Because of this large number of degrees of freedom, almost every movement can be carried out in an infinite number of ways, with an infinite number of combinations of muscle action (Carr & Shepherd 1987). There is not one stereotyped way of getting up from a chair; there are several ways. The therapist will suggest the most appropriate relevant strategy.

The excessive muscle tone (spasticity and hyperactivity of the unaffected side) is the result of a disorder of many interacting systems. It is fascinating to observe the wide field of hypotonicity under the apparent hypertonicity (Ryerson 1993).

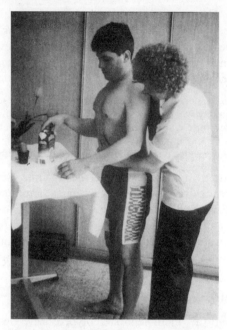

Fig. 3.2 Task: to pour juice into a glass held in the paretic hand and to drink from it. The therapist facilitates selective movements in the left paretic arm and hand by allowing a better dynamic stabilization of the trunk and scapula on the thorax. The therapist stimulates abdominal muscle activity (especially the obliqui) with her left hand and active scapula depression with her right hand.

The hypertonicity or spasticity is not the problem which is treated. The focus of treatment is the situation in which the hypertonicity manifests itself. These situations provide a structure for clinical assessment.

If facing the challenge of spasticity is still relevant, the challenge of hypotonicity could become the next big issue for the therapist. In walking, for example, distal spasticity in toes and fingers can be considerably influenced by the improvement of selective trunk control (dynamic stability of the upper trunk and selective mobility, instead of fixing, of the lower trunk), by adequate weight bearing on the hemiparetic leg after realignment of the joints and muscle fibres and by specific activities providing a better coordination through sensorimotor inputs. Control is based on the quality of the movement and the achievement of the task (Fig. 3.2).

CONCLUSION

Berta Bobath, a creative genius, has given therapists some keys to the 'magic touch' of her hands. It was evident that a large part of the once fashionable neurophysiological model, the hierarchical one, was partially satisfactory. The return to and adaptation of systems models such as Horak's allows a more global vision of the interaction between the art and the science of the

Bobath concept. Considering this new approach to be *the* truth could prejudice the development of the concept; while there is, at this time, no consensus on terminology and definitions of terms it can, however, help us to optimize the 'carry-over' of our patients.

The challenge for the therapist is still to observe a patient's reactions and adapt treatment accordingly. As Hubert Reeves, astrophysicist, said:

Research is nothing but the actual state of the process of exploration of knowledge.

Acknowledgement

My gratitude is extended to Susan Ryerson, senior instructor Bobath/ IBITAH for her assistance in the English translation.

REFERENCES

Affolter F 1981 Perceptual processes as prerequisites for complex human behaviour. Int Rehabil Med 3
Beelen P 1990 Le nouveau panorama. No 5 Kiné 2000, Belgium
Carr J H, Shepherd R B 1987 Movement science foundations for physical therapy in rehabilitation. Aspen, Rockville, p 84
Bernstein NA 1967 The co-ordination and regulation of movements. Pergamon, New York, pp 127, 134
Davies P 1985 Steps to follow. Springer Verlag, Berlin, pp 266–284
Gerber M 1990 Variations de la fréquence cardiaque chez l'hémiplégique adulte lors d'un traitement-type d'après le concept Bobath. Annales de Kinésithérapie 17(9): 421–442
Gerber M, Vaney C L 1994 Verlust Selektiver Rumpfaktivitäten und deren Auswirkungen bei Erwachsenen mit Hemiparese. Krankengymnastik 3: 328–341
Gordon J 1987 Assumptions underlying physical therapy intervention: theoretical and historical perspectives. In: Contemporary management of motor problems. Proceeding of the II STEP Conference, The Foundation for Physical Therapy, Alexandria, Virginia, ch 1, pp 1–30
Horak F B 1990 Contemporary management of motor control problems. Presentation at II Step Conference, Oklahoma
Horak F B 1991 Assumptions underlying motor control for neurologic rehabilitation. In: Contemporary management of motor problems. Proceeding of the II STEP Conference, The Foundation for Physical Therapy, Alexandria, Virginia, ch 4, pp 11–27
Panturin. Unpublished lecture given during advanced course BOBATH/IBITAH, Clinic for Rheumatology and Rehabilitation. Leukerbad, Switzerland
Ryerson S 1993 Clinical assessment of spasticity. Lecture, APTA Annual Convention, Cincinatti, Ohio
Wiard L 1994 Troubles psycho-affectifs de l'hémiplégique gauche. Rôle de l'héminégligence et implications thérapeutiques. Annales Réadaptation Méd Phys 37: 15–23

4. A cognitive approach in the rehabilitation of the upper extremity in hemiplegic stroke patients

J. P. Bleton,   F. Odier

INTRODUCTION

Experimental and clinical studies have suggested a number of possibilities for recovery after hemiplegic stroke.

One such possibility is the anatomopathological restoration of the affected cerebral system which tries to establish compensation by the healthy regions and the opposite cerebral hemisphere (Chollet et al 1991). This plasticity of the central nervous system was also described by Dejerine, who presented the case of a patient affected by infantile hemiplegia who had a hypertrophy of compensation of the pyramidal system on the unaffected side (Dejerine 1901).

A second possibility is the induction of synaptic sprouting, reinforcement of existing neuronal circuits and formation of new polysynaptic connections. Learning allows neuronal connections to be established (Ramon & Cajal 1928).

The third possibility deals with reducing local oedema and necrotic tissue.

The present sensorimotor programmes used by hemiplegic stroke patients are the result of a new functional pathological equilibrium at a lower level. Restoration favours the partial return of normal activities but the lesion frees tonic disturbance and movement disorder.

Review of the literature concerning recovery after a hemiplegic stroke (Thorngren & Westling 1990) reveals that use of the upper limb is regained in 20–30% of cases; however, this usually permits only rudimentary function.

Patients do not easily accept the loss of the use of their affected hand, even when they have recovered a functional independence. They often become disappointed and develop a certain degree of hostility towards their affected hand.

Clinical observation shows that hemiplegic strokes affect not only motor function and muscle tone but also non-motor functions, e.g. proprioceptive and tactile perception. Hemiplegic strokes also affect non-motor and

39

non-sensory functions, e.g. lack of selective attention, visuospatial disorders and mood disturbances (Denes et al 1982).

Hemiplegia with a single motor lesion also evolves into a proprioceptive defect, with a progressive loss of perception on the affected side of the body.

The particular importance that the upper limb has as a means of recognition and action in the immediate surrounding environment has led to the development of a rehabilitation programme including these functions. Encouraged by the results obtained by the Italian school of rehabilitation (Perfetti 1982), the authors have established their own conception of stroke patient rehabilitation, which is the result of their everyday practice and experience. Their established objective is to make cognitive function available as a resource for motor rehabilitation.

ASSESSMENT

Hemiplegic stroke patients must be evaluated from all aspects because other functions besides motor function could be affected.

The assessment is analytical. The tests are performed in different parts of the upper limb. The items are classified into the following three groups: motor function, sensory function and related problems. A fourth and more general group evaluates different aspects of behaviour and mental function. Each item that is inclined to be affected is evaluated in a semiquantitative way according to five progressive degrees.

The different affected functions are transcribed on a histogram and evaluated in a linear fashion, without hierarchical value, showing the profile of the patients' impairment.

The analytical assessment is completed by:

• impairment scales such as 'neurological scale for middle cerebral infarction' (Orgogozo 1983)

• functional evaluation such as the Barthel index (Mahoney & Barthel 1965) and the 'Frenchay arm test' (Wade et al 1983)

• self-assessment of the patient's image of the hand; this scale is constructed by using 10 pairs of Osgood's evaluative adjectives (Van Deusen 1993).

The results of evaluation allow the physiotherapist and the patient, together, to agree on reasonable objectives of rehabilitation.

REHABILITATION STRATEGY

Rehabilitation is based on the use of non-affected learning mechanisms in order to gain new motor functions. It consists of tasks from four progressive levels of difficulty.

Level 1 tasks

This is the phase of recovery of sensory feedback, the aim of which is the restoration of proprioception and kinesthesia in the upper limb.

Objectives are prioritised according to the severity of the perceptual deficit and disorganisation of the body image.

The initial aim is to focus the patient's attention onto the affected upper limb. The exercises are chosen in such a way as to facilitate the patient's awareness of the upper limb and to enable recognition of the hand, fingers, and the various patterns of the limb.

To achieve this awareness, the physiotherapist performs exteroceptive stimuli by mobilising the skin of the fingertips. This is done by applying friction and alternately pressing the extremity of the thumb against the palmar aspect of the other fingers. These rapid movements, particularly in the distal region of the affected limb, reinforce the proprioceptive input from the limb. The physiotherapist ensures the patient's concentration and administers a series of elementary sensory stimuli such as pinpricks, pressure, contact with cold metal objects and localised selective movements. The patient focuses attention on the affected upper limb and becomes aware of the sensory feedback from it.

Exercises

With rare exceptions, where the symptomatology is accompanied by a grasping reflex, the patient is encouraged to stimulate the affected hand frequently during the day by rubbing it with the other hand and placing objects of different textures in it so that it never remains inactive.

By facing up to the physical deficit caused by stroke and the neglect which is exhibited, the patient is taught to rediscover his/her limb in the area of the affected side, to take care of it and to position it correctly.

The 'blind grasping exercise' which entails closing the eyes and catching the thumb of the affected hand with the other hand (as well as other exercises of this type) makes the patient focus attention on the afferent input coming from the affected side and explore body awareness of that side.

During rest periods, the affected limb is placed in different natural positions, avoiding those positions likely to generate articular constraints or overflow of activity. The patient must soon become aware of the quality of correct resting positions of the upper limb, in order to be able to modify incorrect positions.

If the symptomatology is accompanied by hemispatial neglect, a specific rehabilitation programme is adapted at the same time. The objectives of this programme are to encourage the patient to visually explore the affected side in order to become orientated within his/her own environment and to describe complex images and drawings, focusing particularly on the details of those on the hemiplegic side (Seron & Laterre 1982).

Level 2 tasks

This is the phase of assisted exploration of the environment and of the proprioceptive input from joint positions and movements. It allows a veritable base of sensory data to be established.

Manual exploration suggests a motor activity, but the motility is merely a tool of cognitive discovery.

The physiotherapist challenges the patient with various types of sensory stimuli. The patient, eyes closed, is informed of the nature of these stimulations, of the moment of contact and of which area of the limb is being stimulated.

The patient's attention is focused on the recognition of tactile or proprioceptive stimuli. At this stage of recovery, motor function is still weak and is compensated for by the physiotherapist who guides the hand in the zone or the object to be identified, at the same time avoiding the occurrence of overflow of activity. These tactile identifications take place in the form of localised light touching and textural exploration of two or three dimensional shapes. The absence of vision forces the patient to use highly sensitive areas of the hand such as the fingertips, to explore the object to be identified.

The physiotherapist and the patient are seated side by side so that their hands are placed in the same position. Thus, the patient does not need to create a 'mental mirror rotation' by comparing hands.

Exercises

The objective is to ask the patient to interpret sensory information. Motivation is emphasised by the requirement to answer questions dealing with stimulation characteristics. The answers are, in fact, the result of a choice imposed by the physiotherapist, in the form of closed questions, e.g. 'is this stimulation identical to the last one?' or open questions, e.g. 'on which fingers did you feel the stimulation?'. The answers must be explicit. They are always confirmed by the unaffected side, by the physiotherapist's corroboration or by looking. By encountering these experiences, the patient learns progressively to identify the stimuli and gains confidence in his/her analytical capabilities.

The proprioceptive tasks take the form of questions regarding localisation of pressure on the surfaces of the joints, on postures and on segmented movements to which the patient must respond in an explicit away. These kinesthesic identification tasks address as a whole the articulations of the upper limb, but are limited within arm's length.

With the establishment of progressive improvement, the hand is moved at a constant, then a variable, speed, displaced in various directions and placed in different positions. The patient is informed when the movements start and finish.

Level 3 tasks

This is the phase where motor function plays a partial role in the exploration of the environment, thus establishing a cognitive link between the goal of the action and the movement.

The motor programmes persist despite hemiplegia, as their performance in the unaffected side shows (Pailhous & Bonnard 1989). These programmes are not eliminated from the memory but the difficulty lies in finding the means to perform them. Certain motivating situations, which are reminders of past experiences, allow motor function to be re-established (Hauert et al 1989).

Exercises

The method of rehabilitation comprises exploration tasks of progressive difficulty, having a specific effect, most often inadvertently, on motor function. For example, the patient, eyes closed, recognises with the affected hand fairly familiar objects, compares the different components and measures differences between the weight placed in the unaffected hand with that in the affected hand.

While the motor function is inefficient, the movements are guided by the physiotherapist who also prevents any unexpected problems of muscle tone or other movement disorders.

The exercises are adapted to different capabilities of the various areas of the affected upper limb. They take into account the general position of the body. The organisation of these exercises is exaggerated in its accuracy in order to allow the patient to appreciate immediately the degree of ability. The level of difficulty and help provided by the physiotherapist are one reason for the absence of overflow of activity.

The environment and the kind of objects used, i.e. the context in which the exercise is carried out, allow for the modification of equilibrium between the developed internal strength in the patient and the qualitative external forces of the object. For example, among the exercises for rotation of the forearm, the affected hand is placed on a mobile board where the balance is controlled by the muscles of the forearm. The patient, eyes closed, must keep the hand stable despite additional weights which are placed on one side or the other (Fig. 4.1).

The purpose of this exercise is to analyse on which side of the board the successive weights are placed and to compare them with each other, and not to automatically maintain the equilibrium between pronator and supinator muscles. The patient responds to questions such as: 'Is the weight I just placed on the board heavier than the last one? Is it placed more to the front or more to the right?'. This way of proceeding makes the patient analyse his perceptions and express them in an explicit way. The use of light weight, only a few grams, allows the patient to obtain precise muscular

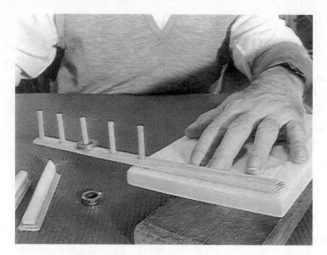

Fig. 4.1 Exercise for rotation of the forearm.

contractions. Even one intense muscle contraction would prevent an exact analysis.

In order to create a progression, the arrangement, size, distance, weight, and degree of freedom of movement, as well as the objects used in the exercise, are modified. It is also often necessary to adapt them in function to the needs of the patients.

Observation shows that the patient often makes mistakes due to the speed, the strength, or the difficulty in coordinating the different body parts called upon in the exercise. Paradoxically, the patient often uses more strength than is needed. In addition, by working at low levels of intensity and speed, it becomes possible to construct complex movements and to diminish abnormal overflow of activity which interferes with the acquisition of new motor function. The overflow of activity is diminished by an action which draws attention to the unaffected hand, e.g. manipulating two balls, or keeping the healthy hand steady on an unstable board. If the derivation task is too easy, the overflow of activity is not mastered.

Level 4 tasks

In this phase the objective is threefold:

- to acquire stable and repetitive motor programmes
- to adapt to exterior constraints as well as to necessities of action
- to adjust in relation to the result.

The motor function can be controlled solely by the patient.

The organisation of the voluntary gesture is explained through models which show the relationship between intention, motor execution and sensory control (Pailhous 1987).

In order to be perfectly executed this motor programmes must be adapted to exterior conditions. The elements to be dealt with come from sensory information. In particular, they concern the context in which the movement should be executed, i.e. spatial characteristics of the situation, the position of the target and the qualities of the objects used. The programme also implies that the subject knows the position of his/her different corporal elements as well as the tension level of his/her muscles. Finally, the subject deals with the information concerning the task to be accomplished, i.e. the precision and the required speed (Paillard & Beaubaton 1978).

Exercises

The physiotherapist chooses the posture, the direction and the speed of the movement. Exercise performance should be as precise as possible, without overflow of activity, and in relation to the patient's skills.

The patient, eyes open, can at each moment see the precision of his/her movement and can modify it if necessary. For example, one exercise is to ask the patient to follow a sinuous drawing with a pointer using only the wrist, the hand resting on a mobile support (Fig. 4.2). The situation is arranged in such way, that body position can be controlled and the affected limb released. Controls, such as spirit levels and sensors sensitive to finger pressure, are placed at the level of the non-affected upper limb, the trunk and the affected fingers. The patient can thus, through vision, proprioception and touch, adjust his/her movement to reach the proposed goal of the exercise.

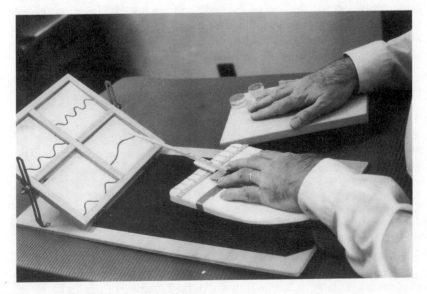

Fig. 4.2   Exercise in precision of movement.

The physiotherapist varies certain elements, e.g. the patient's position, the degree of mobility of the support, the design of the drawing, the size of the pointer, the degree of resistance of the support and the speed of the execution of the movement. The patient must adapt the movement of the wrist to the different constraints. With extreme attention and precise realisation, the patient memorizes the movements and their feedback. He/she can thus perform them at leisure and in less artificial and more functional circumstances.

The progression of difficulty is manifested in three levels:

1. localised exercises for the affected hand
2. exercises demanding a more complete participation of the upper limb
3. bilateral exercises where coordination, rhythm and speed of performance are essential.

The exercises of this level are also useful in the rehabilitation of patients with simple motor hemiplegia. Their sensorimotor quality prevents the loss of feedback and non-use.

Period of rest

The restrictions imposed by such tasks, in monopolising the patient's attention, result in a need for 'between-tasks rests', which also constitute an objective of learning process. The positions in which the affected limb is placed during these intervals are also important. Observation of resting positions of healthy individuals shows that some involve hand contact on the face while others constitute the hands being pressed together. The limbs are often crossed at the midline of the body and fall towards the opposite side as in the sitting position with the arms folded and one leg crossed over the other, or one hand placed on the opposite knee. Re-assuming such positions helps the patient remember past habitual postures.

PRELIMINARY RESULTS

The authors are following the progress of patients whose stroke occurred at least 1 year ago and is of ischaemic origin. In each case the patient had already had conventional rehabilitation in different specialised centres. They are evaluated before and after 2 weeks of daily rehabilitation.

The present results seem to show:

• an improvement of body image and self perception
• an awareness of the attention necessary in relation to the upper limb, particularly in resting positions
• the partial return of sensory feedback
• in a significant number of patients, the return of voluntary analytical movements, notably at the level of the distal extremity of the limb.

The recovered functions are not always used in daily life.
The results are presently being confirmed with a control group.

CONCLUSION

This rehabilitation strategy is based on the use of processes of learning devices in order to acquire new motor behaviour. This approach has not yet been completely refined. The research has been limited to the recovery of the grasping function in the immediate area of the body.

It will also be necessary to study the grasping function in distant space which implies walking.

REFERENCES

Chollet F, Di Piero V, Wise R J S, Brooks D, Dolan R J, Frackowiak R S J 1991 The functional anatomy of motor recovery after stroke in humans: a study with positron emission tomography. Annales of Neurology 29: 63–71

Dejerine J 1901 Anatomie des centres nerveux. Rueff, Paris. Reprint 1980 Masson, Paris, vol 2

Denes G, Semenza C, Stoppa E, Lis A 1982 Unilateral spatial neglect and recovery from hemiplegia. Brain 105: 543–552

Hauert C A, Zanone P G, Mounoud P 1989 Development of motor control in the child. Theorical and experimental approaches. In: Neuman O, Prinz W (eds) Relations between perception and action: current approaches. Springer Verlag, Berlin

Mahoney F I, Barthel D W 1965 Functional evaluation. The Barthel index. Maryland State Medical Journal 14: 61–65

Orgogozo J M 1983 Evaluation des thérapeutiques dans les infarctus cérébraux. In: Dehen H, Dordain G (eds) Neuropharmocologie clinique. Doin, Paris, pp 147–183

Pailhous J 1987 Les fonctions d'organisation des conduites et des données. In: Piaget J, Mounoud P, Bronckart J P (eds) Psychologie, encyclopédie de la pléiade. Gallimard, Paris, pp 902–932

Pailhous J, Bonnard M 1989 Programmation et contrôle du mouvement. In: Bonnet C, Ghiglione R, Richard J F (eds) Traité de psychologie cognitive. Dunod, Bordas, Paris, ch 3, pp 131–197

Paillard J, Beaubaton D 1978 De la coordination visuo-motrice à l'organisation de la saisie manuelle. In: Hecaen H, Jeannerod M (eds) Du contrôle moteur à l'organisation du geste. Masson, Paris, pp 224–260

Perfetti C 1982 Le condotte terapeutiche nella rieducazione motoria dell'emiplegico. Ghedini, Milano

Ramon Y, Cajal S 1928 Degeneration and regeneration of the nervous system. Oxford University Press, London, vol 2

Seron X, Laterre C (eds) 1982 Rééduquer le cerveau. Mardaga, Bruxelles

Thorngren M, Westling B 1990 Rehabilitation and achieved health quality after stroke. A population-based study of 258 hospitalized cases followed for one year. Acta Neurologica Scandinavica 82: 374–380

Van Deusen J 1993 Body image and perceptual dysfunction in adults. W B Saunders, Philadelphia

Wade D T, Langton-Hewer R, Wood V A, Skilbeck C E, Ismail H M 1983 The hemiplegic arm after stroke: measurement and recovery. Journal of Neurology, Neurosurgery and Psychiatry 46: 521–524

5. Orthotic management of stroke patients

E. Condie, D. Condie

A stroke is a clinical syndrome (a collection of signs and symptoms) where there are rapidly developed clinical signs of focal (or global) disturbance of cerebral function, lasting more than 24 hours or leading to death, with no apparent cause other than of vascular origin. (WHO)

THE PROBLEM

The Royal College of Physicians published a report in 1989 entitled *Stroke – Towards Better Management*, which states that stroke is predominantly a problem of the elderly and that 90% of deaths from stroke occur after the age of 65.

Accurate, up-to-date figures concerning this category of patient are extremely hard to unearth; however, most authorities agree that, in the UK, there are 150–200 new cases of stroke per 100 000 of the general population per year. The prevalence of stroke is said to be between 300 and 700 per 100 000 of the population.

CONSEQUENCE OF STROKE

Approximately 30% of patients die within 3 weeks of their stroke, 20–25% are non-hemiplegic and 50% remain dependent on another person (Wade et al 1985).

Of those surviving beyond 3 weeks (and who are admitted to an acute hospital), 20% never return home. 30% go home and lead a restricted life, and the remainder, i.e. 50%, make a good, functional recovery (Royal College of Physicians, 1989).

CLINICAL PRESENTATION

This is widely variable; however there are some commonly encountered features:

- paralysis or paresis leading to loss of selective movements
- changes in resting tone: hypertonicity (spasticity), hypotonicity or combination of both

- postural disorders
- sensory deficit
- communication disorders
- emotional and intellectual impairment.

The first three of these clinical features, probably in combination with one or all of the others, lead to loss of coordinated patterns of movement. This, in turn, leads to considerable difficulty with walking and, as a result, can produce loss of independent mobility. It is very likely that this loss of independent mobility will exert a strong influence on whether or not a patient can return to his/her own home.

It is therefore clear that anything which can be done to assist the patient to regain independent mobility is to their considerable advantage. The therapist's key role within the rehabilitation process is covered in other chapters; however, it is perhaps worthwhile summarising the aims of the wide variety of treatment programmes which currently exist.

These are:
- to assist the patient to achieve a functional recovery
- to re-establish normal movement, where possible.

However, despite the best efforts of skilled therapists, many stroke patients will have considerable locomotor difficulties.

A physical examination of the patient will normally demonstrate a typical pattern:

- Imbalance of subtalar musculature with weakness of invertors and/or spasticity of invertors.
- Imbalance of ankle musculature with weakness of dorsiflexors and/or spasticity of plantar flexors.
- Imbalance of knee musculature with weakness of flexors and/or spasticity of extensors.

In addition, weakness of hip flexors, abductors and hip extensors is commonly present in isolation or combination.

Some of the most severe locomotor problems are related to the presence of extensor synergy which manifests itself as:

1. Plantar flexion of the foot during stance (sometimes known as equinus'). This is possible cause of knee hyperextension.
2. Inversion of the foot on weight-bearing (sometimes known as 'varus').
3. Plantar flexion of the foot during swing phase (with or without inversion) causing foot or toe clearance difficulties.

All of the problems identified above can be managed by the application of a properly fitted ankle–foot orthosis.

Note

It is of fundamental importance that any orthosis must be individually made for each patient by an appropriately skilled individual. The use of 'off-the shelf' orthoses which are not custom-made is not recommended for stroke patients.

BIOMECHANICAL CONSIDERATIONS AND ORTHOTIC DESIGN

Equinus

The equinus position of the foot is generally caused by spasticity of the plantarflexor group of muscles (Fig. 5.1A). It follows that the orthosis supplied to overcome this problem will be required to generate a dorsiflexion moment about the ankle joint. This will necessitate the application of a three-point force system posteriorly on the calf, anteriorly at the level of the ankle joint and distally on the plantar surface of the foot (Fig. 5.1B).

In theory, at least, is is not necessary to immobilise the ankle completely. Thus the specifications of the ideal orthotic joint for this group of patients might read 'resist plantar flexion/free dorsiflexion'.

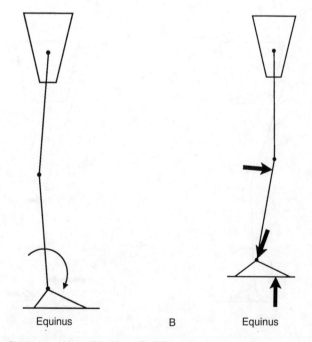

A   Equinus   B   Equinus

Fig. 5.1   A. Equinus position of the foot. **B**. Three-point force system.

Varus

The varus position of the foot is also a result of spasm in the calf musculature, notably the triceps surae, which is a powerful supinator of the foot (Fig. 5.2A). The orthosis supplied to overcome this problem will be required to generate a pronating movement about the subtalar joint. This will require the application of a three-point force system proximally on the medial aspect of the calf, laterally just above the lateral malleolus and distally on the medial aspect of the foot (Fig. 5.2B).

Theoretically, as with the ankle, there is no need to immobilise the subtalar joint and the specification for the ideal orthotic joint for this group of patients might read 'resist supination/free pronation'.

Conventionally constructed orthoses for equinus and varus consist of bilateral below-knee irons incorporating an ankle joint with some form of stop to limit plantar flexion, and a T-strap to prevent supination (inversion). Normally, these designs of orthoses totally eliminate plantar flexion and all subtalar motion.

The most commonly employed contemporary design of plastic orthosis is the simple polypropylene ankle–foot orthosis (AFO) (Fig. 5.3). As with the metal and leather orthosis, this tends to virtually eliminate all ankle and subtalar motion; however, some practitioners are now employing articulated polypropylene AFOs which do allow free dorsiflexion.

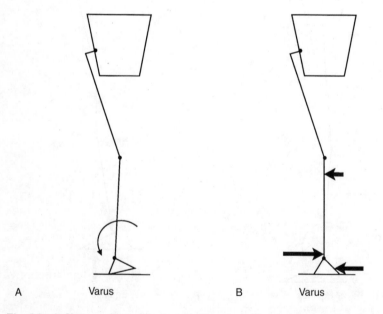

A   Varus   B   Varus

Fig. 5.2   A. Varus position of the foot. B. Three-point force system.

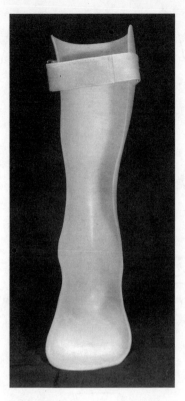

Fig. 5.3   Polypropylene ankle–foot orthosis.

There is, as yet, no published research involving large numbers of patients which examines the effect (good and bad) of these articulated devices on the gait of stroke patients.

Hyperextension of the knee

Two orthotic approaches to this problem require to be considered.

Some hyperextension problems of the knee are simply a reflection of the equinus position of the ankle. If this is treated (perhaps by the use of an AFO) the hyperextension problem may also be eliminated (Fig. 5.4A,B).

In other cases, the hyperextension is, at least in part, attributable also to spasticity in the knee extensors, and in these circumstances this approach will not be effective (Fig. 5.4C). The alternative approach necessary in these instances is to apply the orthotic treatment directly to the knee joint. Thus the orthosis for this problem will need to apply a knee flexion movement. This may be achieved by the application of a three-force system anteriorly, proximally and distally on the leg; and posteriorly, just below the knee joints (Fig. 5.4D). If this three-force system is required to control the equinus, the

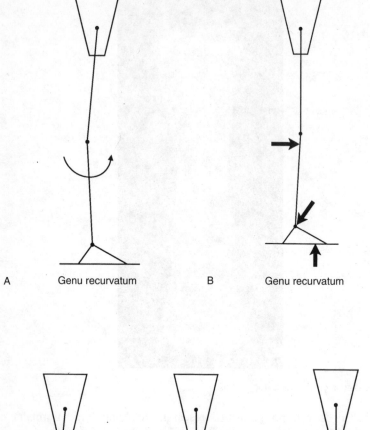

A   Genu recurvatum   B   Genu recurvatum

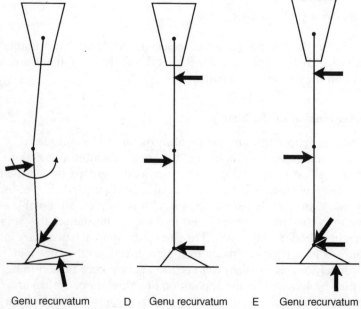

C   Genu recurvatum   D   Genu recurvatum   E   Genu recurvatum

Fig. 5.4A–E Hyperextension of the knee.

resulting combined orthotic force system comprises four forces located as illustrated (Fig. 5.4E).

The specification for the orthotic joint used in this application may be defined as 'limit extension/free flexion'.

The most commonly used knee–ankle–foot orthosis employed in this situation comprises polypropylene thigh and foot/ankle sections linked by appropriate orthotic knee joints.

It is worthwhile remembering that following successful fitting of an ankle–foot orthosis it *may* be possible to achieve further improvement in the gait pattern if the patient is able to reduce secondary or compensating measures such as circumduction and hip-hitching.

TIMING

There remains the major question of the timing of orthotic applications in relation to conventional therapy.

Broadly speaking, there are two options:

1. The orthosis can be supplied when physiotherapy has been discontinued to control any residual gait problems. This is reasonably widely accepted practice.
2. The orthosis can be employed in parallel with therapy during the initial mobilisation of the patient.

Many authorities refer to the importance of early weight-bearing and suggest that the balance mechanism and proprioceptive feedback may, as a consequence, be stimulated. It is also widely believed that standing may well inhibit the development of contractures in the calf muscles. Indeed there is considerable evidence from many centres worldwide of this effect following the fitting of AFOs to children with cerebral palsy.

Surprisingly, there is a distinct lack of reference to, or support for, the use of orthoses in contemporary textbooks on stroke management written for and by therapists and doctors in connection with this early stage of management. Many advocates of early weight-bearing through the affected leg and balanced standing make only the briefest and unenthusiastic comments on these devices.

Many clinicians would now agree that their experience of the effect of the provision of a properly fitted ankle–foot orthosis to many stroke patients in the early stages of recovery is much more positive. These effects are summed up well by a senior member of the physiotherapy profession in Scotland who worked for many years with cerebral palsied children, and who, regrettably, suffered a stroke with a resulting left-sided hemiplegia. At her own request, she was fitted with an ankle–foot orthosis approximately 6 weeks after the stroke.

One year later she was invited to comment on her AFO and its effects; and her comments are summarised as follows:

- 'prevents contracture'
- 'inhibits primitive total reflex patterns'
- 'gives opportunity to develop postural control and balanced standing'.

These beneficial effects have been observed over a period of several years on many other patients from specialist centres worldwide who have been fitted an AFO within weeks or even days of the stroke occurring.

There is, however, no scientific evidence to support the view that this practice would improve the outcome of stroke rehabilitation because, in spite of the vast quantity of literature published on the subject of hemiplegic gait and its management, remarkably few publications provide quantitative evidence of the effectiveness of orthotic treatment.

The use of an orthosis as an adjunct to a professionally delivered therapy programme may well offer the best prospects of recovery from locomotor difficulties following stroke. Any attempt to investigate properly the use of ankle–foot orthoses in this way is to be warmly welcomed and is long overdue.

REFERENCES

Royal College of Physicians and Surgeons 1989 Stroke – towards better management. RCPS, London
Wade D et al 1985 Stroke – a critical approach to diagnosis, treatment and management. Chapman & Hall, London

6. Functional electrical stimulation in stroke rehabilitation

D. J. Maxwell, A. C. B. Ferguson, M. H. Granat,
J. C. Barbenel, K. R. Lees

INTRODUCTION

Functional electrical stimulation (FES) as an alternative to conventional orthotic support is an increasingly popular treatment for the hemiplegic stroke patient. However there is a lack of statistically valid evidence for its efficacy (Wagenaar & Meijer 1991a, b).

Electrical stimulation (ES) has been proposed for many conditions that have resulted in paresis. ES has been applied in stroke rehabilitation for the treatment of shoulder subluxation (Faghri et al 1994), spasticity (Stefanovska et al 1991) and, functionally, for the restoration of function in the upper and lower limb (Kralj et al 1993).

The most successful application of FES has been a single channel of stimulation applied to the peroneal nerve to provide correction of drop foot during the swing phase of gait. The peroneal stimulator (PS) consists of a stimulator, worn either on the shank or at the waist, a pair of stimulating electrodes and a heel switch. Electrode position and polarity are crucial for effective operation. Surface electrodes are positioned over the common peroneal nerve around the head of the fibula where the nerve is most superficial. Stimulation at this site results in eversion and dorsiflexion of the foot. The relative magnitude of these movements at the ankle is responsive to subtle changes in electrode position. The timing of the stimulation is controlled by a switch worn under the heel of the affected leg. From heel off to heel strike, stimulation is on resulting in dorsiflexion and eversion of the foot.

This application of FES was first demonstrated by Liberson et al in 1961. The technique has been widely applied in the former Yugoslavia (Slovenia) but it has not become widely accepted in other parts of the world.

It has been suggested that in some cases FES can provide both therapeutic and orthotic benefits to the user. As the PS assists in a functional movement it has an obvious orthotic action. It may also have a therapeutic effect as, unlike conventional orthotics which have only a passive function, it acts through the neuromuscular system with the possibility of producing a trophic or retraining effect which results in improved function when the device is not operating.

There are a number of possible reasons why the PS has not become more widely used:

• The articles which have been published on the use of the PS have not demonstrated its clinical efficacy.
• The PS can be difficult for the patient to apply correctly.
• The PS is not widely available and the most popular PS has a high retail price (Microfes manufactured by Gorenje, Jozef Stefan Institute, Ljubljana, Slovenia, with a retail price of greater than £600).

To address some of these points a study of the role of the PS in stroke rehabilitation was undertaken.

AIM

The aim of the study was to determine the orthotic and therapeutic benefits of the PS for stroke patients (more than 3 months post-stroke) using objective outcome measures and appropriate control measurements.

SELECTION CRITERIA

To be accepted for the study the patients had to meet the following criteria:

• have hemiplegia as a result of stroke
• be more than 3 months post-stroke
• have spastic drop foot which can be corrected by the PS
• be able to walk independently with the PS
• have sufficient communication skills to learn the use of the PS
• be able to operate the PS (with the help of a carer if required).

19 patients were selected for the study of which 2 subsequently dropped out prior to the treatment period. Another patient could not be included in the statistical analysis as he was unable to walk without wearing an ankle-foot orthosis (AFO) or the PS. The remaining 16 patients (15 male, 1 female) had an average age of 56 (min 43, max 66) and were an average of 7 months (min 3, max 24) post-stroke. There were a variety of lesion sites and a broad range of functional capabilities (Barthel index: average 81, min 51, max 100).

EXPERIMENTAL PROTOCOL

The protocol of testing involved assessing the patient's gait over a period of 1 week; these measurements were repeated three times over a 12-week period. An interval of 4 weeks occurred between each of these testing sessions. The PS was not introduced until the second testing session. During this second session the subject was instructed in the use and application of the PS. No measurements were taken of the patient walking with the PS during this session. For the following 4 weeks the patient used the PS at all times. When patients returned for the third testing session measurements were taken both with and without the assistance of the PS. In order to make the laboratory measurements more sensitive to the patients' mobility problems, their walking was assessed on three different surfaces. The surfaces used were linoleum, carpet and uneven ground (simulated by irregularly spaced battens under a thin carpet).

The Barthel index (BI) was used as a measure of overall functional ability and this was reapplied at each testing session.

While the patient was using the PS at home he was visited each week to ensure the PS was applied correctly.

Gait measurement system

The gait assessment was performed by recording the temporal parameters of the patient's gait using instrumented insoles as he walked a set distance across each of the three surfaces (Granat et al 1994). The instrumented insoles comprised four switches; one under the heel, another under the big toe and the other two under the first and fifth metatarsals. The activity of the switches was recorded at a sampling rate of 50 Hz. Post-test processing of these data generated the gait parameters.

The action of the PS will have a direct effect on the duration of heel strike and the degree of inversion. It may indirectly influence the speed and symmetry of the gait. These four parameters were chosen as best illustrating the effects of the PS. Speed was calculated from the time to traverse the walkpath. Swing symmetry was the ratio of the swing time of the affected leg to the swing time of the contralateral leg. Heel strike was the percentage of the stance period of the affected leg when there was only heel contact. Inversion was the proportion of midstance for which the affected foot was inverted.

The PS used by the patients had the facility to log the length of time for which stimulation was delivered. Additionally, as a safety feature, the stimulator would remain active for only four seconds after which it would require to be retriggered by the action of the heel switch. Consequently it was not possible to inadvertently leave the PS delivering stimulation. This also ensured that time logged by the stimulator was a true representation of the level of activity of the user.

ANALYSIS

The final session of gait testing allowed the orthotic benefit of the PS to be determined by comparing the measurements obtained both with and without the PS.

The therapeutic benefit of the PS was calculated by comparing the change between the first and second testing sessions (control period) with the change found between the second and third sessions (treatment period).

If the improvement over the treatment period was greater than the improvement over the control period then there had been a therapeutic benefit. This study design allowed each patient to act as their own control.

RESULTS

Orthotic benefit

The results were determined both for the group as a whole and for each individual. For the whole group an improvement was found in each of the four gait parameters. However, the only result which was statistically significant (ANOVA, $p < 0.05$) for the group as a whole was the reduction in inversion of the affected foot.

Although the patient group being dealt with all met the selection criteria they were in fact quite heterogeneous, as is common in stroke populations. Examination of the individual results showed the emergence of subgroups of patients with similar effects. The individual results for speed and inversion are displayed in Figure 6.1. Significant improvements (paired t-test, $p < 0.05$) in inversion were seen in nine patients. These same patients also tended to show improvements in most of the other parameters.

Using the criterion of speed it was found that those patients in the midrange of walking speed (0.1 ms^{-1} to 0.6 ms^{-1}) were the most likely to show significant improvement with the PS. Slower walkers have more severe gait problems and the PS has too small an impact on their overall condition to provide significant improvement. Faster walkers tend to have sufficient recovered function to allow them to walk at their speed of choice without the assistance of the PS. It should be noted that in nine of the patients in which speed did not significantly improve at least one other parameter did

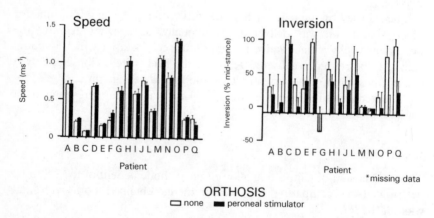

Fig. 6.1   Results (average plus standard deviation) from 16 hemiplegic patients for speed and inversion of the foot (affected side) with and without the assistance of the PS. Subject K is excluded from this analysis as he was unable to walk without an orthosis.

improve significantly. This suggests that speed alone is not an adequate outcome measure for gait therapy.

In general, the effect of testing the subjects on different surfaces was to exaggerate the individual differences between the subjects with the simulated uneven ground giving the greatest difficulty.

Figure 6.2 shows the estimated average daily walking distances for each of the subjects and each subject's BI at the third testing session. The greater a subject's BI the further he tended to walk. However, some subjects appeared a great deal less active than other subjects with a similar BI score. Specifically, in the case of subjects F and M, they both experienced difficulty in applying the PS independently.

The PS used was technically reliable but most patients experienced difficulty in using it. Eight of the patients were able to apply the PS independently. However in some cases its effectiveness was compromised by poor electrode placement. If patients are to use the PS successfully at home they require to have the use of the PS incorporated into their gait re-education programme.

Therapeutic benefit

For the group as a whole no significant therapeutic effects were found for the PS. It should be noted that no significant deterioration was found in the subjects' unassisted gait after having used the PS exclusively for 4 weeks. Two subjects (K and P) were dependent on their AFO, due to mediolateral ankle instability, at their entry to the programme. Both subjects were able to use the PS successfully for the whole treatment period and both preferred using the PS. After the treatment period subject P had recovered sufficient

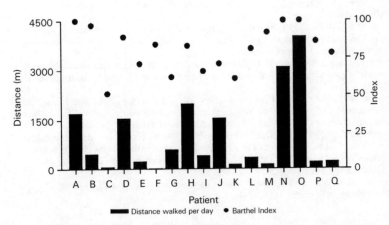

Fig. 6.2 Average daily distance walked by each patient using the PS and each patient's Barthel index at the third testing session. The average daily distance was calculated from stimulator use time and average walking speed.

ankle stability to walk without his AFO demonstrating, for him, a clear therapeutic benefit.

CONCLUSION

The results of this study have shown that the PS is most suited to the treatment of the problem of spastic drop foot with inversion in adult hemiplegia. From the orthotic improvements that were measured it would appear that the most benefit from the PS would be received by a subpopulation of the adult hemiplegic community who suffered from drop foot with pronounced ankle instability.

Nine of the patients in the study had in the first instance been admitted to the Acute Stroke Unit, Western Infirmary, Glasgow. This unit dealt with approximately 400 patients (from a catchment population of 226 000) during the year of the trial. Of the nine patients, seven showed a significant improvement in their gait when using the PS. This represents 2% of the patient intake of the unit. If the initial selection criteria were revised in light of the result of this study it should be possible to identify those patients who would benefit most from using the PS.

This study was unable to show an overall therapeutic benefit from the use of the PS when applied 3 months post-stroke. However, it should be noted that one subject did show a recovery of function after using the PS.

This work was funded by a grant from the Scottish Office Home and Health Department (K/CRED/4/C164).

REFERENCES

Faghri P D, Rodgers M M, Glaser R M, Bors J G, Ho C, Akuthota P 1994 The effects of functional electrical stimulation on shoulder subluxation, arm function recovery, and shoulder pain in hemiplegic stroke patients. Archives of Physical Medicine and Rehabilitation 75: 73–79

Granat M H, Maxwell D J, Bosch C J, Ferguson A C B, Lees K R, Barbenel J C 1994 A body-worn gait analysis system for evaluating hemiplegic gait. Medical Engineering and Physics (accepted for publication)

Kralj A, Acimovic R, Stanic U 1993 Enhancement of hemiplegic patient rehabilitation by means of functional electrical stimulation. Prosthetics and Orthotics International 17: 107–114

Liberson W T, Holmquest H J, Scott D, Dow A 1961 Functional electrotherapy: stimulation of the peroneal nerve synchronized with the swing phase of gait of hemiplegic patients. Archives of Physical Medicine and Rehabilitation 42: 101–105

Stefanovska A, Rebersek S, Bajd T, Vodovnik L 1991 Effects of electrical stimulation on spasticity. Critical Reviews in Physical and Rehabilitation Medicine 3(1): 59–99

Wagenaar R C, Meijer O G 1991a Effects of stroke rehabilitation (1). Journal of Rehabilitation Sciences 4(3): 61–73

Wagenaar R C, Meijer O G 1991b Effects of stroke rehabilitation (2). Journal of Rehabilitation Sciences 4(4): 97–109

7. Proprioceptive neuromuscular facilitation (PNF) in stroke rehabilitation

M. Heideman

INTRODUCTION

The main emphasis of this chapter is focused on how the concept of proprioceptive neuromuscular facilitation (PNF) can help a hemiplegic patient on his/her way during rehabilitation. To ensure effectiveness of treatment it is necessary for physiotherapists to continue developing their ability to evaluate the handicap of the hemiplegic patient in the most efficient way.

THE PNF CONCEPT

The PNF concept is based on a *basic philosophy* as stated by Dr Herman Kabat: all human beings, including those with disabilities, have untapped existing potential.

It seems that there is sufficient experimental evidence that central mechanisms (networks) are indeed far more flexible and fluid than was previously thought (Goldberger 1980, Sejnowski 1988). This type of adaptive plasticity is not a local function but a distributed function in which numerous centres of the brain participate and which depends also on the central state of the brain (Mulder 1994).

The adult patient with hemiparesis should be observed as a whole person. The different treatment procedures should be applied relative to the status of the patient after analysis of potentially normal and pathological movement. Evaluation and treatment should be a circular process.

Tools of the PNF concept

The 'tools' of the PNF concept are:

• PNF philosophy: the main point of which is the 'positive approach'. This means looking for good potential using it in a proper way via predictable irradiation. For hemiplegic patients a PNF treatment, for example, will start with the uninvolved side which is always affected as well.

• Basic principles, to be followed strictly.

• Patterns, created by the analysis of normal movement, which are multidimensional and therefore much more functional.

• Techniques, as special procedures within the patterns of movement for either inhibition or facilitation. These depend on the specific problems of different structures, e.g. joints, muscles, soft tissue, sensibility, perception.

• Stages of motor control: mobility, stability, controlled mobility and skill. All of these can be combined in transitional levels. This should be considered during evaluation and treatment.

Pillars of treatment

The main pillars of treatment are:

• Vital functions such as breathing, facial expression, chewing and swallowing.

• Mat activities for activities of daily living (ADL) and functions such as postural activities.

• Gait for human specific locomotion.

• 'Table' treatment for specific problems such as pain, strength, range of motion (ROM), selective motor control.

• Self-care for independence and skill in the real world environment. This means from the 'muscle-level' to the 'movement-level' to the 'real task-specific level' of ADL. This is achieved by helping the patient to acquire skill in meaningful and realistic tasks.

• Home programme for automobilization and stabilizing the level of recovery.

The PNF concept should be applied properly to all three stages of the recovering stroke patient: the initial, intermediate and advanced stages.

THE INITIAL STAGE

In the initial stage the short-term goals are:

• to improve respiratory and feeding function
• to increase body awareness
• to improve trunk and proximal control; this is the most important goal at this stage of recovery
• to increase ability to cross the midline
• to maintain mobility of scapula, shoulder, elbow, wrist, hand and ankle joints
• to normalize tone
• to begin reversals of the antagonists
• to improve functional abilities, e.g. rolling, side lying to sitting.

It is important to highlight the third goal for the initial stage. Knott always placed emphasis on the trunk as the key to normal motor control. These days, more than ever before, empirical work is being confirmed and underpinned by scientific findings.

TRUNK FUNCTION

Analysis of trunk function

According to normal motor development a cephalocaudal as well as a proximal–distal and finally a distal–proximal direction of motor control can be observed (head control before trunk control, proximal dynamic stability before distal coordination). This means that, as long as the patient is unable to dynamically stabilize his/her trunk properly, no skilful, distal coordinated movement can be expected. Trunk function is the main means whereby the necessary flexible background for movement in space is provided. If stability is not present, influencing forces created by extremity movement would disturb balance and posture. PNF extremity patterns indicate distal to proximal timing. They can only be used once head and trunk control is established. The resisted mat activities of the PNF concept are used to improve this proximal control. In addition, special techniques are applied for strength, flexibility, stability, control of movement, reversal of movement and coordination in order to improve trunk function. For all treatment procedures, stages of motor control, such as mobility, stability, controlled mobility and skill, have to be considered.

The trunk and proximal areas of the extremities are controlled ipsilaterally and contralaterally by the descending system, the corticospinal tract. Therefore, these areas recover earlier than the distal components and this can very often be seen in clinical work. On the other hand, in the motor cortex the trunk and proximal areas are poorly represented compared to the distal extremities and the face. This tells the physiotherapist that the trunk must be worked very intensively and with all the possibilities which are available, in order to achieve the goal of dynamic stability in this part of the body.

The work of Astryan & Feldman (1965), Belen'kii et al (1967) and Lee (1980) showed that postural adjustments take place before movement starts.

How does PNF facilitate trunk function?

Some examples are listed below:
- By assisting and facilitating expiration to correct the position of the patient's thorax as the abdominal muscles work optimally only in the case of an adequately stabilized thorax. A lack of efficient contraction of the obliqui results when they are approximated, which occurs with increased thoracic kyphosis.
- By assisting upper trunk control, e.g. using chopping.

• By assisting lower trunk control, using lower trunk rotation (LTR) and bilateral lower extremity patterns.
• By assisting rolling, using scapula and pelvis patterns.
• By using sitting as a functional activity.

Lower trunk rotation (LTR). In supine lying, segmental trunk movement that incorporates lower extremity movement can be performed. The activity of LTR can be used to achieve different goals, as there are:

• Extremities crossing the midline.
• Muscles, which are bilaterally activated to promote an integration of the two sides of the body.
• Flexor and extensor phases of movement and interaction of antagonists.
• Possible reductions in hypertonia and, as in side lying, there will be promotion of the forward rotational movement of the pelvis, which is necessary for ambulation.

Additional techniques such as rhythmic initiation, dynamic reversals and repeated contractions may facilitate the performance of LTR.

The upper extremities should be positioned at the patient's side out of synergetic patterns.

Bilateral lower extremity patterns. As with LTR activity, contact between the lower extremities will improve sensory feedback and provide a 'tracking' or following response in the involved limb. The lower trunk patterns incorporate a rotational component, but the emphasis at this stage is on the mass flexion and mass extension movements of the extremities to facilitate the lower trunk flexors and extensors. To avoid movement into a synergistic pattern, the involved leg should perform a flexion/adduction (flex/add) and extension/abduction (ext/abd) pattern.

How much of the range of the extensor pattern is used depends on the patient's reaction. In practice, the patterns are performed in lengthened, middle or shortened range. If the extensor tone in the lower limb or in the low back is dominant, as often occurs in the later stage, then emphasis is placed on the flexor phase of the lower trunk, which will promote a balance of tone. As flexor control increases, movement can be initiated from more lengthened ranges, in which case the effects of gravity and the length of the lever arm are increased. For patients who have a generalized decrease in tone or a predominant flexor withdrawal response, the extensor phase rather than the flexor phase should be emphasized.

For all hemiplegic patients, the combination of hip extension with abduction is important for the stance phase of gait and can be enhanced by facilitation of isometric contraction in the shortened range of the trunk extensor pattern. At this stage the trunk is facilitated in combination with the extremities. Nevertheless, the final goal should be the ability of the patient to move the trunk segmentally and to use it as a stabilizing background for independent activity of the extremities.

THE INTERMEDIATE STAGE

In the initial stage of treatment, trunk and proximal areas are promoted as well as movement out of synergy. These goals may be further emphasized in the intermediate stage. Treatment goals appropriate to this middle stage are:

• To promote a balance of antagonists, inhibition of spasticity and facilitation of reversal movements.
• To promote advanced patterns and unilateral patterns.
• To enhance control of proximal musculature during performance of higher level activities such as bridging.
• To promote initial stages of motor control in the intermediate joints.

Mobilization of proximal extremity joints decreases tone by using scapula–arm patterns and pelvic-leg patterns. Once tone decreases, the elbow and the knee can be included in the extremity patterns.

Static dynamic activity in the quadruped position or modified plantigrade position (standing supported by hands on table) will enhance the weight-bearing ability of the involved limbs.

THE ADVANCED STAGE

The advanced stage should include the following goals:

• To promote the skill level of motor control by:
  — improving function of the distal segments
  — improving eccentric control with the 'combining of isotonics' technique
  — increasing speed and endurance of movement
  — improving reciprocal movement
  — facilitating normal timing of movement.
• To improve the gait pattern.
• To improve the patient's ability to perform ADL; this means consistency in achieving an action-goal with some economy of effort by knowing how to match his/her ability to features of the environment.

Of these goals, the ability to perform ADL is the most important overall aim. The patient has to deal with a new situation, and has to return to real life with all its advantages and obstacles. Therefore, the emphasis of treatment at the advanced stage should be on a shift from neurotherapy to a functional or task-orientated approach. What does this mean?

Assumptions

Some assumptions are listed below (Gentile 1994):

• Location of control is distributed across several concurrently-active neural subsystems and shifts with task demands. (Are these subsystems really covered by exercising a leg pattern for gait?)

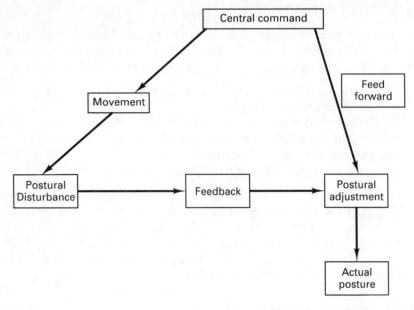

Fig. 7.1   Shaping of movement by input during performance.

• Posture and movement are planned in advance and emerge as a consequence of the dynamic interaction among neural subsystems. (Is this feedforward mode attained by telling the patient what to do?)

• Input during performance is used to shape the ongoing movement (feedback mode) and to influence future movement by adjusting motor plans in advance of an anticipated disturbance (feedforward or predictive mode) (Fig. 7.1). (Are therapeutic situations created with these conditions?)

• Recovery after damage involves 'adaptive rewiring' among neural subsystems brought about by *actively* adapting to environmental demands.

• Responsibility for the organization of adaptive behaviour rests on the patient and his/her active problem-solving. The therapist assists in this process by selecting appropriate tasks, structuring the performance and environment and by guiding the patient's problem-solving. The therapist needs to be very good at task analysis. It is helpful to use the *Taxonomy of tasks,* developed by Gentile (1994).

• Practice in organizing movement (Fig. 7.2) to meet task demands and successfully attaining action-goals leads to skill in functional activities.

• With practice, environmental events become familiar.

Application of PNF

The PNF concept is quite successful in meeting these demands to improve the skill level. As the PNF patterns activate the physiological muscle chains they can be used to facilitate the complexity of motion that is required, e.g.

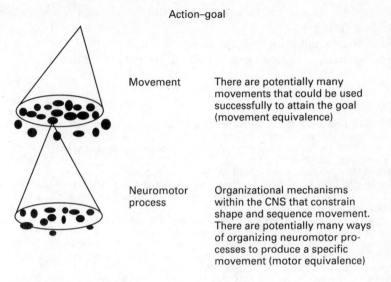

Action–goal

Movement — There are potentially many movements that could be used successfully to attain the goal (movement equivalence)

Neuromotor process — Organizational mechanisms within the CNS that constrain shape and sequence movement. There are potentially many ways of organizing neuromotor processes to produce a specific movement (motor equivalence)

Fig. 7.2 Organizing movement.

for getting dressed or for brushing the teeth. If necessary, the physiotherapist could apply 'hands on' to increase proprioceptive and exteroceptive input which can help to adjust posture and movement during performance.

Some points to consider are as follows:

- Structure the environment for practice (do not brush teeth without toothpaste).
- Avoid goal confusion (do not interrupt with verbal adjustments).
- Promote patient's self-efficacy (choose tasks that are achievable).
- Therapist observes the patient's performance if necessary with hands on (do not talk).
- Consider the delay of augmented feedback by at least 5 seconds.

The physiotherapist must always remember, that **learning takes place in the patient**.

CONCLUSION

The PNF concept provides a functional approach to the patient's needs and requirements, namely to use the body in the way it works best. The physiotherapist starts by working the patient's good potential. This means that the uninvolved parts influence the involved body parts, via 'irradiation', with all the 'tools' PNF has to offer.

According to normal developmental motor control the patient is treated in a proximal to distal direction first and later in the distal to proximal direction. Trunk patterns are used to build up postural stability as necessary background leading on to independent extremity patterns for gait and handling function.

Finally, the patient is asked to achieve ADL in a skillful way and in real circumstances, in order to give impetus to the patient's independence.

REFERENCES

Astryan D, Feldman A 1965 Functional tuning of the nervous system with control of movement and maintenance of a steady posture. Biophysics 10: 925–935

Belen'kii U Y, Gurfinkel V S, Pal'tsev Y I 1967 Elements of control of voluntary movements. Biophysics 12: 135–141

Davies P M 1990 Right in the middle. Springer Verlag, Berlin

Gentile A M 1994 Motor learning, therapeutic concept and approaches. Own handwritten notes, taken during course in Bad Ragaz, Switzerland. Teachers College, Columbia University

Gerber M, Vaney C 1994 Verlust selektiver rumpfaktivitaeten und deren auswirkung bei erwachsenen mit hemiplegie. Krankengymnastik KG, Nr. 3

Goldberger M E 1980 Motor recovery after lesions. Trends in Neurosciences 3: 288–291

Lee W A 1980 Anticipatory control of posture and task muscles during rapid arm flexion. Journal of Motor Behaviour 12: 185–196

Markos D, Minor D, Sullivan P E 1982 An integrated approach to therapeutic exercise. Reston, Virginia.

Mulder T 1994 The learning machine. Ideas about adaption and learning following nervous system damage. Proceedings of the third symposium of the Graduate Institute of Human Movement, pp 29–44

Observational Gait Analysis 1993 The pathokinesiology service and the physical therapy department, Rancho Los Amigos Medical Center (author not known)

Sejnowski T J 1988 Open questions about computation in cerebral cortex. Psychological and Biological Models: 372–389

8. The recollection of my whole body in my brain: physiotherapy based on aspects of the Affolter concept

K. Nielsen

INTRODUCTION

Research findings suggest a model of development in which sensorimotor learning establishes a pool or 'root' of experiences that continues to grow throughout life. This model provides an explanation for the success of using tactile–kinaesthetic input in therapy for adults with perceptual problems caused by brain injury. Through working on the root, this can be rebuilt and strengthened to form a base for redevelopment and for learning.

One can compare such a rehabilitation model with a growing tree. A tree will only live and sprout branches if the root is healthy and flourishing. A brain injured patient will develop and learn to master the challenges of daily living if his root of development is organised and strong.

Therapists use their knowledge and understanding to ensure that the patient receives tactile–kinaesthetic information in a way that will be as useful as possible. All sensory input in relation to the problem to be solved has to be sorted out and organised. The treatment will enable the patient to solve problems in daily living such as how to open a door, sitting in a wheelchair, or how to walk to the kitchen to take a glass out of a high cupboard.

Children actively seek out challenges or 'problems' and try to solve them; they touch, explore and change topological relationships between objects, persons, support and themselves. Problem-solving on a high level in a complicated adult world, e.g. to prepare and cook a meal or to arrange a holiday, is based on the ability to organise all incoming information and problems. Adults use their pool or root of experiences all the time. Information that is new and necessary will be searched for and constantly added and connected.

THE AFFOLTER APPROACH

The Affolter approach is designed to help the patient make use of their tactile–kinaesthetic abilities to solve problems. The tactile–kinaesthetic

71

system is used extensively in the early development of the root. Interaction defined as topological change between person and environment is impossible without tactile–kinaesthetic information. The child literally needs to 'get in touch', in order to interact and to experience, and so it is with patients. What one is seeing, hearing, smelling or tasting is inextricably linked with knowledge based on tactile–kinaesthetic experience.

Some patients can describe their difficulties in obtaining and using tactile–kinaesthetic information, but the majority are unable to do so. They express their difficulties in an indirect way; e.g. when requested to carry out a task, their reply may be: 'Not to day, I will try tomorrow' or 'I have to go to the toilet'. The following observations were made by different stroke patients and point to perceptual problems and dislocation between the patient and his/her environment.

Observations

'I see there is a world to my right side, but when I begin to move, it disappears and I get scared and spastic.'
   This patient did not move very much, and was classified as unmotivated.

'I see and move my left side, but I do not feel it belongs to me. I do not feel whether I am sitting, standing or walking. I am afraid to cross an open space.'
   This 42-year-old patient has had two strokes. She had very little motor deficit. Doctors and therapists assumed that she was not willing to go back to work. However, after a few weeks of adequate treatment for her perceptual problems, she literally succeeded to find her body again, and she was happy to resume her work as a nurse.

'I have to stamp my feet on the floor several times to be sure that I'm standing and not still lying down.'
   Luckily this patient found a kind of solution herself.

'My physiotherapist cannot help me anymore. She says I know how to control the muscle tone and I can move almost normally; but when I try to use my right arm in everyday life, I lose control of it completely. In fact I'm one-handed.'
   Therapists can often become frustrated when working with such patients. They may even accuse the patient of not wanting to use his/her hand.

'When I start to move, I have to stop thinking; when I am thinking, I stop moving.'
   If therapists are aiming for better function, they should consider that a function always has a cognitive component.Observations made by patients on their inability to grade muscle strength when manipulating objects, or to accurately judge spatial relationships, also indicate perceptual disorders; as also do problems in dressing or using tools of daily living, e.g. toiletries.

Techniques of the approach

With the Affolter approach one can help the patient overcome such difficulties. By physically guiding the patients' hands and bodies in real situations of everyday life, one can help them to perceive their bodies and their environment, and to sequence activities and events. Because the therapist's hands are directly guiding the patient, the therapist receives explicit information about each patient. The therapist feels the patient's ability to attend to tasks, anticipate and sequence events, solve problems and adjust muscle tone.

Activities selected for this therapy approach must have a clear purpose (goal) and require participation, and should allow the brain injured patient to relate information to their previous experiences. Guiding techniques are used to enable the patient to find and maintain their body's stability ('Where is the world? Where is my body?') and to discover cause and effect in relationships.

With this method, one is aiming for:

1. The retrieval of past experiences.
2. The storing of interactive experiences to rebuild and strengthen the root.

Consequently, the aim for the patient is to:

• Attain better organisation of input (the patient shall first of all learn to organise his/her changed body in relationship to the environment).
• Achieve more normal muscle tone.
• Be able to take control of his/her own movement.
• Transfer specific tactile–kinaesthetic experiences to other performances.
• Improve attention, concentration and memory.
• Achieve the realisation of body and mind as a whole.

Three different kinds of guiding are used: 'nursing', 'assisting' and 'intensive' guiding.

NURSING GUIDING

This is used by nurses and others when handling a patient who is inactive or even unconscious, e.g., when dressing the patient in bed. It can also be very helpful for agitated and restless patients.

When, for instance, the right leg has been moved, the search for tactile information begins at the right foot, continues along the leg to the hip, and further to the pelvis and the right side of the trunk. With both hands the guider enables the patient to be in good contact with the surface of support. Then, the guider can move the patient's left leg towards a new place on the support. Again, the guider helps the patient to gain tactile information about the leg's new position, this time with the left side of the body. Subsequently, the right leg can move and so on.

This routine can be used to dress the legs (trousers, socks and shoes) and to bend the knees up to lift the pelvis (bridging). The aim is for the patient to feel the resistance of the firm support. The mattress should be firm in order to give the patient good tactile information, and so that its stability can be trusted.

ASSISTING GUIDING

This is used with patients who have some motor function and can make use of some tactile information, but who do not act spontaneously in a given situation and/or are unable to integrate left and right sides of their body.

When difficulties arise during a task, the patient's hands and body are guided to solve the problem together with the patient, in the case, for instance, of a bottle which needs to have the top unscrewed in order that the patient may have a drink. If the patient takes over the action, the guiding can stop but is resumed again if he/she cannot complete the activity sequence. However, if necessary, the patient can be guided throughout the entire sequence.

As far as possible, guided movements will alternate between left and right sides of the body, so that the patient experiences and becomes aware of both sides. Movements through space with both sides of the body, e.g. moving both arms at the same time, is avoided. Instead, one side of the patient's body always has a stable reference point, which may be a tabletop or a wall.

INTENSIVE GUIDING

There are three stages for every action and there is always a meaningful goal for the patient.

The guider's body feels the patient's body, the guider's fingers lie exactly over the patient's fingers ... thumb on thumb ... forefinger on forefinger ... shoulder on shoulder ... trunk on trunk (see Fig. 8.1A,B).

Stage 1

This involves a search for information about the relationship between the patient and the stable environment in relation to the goal:

• 'Where is the world?'
• 'Where is my body?'

The search for tactile information begins on one side of the body, e.g. the right side. With the therapist's hand placed over the fingertips and following to the hand, wrist, forearm and elbow, the patient feels the surface of a stable tactile reference, e.g. a table. The tactile information is gained through small, almost invisible, searching movements on the surface. The search for information continues, still on the right side, at the shoulder, then along the trunk against the edge of the table placed in front of the patient. The search is extended to the right hip so that the patient can feel (perceive) the stool upon which he/she is sitting. Then searching continues along the thigh to the foot. Here again, the patient can feel his/her own foot on the floor.

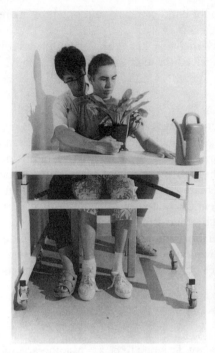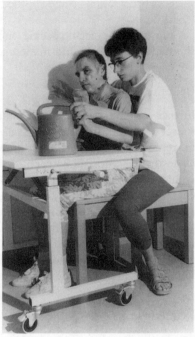

A   B

Fig. 8.1 Intensive guiding. A plant is going to be watered. The patient is sitting on a stool at a table; her right side is close to the wall. The therapist is sitting behind the patient on another stool at the same level. **A.** A search for tactile information in relation to the flowerpot, table, stool and floor on the right side from the fingertips along the hand, forearm, trunk, hip, thigh to the foot. **B.** Following the movement of the left hand to the watering-can the search for tactile information is carried out on the whole left side. (43-year-old patient with right hemiplegia after a cerebral haemorrhage.)

Stage 2

This involves preparing and planning the next movement itself:

- 'Is everything all right?'
- 'Do I feel secure on the right side?'
- 'Is the environment on the right side reliable enough to allow a movement with the left side?'
- 'Where is the goal?'

Stage 3

This is the performance stage. One movement takes place towards the goal. Following the example above, the left arm is moving.

It is now the turn of the left side to obtain information about its relationship to the environment in its new position. This is achieved in a way similar to the procedure on the right side (repeat stage 1). After the stage of preparation (stage 2), the right hand can carry out one movement (stage 3).

Step by step each specific movement of the task is completed by alternating the tactile information received through each side of the body.

Benefits

Intensive guiding enables the patient to experience the change between sources of information, especially the alternation between touch and movement, i.e. between tactile information received via skin surfaces and kinaesthetic information received through muscles and joints. Visual and auditory information will also be organised. Moreover, intensive guiding enables the patient to experience goal-orientated movements with the left and right sides interrelating with each other. Providing that an appropriate goal has been chosen for the individual patient, and that the therapist guides in the correct way, the patient will attend, concentrate and actively participate. The muscle tone becomes normalised and he/she is building the foundation for recovering function in the paretic side.

ENDNOTE

Originally, the Affolter approach was not designed to be a physiotherapeutic treatment. Dr Affolter is a teacher for handicapped children, a psychologist and a speech-scientist. However, many physiotherapists have found that this treatment has a very positive affect on movement difficulties and that the principles of the concept can be integrated very well in physiotherapy with brain injured patients.

FURTHER READING

Affolter F 1987 Wahrnehmung, Wirklichkeit und Sprache. Neckar-Verlag, Villingen-Schwenningen
Affolter F 1991 Perception, interaction and language. Springer Verlag, Berlin
Affolter F, Bischofberger W 1993 Wenn die Organisation des Zentralen Nervensystems zerfällt und es an gespürter Information mangelt. Neckar-Verlag, Villingen-Schwenningen
Affolter F, Stricker E 1980 Perceptual processes as prerequisites for complex human behavior: a theoretical model and its application to therapy. Huber, Bern
Bischofberger W 1989 Aspekte der Entwicklung taktil–kinaesthetischer Wahrnehmung. Neckar-Verlag, Villingen-Schwenningen
Davies P M 1985 Steps to follow. Springer Verlag, Berlin
Davies P M 1994 Starting again. Springer Verlag, Berlin

9. The motor relearning programme

M. Thorsteinsdottir

THE MOTOR LEARNING MODEL

Over the last 10 years or so, the Australian physiotherapists Janet Carr and Roberta Shepherd, professors at the University of Sydney, have been developing a theoretical framework for rehabilitation which they have called the motor learning model. The motor relearning programme for stroke is an illustration of how the model can be applied to stroke rehabilitation. The model is, however, applicable to the rehabilitation of other movement-disabled people, i.e. to the training of any individual who needs to improve his or her motor performance (Carr & Shepherd 1987a).

The model has been developed by a deductive process out of research into motor behaviour, from the broad area of movement science. The need for rejuvenation of the therapeutic approach in neurological rehabilitation has led to a renewed search for knowledge in the basic sciences and other disciplines associated with movement (Nativ 1993). Considerable changes in the understanding of motor behaviour and motor control have taken place during the last few decades. At the same time, an increasing effort has been made to pool resources and theoretical perspectives of movement and action from different fields, e.g. neurophysiology, muscle biology, biomechanics, cognitive psychology and motor learning, under the umbrella of movement science. Contemporary motor control research thus involves a multidisciplinary effort (Gordon 1987, Winstein & Knecht 1990). Carr & Shepherd have made an important contribution to physiotherapy by illustrating how physiotherapists can derive implications from scientific knowledge and plan therapeutic strategies thereby showing the potential usefulness of movement science to physiotherapy. Winstein & Knecht (1990) consider that the relationship might be mutually beneficial, i.e. physiotherapy can contribute to the knowledge base of movement science.

It is important to be aware of the fact that the model is based on concurrent assumptions about how movement is controlled, how the organism functions in the environment, and about the effects of brain damage, and the capacity of the system to recover. These assumptions and, consequently, the treatment approach are liable to change with increased understanding and new knowledge (Carr & Shepherd 1987b).

ACQUISITION OF SKILLS

As suggested by the name of the model, the authors are, as are many others, proponents of a more cognitively-orientated approach to recovery. They propose that the emphasis should be on the active participatory 'learner' role of the movement-disabled person in contrast to the more passive 'patient' role (Carr & Shepherd 1990). The principles and process of motor skill acquisition, which is the cornerstone of this approach, are assumed to be valuable to the acquisition of functional skills – or motor relearning – of the movement-disabled person. Movement-disabled individuals are considered to have the same needs with regard to learning as non-disabled individuals, i.e. they need, for example, to understand the goal, have the necessary opportunity to practise, and be informed about their performance. Motivation, positive attitudes, reinforcement from staff, relatives and friends, and an environment which encourages the patients to be active learners and provides the opportunity to practise are necessary requirements for successful results (Carr & Shepherd 1987b).

Stages of skill acquisition

According to some authors (Fitts & Posner 1967, Gentile 1987), skill acquisition occurs in stages. The first stage is the cognitive stage, wherein the learner needs explanations, demonstrations, guidance, and feedback. Later stages involve further practice and refinement, with modification of the environment to ensure maximal repetition and adaptability, leading gradually to an automatization of the learned skill.

Physiotherapists can make use of scientific knowledge concerning the best way of teaching/learning, e.g. how to identify the goal, the most efficient way of using extrinsic feedback, or how to arrange practice. The significance of the necessary amount of practice is emphasized. There is a striking contrast between the relatively brief practice time of patients (Turnbull & Wall 1989) and, indeed, the time actively spent, even in a rehabilitation centre (Keith 1980), and the amount and intensity of practice which is normally considered necessary for skill acquisition. At least one study has shown the value of intensive rehabilitation of stroke patients (Sivenius et al 1985).

APPLICATION OF THE PROGRAMME

The motor relearning programme consists of four steps which demonstrate the application of the motor learning principles discussed above. Step 1 concerns analysis, where the patient's motor performance is compared with a normal model based on results of biomechanical studies, and the underlying problem is analysed. Steps 2 and 3 concern the motor training of missing components and the whole task respectively. Preferably, the whole task should be practised, e.g. standing up or reaching to grasp an object. If the patient, however, cannot control necessary muscle activity or other essential components of the task, specific training of that component or modification of the task or the environment may be necessary. In either case, the principle techniques are explanations which help the patient to grasp the idea of the movement and understand the goal, instructions, verbal and/or manual guidance, feedback (specific and accurate information about results) and error correction.

Step 4 involves transference of training and emphasizes factors such as organizing the environment and the 'routine' of the patient in order to provide context-specific, consistent practice, both self-monitored (by the patient) and with the involvement of staff, relatives and friends (Carr & Shepherd 1987a). This approach to rehabilitation requires that the therapist is skilled at teaching and directing. The therapist becomes a designer of learning situations (Nativ 1993).

FUNCTIONAL TRAINING

Tasks

The motor learning model is aimed at enabling the movement-disabled person to relearn how to perform and become skilled at everyday actions such as reaching, sitting, standing up and walking, or other motor tasks relevant to the individual. Training of functional tasks is considered to be remedial in itself. Task-specific training is in contrast to therapeutic models in which facilitation of certain reactions and movement patterns are considered to carry over into improved function. The fact that this does not always happen is known to physiotherapists. It is generally believed that we learn what we practise. This indicates that training should be task- and context-specific. In other words, practice of a particular action is assumed to promote learning of that action and, thereby, the necessary neural adaptation. What is learned are the muscle activation patterns which make up that action (Carr & Shepherd 1990).

It is therefore suggested that the relearning of the most basic and essential functional tasks should start as soon as possible after stroke. There is reason to believe that training of everyday tasks will be seen as relevant by the patient as well as by the staff and will, therefore, be more easily transferred into the daily routine than particular exercises, the purpose of which may only be understood by the physiotherapist.

Skill in motor tasks is achieved by a successful linking of joint movements into coordinated synergies (Bernstein 1967). According to Bernstein, the synergies evolve as the central nervous system, interacting with the musculoskeletal system and the environment, solves the problem of each specific motor task. The 'solution' depends on the purpose of the task and the environment in which the task is performed. When one reaches out to grasp an object, the hand is shaped to the object; the reaching movement is shaped to the environment, e.g. the placement of the object, and to the initial body position, as are postural adjustments, which are also task-specific. Movements must also be shaped to the temporal features of the environment, such as the speed of a ball one is trying to catch (Gordon 1987).

Problem-solving

Skill acquisition is thought to be best ensured by practice which involves active problem-solving by the learner, enabling him/her to gain control of necessary muscle activity and of the spatiotemporal components of the action. If standing up is taken as an example, that action has specific temporal and spatial movement characteristics, the main components being trunk flexion at the hip and ankle dorsiflexion moving the body horizontally, followed by extension of hips, knees and ankles. To be efficient, these movements have to be performed with appropriate angular displacements, timing, and in a sequence (Carr 1987, Carr & Gentile 1994, Shepherd & Gentile 1994).

Modifications

It is often necessary to practise a modified version of a task while the patient still lacks adequate control and strength. Standing up from a higher chair thus reducing the force requirement of the action (Rodosky et al 1989), or supporting the arm on a table while practising reaching, are examples of such modifications. These may play an important role in the prevention of compensatory strategies which are thought to interfere with recovery. LeVere (1980) has suggested that if compensation is allowed to occur, there will be no stimulus to the system to recover. Compensation by the intact side may reinforce what has been described by Taub (1980) as 'learned non-use' of the affected side and is difficult to overcome (see Appendix 4 in Carr & Shepherd 1987a).

Examples of compensatory strategies are: reaching forward by abducting and internally rotating the shoulder joint, elevating the pelvis during the swing phase of walking due to lack of knee flexion, and taking the weight onto the intact leg while standing up. These strategies emerge as they provide the most biomechanically advantageous solution to a motor problem given the effects of the lesion and the condition of the musculoskeletal linkage. They are therefore functionally preferred and there is a strong tendency for these strategies to become learned (Shepherd & Carr 1991). Most people have probably experienced how difficult it is to change or unlearn movement patterns which have been practised. This may be even more difficult or complex for a stroke patient to achieve.

Obviously, task-specific training involves, besides motor learning principles, the application of kinesiological principles, i.e. biomechanics, knowledge of muscle action and muscle adaptability. This is emphasized by Carr and Shepherd.

Analysis

Appropriate analysis of the altered biomechanics or the movement components with which the patient has problems, which is the basis of correct decision-making regarding therapy, demands sound knowledge and understanding of biomechanics.

When starting to develop a theoretical framework for rehabilitation, Carr and Shepherd found a poverty of kinematic or kinetic studies of actions such as standing up. In fact, descriptions of everyday actions have, until recently, been rather limited, except in the case of walking. Now there are many studies which can be used to improve the understanding of tasks and develop normal models on which analyses and treatment can be based. Carr and Shepherd have described the critical observable features of everyday actions which have been called essential components and are developed from biomechanical studies.

Analysis of the patient's problems, most often done by observing attempts to perform the task, involves identifying the cause of these problems. If, for example, the patient hyperextends the knee when taking weight through the lower limb, the therapist has to ask 'why does it happen?' Is it because the quadriceps lacks control of the eccentric and concentric activity in the $0-15°$ of extension; is it due to shortened and hyperreflective plantarflexors; or is it caused by malalignment at the hip? Similarly, difficulties in standing up may be due to failure to place the feet backwards which causes inappropriate ground reaction forces; the reason might also be decreased movement of the trunk forward (Shepherd & Gentile 1994), or lack of muscle strength in the affected lower limb.

Clearly, some of the components are not easily observable. Therapists can infer muscle activation patterns and generation of forces by observing the key kinematic features of the action, and can confirm their characteristics by the use of data from electromyography (EMG), force plate and video (Carr & Shepherd 1989). The motor relearning programme for stroke provides guidelines for the analysis of each task, in which common problems are described as well as the predictable compensatory strategies.

Postural adjustments and balance

A very important issue concerning functional training, and a good example of the need to rethink therapeutic strategies as new information emerges, relates to postural adjustments and balance.

First, postural adjustments have been shown to be anticipatory as well as ongoing and, therefore, not solely dependent on feedback. Secondly, they have been shown to be specific to each task. Many investigators have demonstrated that postural adjustments are pre-planned and organized with volitional movement such as rapid arm raising in standing (Lee 1980). Task-specificity of postural adjustments suggests that a carry-over between different actions should not be expected. It also suggests that balance and actions are interrelated and should not be treated separately.

On the contrary, patients should be assisted to relearn the interdependent task movement and postural adjustments by practising self-initiated actions. In normal daily function, balance is most often needed in connection with such actions, e.g. looking around, reaching, moving objects and walking. Postural responses to external perturbations are also context-specific and may, for example, be dependent on the conditions of support or the intention (Nashner & Cordo 1981).

Recent developments in the understanding of balance and postural adjustments are bound to make all therapist examine critically how balance problems are treated and the theoretical rationale upon which techniques such as rhythmic stabilization and facilitation of equilibrium reactions are based.

Good control of balance is characterized by muscular control and correct timing in order to maintain alignment. Balance is considered dynamic, involving intermittent correction with as little expenditure of energy as possible (see Appendix 5 in Carr & Shepherd 1987a). Accordingly, treatment techniques which aim at increased stiffness and/or co-contraction may well be contraindicated as these qualities are seen rather as compensatory solutions by those who have balance problems.

Spasticity

Another issue which is being critically examined by several authors is spasticity. Spasticity has commonly been viewed as the major cause of dysfunction after stroke, and is considered to be a direct effect of the central lesion. Consequently, the main emphasis in treatment has been on 'inhibiting' spasticity.

Recently however, authors have pointed out that the major defects in function of patients after stroke are weakness, loss of dexterity or loss of fractionation (Burke 1988, Nativ 1993).

Loss of fractionation

This is fundamentally a disorder of voluntary control; patients are unable to shape their movements to the environment and to the task, as they lack the ability to selectively modulate the muscle activity within the synergy (Gordon 1990). For example, a patient may not be able to reach forward by flexing at the shoulder joint without also flexing at the elbow. An abnormal temporal sequence of muscle activation has also been demonstrated in spastic patients. For example, Nashner (1985) compared postural adjustments of spastic children with normal adjustments and found reversals in the normal temporal (distal to proximal) sequence of muscle contractions in the spastic legs.

Carr & Shepherd (1989) have pointed out that those muscles that are apparently more spontaneously activated than their antagonists, are muscles that are shortened and most often 'rest' in a shortened position.

Experimental evidence suggests that both active and passive shortening of muscle will increase its stiffness and facilitate the stretch reflex, while the opposite happens with lengthening. This is discussed by Hoessly (1991), who describes how flexion at the knee can be improved by repeated eccentric work of a spastic quadriceps. A maintained shortened position will lead to a change in the resting length of the muscle, the connective tissue will undergo remodelling and the muscle will become stiffer. Hence, the muscle will change its response to passive lengthening, which is how we clinically evaluate hypertonia.

Mechanical factors

There is now quite convincing evidence to suggest that the excessive stiffness, which often is defined clinically as spasticity, may partly be explained by changes in the mechanical properties of the contractile elements within the muscles and/or increased connective tissue stiffness (Carey & Burghardt 1993). These authors suggest that scientific attention must expand beyond the reflex and neural control components of lesions of the central nervous system to address possible mechanical factors as well.

Dietz and his colleagues have found that the observed limited dorsiflexion in walking is not associated with electromyographical activity in the antagonistic calf muscles, but is due to plantarflexor stiffness stemming from changes in the mechanical properties of the contractile element within the muscle. The authors theorized that with impaired supraspinal input, unique muscular adaptation will take place with a shift to a more mechanical control from the normal neuronal control (Dietz & Berger 1983). Such adapted control could be viewed as a form of compensation, as the patients would gain better stability, similar to the case of increased postural stiffness being a form of compensation for poor control of balance. This will, however, be at the expense of mobility and movement speed.

Training strategy

Carr & Shepherd (1987a) suggest that with appropriate training strategies the development of muscle imbalance and contracture which is typically seen after stroke, can be affected. The training strategy should involve:

- active regaining of motor control
- maintainance of soft tissue length by both active and passive means.

The emphasis is thus on muscle control which involves modulating stiffness, e.g. during eccentric or lengthening activity. Care should be taken in avoiding muscle imbalance and the patient should learn to control unnecessary muscle activity. It is pointed out that functional training, such as standing up, is a good method for the prevention of muscle shortness, although in some cases additional stretching methods are required.

There are still many unanswered questions concerning the neurophysiology of spasticity. There is, however, enough evidence to suggest that we should review existing methods of therapy. This involves reviewing the rationale against resistance training (Nativ 1993).

CONCLUSION

The motor learning model – a theoretical framework for rehabilitation – proposes early task- and context-specific training incorporating motor learning and biomechanical principles. The importance of measuring the effects of the therapeutic model has been emphasized by Carr and Shepherd. For that purpose they have developed a functional scale, the motor assessment scale, whereby particular functional activities are graded on a point scale, but they also point out that there are many means of measuring specific aspects of motor performance (Carr & Shepherd 1987b).

In this introduction of the model, emphasis has been placed on its theoretical background and the main theoretical assumptions upon which it is based, rather than on describing the treatment methods or practical details. Gordon (1987, p 2) said:

In order to develop a meaningful critique of our therapeutic approaches, it is first necessary to identify the assumptions on which they are based.

For further information about the model and its use, publications by Carr & Shepherd (see References) are recommended, but as the authors point out, in order to use the model, physiotherapists will need to read widely in the movement science field.

REFERENCES

Bernstein N 1967 The coordination and regulation of movement. Pergamon Press, Oxford
Burke D 1988 Spasticity as an adaptation to pyramidal tract injury. In: Waxman S G (ed) Functional recovery in neurological diseases. Advances in Neurology, 47: Raven Press, New York
Carey J R, Burghardt T P 1993 Movement dysfunction following central nervous system lesions: a problem of neurologic muscular impairment. Physical Therapy 73 (8): 538–547
Carr J H 1987 Analysis and training of standing up. Proceedings of the 10th International Congress of the World Confederation for Physical Therapy, Sydney 1: 383–388
Carr J H, Gentile A M 1994 The effect of arm movement on the biomechanics of standing up. Human Movement Science 13: 175–193
Carr J H, Shepherd R B 1987a Motor relearning programme for stroke, 2nd edn. Butterworth-Heinemann, Oxford

Carr J H, Shepherd R B 1987b A motor learning model for rehabilitation. In: Carr J H, Shepherd R B (eds) Movement science: foundations for physical therapy in rehabilitation. Aspen, Maryland

Carr J H, Shepherd R B 1989 A motor learning model for stroke rehabilitation. Physiotherapy 75(7): 372–380

Carr J, Shepherd R 1990 A motor learning model for rehabilitation of the movement-disabled. In: Ada L, Canning C (eds) Key issues in neurological physiotherapy. Butterworth-Heinemann, Oxford

Dietz V, Berger W 1983 Normal and impaired regulation of muscle stiffness in gait: a new hypothesis about muscle hypertonia. Experimental Neurology 79: 680–687

Fitts P M, Posner M I 1967 Human performance. Brooks/Cole, California

Gentile A M 1987 Skill acquisition: action, movement, and neuromotor processes. In: Carr J H, Shepherd R B (eds) Movement science: foundations for physical therapy in rehabilitation. Aspen, Maryland

Gordon J 1987 Assumptions underlying physical therapy intervention: theoretical and historical perspectives. In: Carr J H, Shepherd R B (eds) Movement science: foundations for physical therapy in rehabilitation. Aspen, Maryland

Gordon J 1990 Disorders of motor control. In: Ada L, Canning C (eds) Key issues in neurological physiotherapy. Butterworth-Heinemann, Oxford

Hoessly M 1991 Use of eccentric contraction of muscle to increase range of movement in the upper motor neurone syndrome. Physiotherapy Theory and Practice 7: 91–101

Keith R A 1980 Activity patterns of a stroke rehabilitation unit. Social Science and Medicine 14A: 575–580

Lee W A 1980 Anticipatory control of postural and task muscle during rapid arm flexion. Journal of Motor Behavior 12(3): 185–196

LeVere T E 1980 Recovery of function after brain damage: a theory of the behavioral deficit. Physiological Psychology 8: 297–308

Nashner L M, Cordo P J 1981 Relation of automatic postural responses and reaction-time to voluntary movements of human leg muscles. Experimental Brain Research 43: 395–405

Nashner L M 1985 A functional approach to understanding spasticity. In: Struppler A, Weindl A (eds) Electromyography and evoked potentials. Springer-Verlag, Berlin

Nativ A 1993 Kinesiological issues in motor retraining following brain trauma. Critical Reviews in Physical and Rehabilitation Medicine 5(3): 227–246

Rodosky M W, Andriacchi T P, Andersson G B 1989 The influence of chair height on lower limb mechanics during rising. Journal of Orthopaedic Research 7: 266–271

Shepherd R, Carr J 1991 An emergent or dynamical systems view of movement dysfunction. Australian Physiotherapy 37(1): 4–5

Shepherd R B, Gentile A M 1994 The effect of varying initial trunk position on the biomechanics of standing up. Human Movement Science, in press

Sivenius J, Pyörälä K, Heinonen O P, Salonen J T, Riekkinen P 1985 The significance of intensity of rehabilitation of stroke – a controlled trial. Stroke 16: 928–931

Taub E 1980 Somatosensory deafferentation research with monkeys: implications for rehabilitation medicine. In: Ince L P (ed) Behavioral psychology in rehabilitation medicine: clinical implications. Williams & Wilkins, Baltimore

Turnbull G I, Wall J C 1989 Gait re-education following stroke: the application of motor skills aquisition theory. Physiotherapy Practice 5: 123–133

Winstein C J, Knecht H G 1990 Movement science and its relevance to physical therapy. Physical Therapy 70(12): 759–762

10. Neurodynamics related to the treatment of patients following a cerebrovascular accident

H. McKibbin

INTRODUCTION

The purpose of this chapter is to emphasize the importance of considering neurodynamics from both the biomechanical and physiological aspects when treating stroke patients.

Adverse neural tension (ANT) and adverse mechanical tension (AMT) have been terms used to describe an abnormal physiological or mechanical response produced by nervous system structures when their mechanics are tested. It is important to remember that this describes a situation where pathology has occurred. In the musculoskeletal field where the concept has been developed, notably by Elvey (1986), Maitland (1979) and Butler (1991), the patient's primary presenting problem may be in part, or even wholly, the result of pathology disrupting normal neurodynamics. Patients referred with central nervous system (CNS) lesions may have subclinical ANT but this is not their primary reason for referral.

Physiotherapists treating neurological patients should therefore not consider ANT only when it has developed and is limiting rehabilitation at a later stage. Instead an awareness of normal neural biomechanics and physiology applied from the first treatment could prevent or reduce the development of such pathology.

This obviously necessitates an appreciation of normal neurodynamics in the same way that a physiotherapist working in neurology will pursue an understanding of normal movement. Applying such a knowledge, even in the absence of pathology, will help achieve maximally effective treatments. The development of ANT will not, however, always be preventable in neurological patients due, for example, to prolonged abnormal posturing preventing the nervous system completing normal excursion. This must be recognized, considered during other treatment and also treated directly.

It is not the purpose of this chapter to explain in detail the concept of neurodynamics or the various pain mechanisms involved in pathology, but there is a list of suggested reading at the end of the chapter.

OUTLINE OF NEURODYNAMICS

Broadly, the concept addresses the mobility within and between the two types of nervous tissue, i.e. conducting tissue such as axons and myelin, and connective tissue – endo-, peri- and epineurium and also dural tissues. In addition, it looks at the movement relationship between the epineurium and dura and their closest neighbouring structure which is called the mechanical interface.

THE NERVOUS SYSTEM

The central and peripheral nervous systems (CNS and PNS) must be viewed as a continuum and not as two separate entities. They are continuous electrically via impulses, chemically via axoplasmic flow and mechanically via connective tissue. Where normal neurodynamics exist, tension or movement of the nervous system in one part of the body affects tension or causes movement in other areas, thus allowing the system to adapt to the position of a gymnast, for example, without interruption of conduction or even damage. Tissues will move on each other and funiculi which are undulating at rest will straighten, generating tension.

Pathology

The concept also recognizes the necessity of normal nerve physiology in maintaining the neurone and its target tissue. Pathology affecting the neural tissue itself or the movement of connective tissue within the nerve, e.g. sliding of bundles of fascicles on each other, is referred to as intraneural pathology. Pathology affecting movement between the nerve as a whole and its mechanical interface is described as extraneural pathology. Presenting signs and symptoms can indicate the proportion each type of pathology contributes to the patient's problem and this in turn influences treatment selection.

Symptoms

Symptoms that implicate the nervous system as a source include unfamiliar patterns of pain, often vague, wandering and not necessarily corresponding to dermatomes. It may involve the whole limb or present in clumps or lines, particularly along the course of a nerve, or there may be a catch of pain from a combination of movements unique to that patient.

Neurological therapists may have, in the past, attributed such symptoms solely to fluctuations in tone and altered sensation or perception, or blamed their own handling skills for causing pain when mobilizing a shoulder girdle with increased tone.

Neural mechanics

A knowledge of nerve anatomy enables physiotherapists to appreciate which nerves are under tension in different positions.

ULTT1

Upper limb tension test one (ULTT1) developed by Elvey was called the straight leg raise (SLR) of the upper limb for its effect on the brachial plexus and especially on the median nerve. Its components are a combination of shoulder girdle depression, abduction, lateral rotation, supination, elbow extension, and wrist and digit extension. Test components may be added in any order.

This is not dissimilar to positions used to mobilize shoulder girdles and upper limbs.

Shoulder girdle depression

Considering that the normal range of elbow extension without shoulder girdle depression (SGD) is $+16.5°$ to $+53.2°$ short of full extension (Pullos 1986), it is essential to be aware of normal neural mechanics and responses before positioning patients who do not have full sensation and normal protective muscle response or active movement.

SGD moves the C5, C6 and C7 nerve roots in particular, in a caudal direction and if these have already been tensioned as in some patterns of spasticity, the excursion of the upper limb into ULTT1 is more restricted than without SGD.

It could be hypothesized that improved neurodynamics are in part responsible for release of flexor tone in the upper limb of a neurological patient when a shoulder girdle that has been held in depression is mobilized, as tension is released proximally, allowing more nerve excursion distally.

The other extreme is overzealous supporting of the hemiplegic upper limb for prolonged periods causing shortening of neural and other soft tissues restricting head and upper limb movement.

Differentiation of symptoms

To differentiate symptoms or signs such as decreased range of movement to the nervous system as opposed to local soft tissue or joints, sensitizing manoeuvres are used, which alter neural tension and the relationship of the neural tissue to its mechanical interface in the affected area by movement of the nervous system elsewhere. This does not mean, therefore, that symptoms must become worse to implicate the nervous system.

While cervical spine side flexion could normally be used to differentiate forearm symptoms to the nervous system, movement of the head in a hemiplegic patient may influence the tone and hence signs or symptoms in the arm. However, on the basis of the nervous system being a continuum, the sound arm could be used instead to differentiate, although the work of Rubenach should be noted (Rubenach 1985). This demonstrated that adding the opposite ULTT1 eased the original symptoms in 77% of 116 normal subjects. Again this shows that it is an alteration rather than an increase in symptoms that is significant.

If moving the opposite arm could possibly have a mechanical effect on the neural tissues of its counterpart, then maybe one should specifically aim to do so in patients with dominant patterns of tone preventing movement of a limb. Some neural tissue movement in a persistently flexed upper limb could reduce the extent of ANT development and interfere with later rehabilitation.

Trunk neuromobilization techniques can reduce upper limb flexor tone without touching the limb but this may well also simultaneously mobilize the brachial plexus via movement of the dura.

Trunk tone and position

Treatment of the neurological patient aims at normalizing tone and may include 'trunk mobilization techniques'. It is interesting to note that an area of the thoracic spine prone to altered neurodynamics (T6 tension point) which receives particular attention from musculoskeletal physiotherapists is close to the central key point.

The Bobaths observed some years ago that the trunk tone and hence position was an important influence on tone of the limbs, and this could affect the limb movement available. From a musculoskeletal standpoint it is also recognized that trunk position affects limb range of movement, but as a result of neural biomechanics rather than tone. However, since neuromobilization of the trunk also produces a very effective Maitland grade II+ or III of the neuroaxis, it is impossible to mobilize tone without affecting neurodynamics.

Incidentally, when positioning a neurological patient across the corner of the bed to simultaneously mobilize adductors and the trunk, the patient is actually in the position used for tensioning the obturator nerve. The dura is tensioned by slumping the trunk, so if this has occurred, the amount of abduction available could be restricted. Alternatively, if the patient has first been taken to full abduction, trunk flexion could appear reduced with resistance to the movement. The position of the trunk and therefore the tension in the neuroaxis could also affect the amount of head on trunk movement.

Another position frequently used in the treatment of stroke patients is prone standing. This again demands good neurodynamics as it could be equated to a bilateral straight leg raise (SLR) with dorsiflexion, which primarily tensions the sciatic plexus, followed by truncal slump to varying degrees. The patient who insists on lifting their head may in fact be attempting to reduce tension on their neural tissues and posterior thigh symptoms could have a neural and/or hamstring origin.

The dura is of course highly innervated except in the dorsal midline, by the sinu vertebral nerves. This means that in the same way as the connective tissue of the PNS, which is innervated by the nervi nervorum, it can be a source of symptoms when its mobility and excursion are restricted.

Tension is transmitted from the spinal cord to the brainstem and the spinal dura to the cerebral meninges during slumping of the trunk and SLR. It could be hypothesized that extended periods of sitting in bed will be of particular irritation to those who have recently had a cerebral lesion and have raised intracranial pressure.

Sympathetic nervous system

The normal neurodynamics of the sympathetic nervous system can also be disturbed by the flexed thoracic spine and poking chin postures observed in poorly seated stroke patients, and those lacking truncal control. This is because the sympathetic chains run posterior to the axis of flexion and extension in the thoracic spine and anterior to it in the cervical spine.

Signs and symptoms

Signs and symptoms indicative of the sympathetic nervous system are often evident in a stroke patient's painful hemiplegic arm. Oedema due to a dependent position or reduced active movement of the limb may predispose it to an entrapment syndrome. Diabetes which is 2–4 times more common in stroke than a normal population (Poulter et al 1993) will raise the intrafascicular pressure within nerves (Myers & Powell 1981) so a stroke patient's nervous system may already be more susceptible to pathology.

Physiological aspects

The physiological aspects of the concept of neurodynamics are as important, if not more so, than the biomechanics.

Pressure

In relation to stroke patients the vascular supply to the nervous tissue could already be impaired by vascular disease, and in addition could be reduced by the pressure on nerves of passing under or through a spastic muscle which has become an unyielding mechanical interface. An example could be spastic pectorals, biceps or pronators, or tension of prolonged abnormal postures, such as wrist flexion reducing the lumen of the vessel. Extraneural tethering may mechanically restrict the movement of blood vessels supplying nerves.

Sunderland (1976) describes a pressure gradient, Sunderland's law, that must be maintained for adequate intrafascicular circulation, which is a prerequisite for normal neural function. If this is interrupted, impaired venous drainage will ensue.

Sunderland applies his law to carpal tunnel syndrome where the pressure in the tunnel may rise to around 30 mmHg. It could equally well be applied, however, to other examples of pressure such as spastic muscle. It describes three stages of pathology: hypoxia – causing pain; oedema, which remains because the perineurium is not crossed by lymphatics; and finally, fibrosis – causing intraneural pathology. It is this oedema that initially impairs gliding of fascicles; the nerve fibres become increasingly fixed as fibrosis develops (intraneural pathomechanics and pathophysiology). This creates a stretching force and friction not only at the initial site of pathology but also elsewhere along the course of the nerve, due to the altered neurodynamics; this in turn may lead to further epineurial oedema or even bleeding and therefore inflammation. This is a postulated mechanical cause of the 'double crush' syndrome, described initially by Upton & McComas in 1973.

Rydevik (1981) and Ogata & Naito (1985) used an intravital microscope and hydrogen washout technique respectively, to measure bloodflow in rabbit sciatic and tibial nerves under varying amounts of pressure. The results were similar with a pressure of 20–30 mmHg causing retardation of venous blood flow in the epineurium. Increasing pressure reduced the flow in the supply arterioles and endoneurial capillaries until flow was arrested at 70–80 mmHg or 60–80% of the mean arterial pressure.

Lundborg et al (1983) measured endoneurial fluid pressure (EFP), which parallels the occurrence of an endoneurial oedema, and may interfere considerably with endoneurial capillary bloodflow. Local compression of 30 or 80 mmHg was applied to a rat sciatic nerve for between 2 and 8 hours. The pressure increased threefold at either compression for 8 hours, and remained the same at 24 hours after it was removed, indicating no significant drainage of the intrafascicular oedema. Marked endoneurial oedema, separation of nerve fibres and varying degrees of nerve fibre injury were observed in the zone beneath the perineurium in association with the raised EFP. These signs were still evident 28 days after the compression period (Powell & Myers 1986). Injury varied according to the pressure.

While any compression of a nerve under a spastic muscle is more likely to occur over a short distance than at a specific point, the effects of the subsequent pathology should be considered as possible until work confirming the pressures is completed. If the physiology of nerves does prove to be affected by the pressure from increased tone, the duration of pressure will exceed that of any experimental work. The latter has found that damage is proportional to the magnitude and duration of the compression, which in turn influences the reversibility.

Axoplasmic flow

Local energy from capillaries in the endoneurial space is required for both impulse transmission and axonal transport. Dahlin & McLean (1986) found a pressure of 30 mmHg induced a slowing or cessation of fast and slow antegrade and also retrograde flow, with reactive changes in the nerve cell body. Reduced axoplasmic flow is the other postulated mechanism responsible for the double crush phenomenon of Upton & McComas (1973). They suggest that the altered flow predisposes other vulnerable sites of the nervous system to pathology. Could this explain the nature of shoulder–hand syndrome in some patients?

Neural stretch

Another possible neurophysiological cause of painful shoulders could be excessive neural stretch from subluxation. Ogata & Naito (1986) found that elongation of a nerve by 15.7% caused a complete arrest of the circulation. When neurotherapists see feet in plantar flexion and inversion or subluxed shoulders, they should aim not only to correct tone but to prevent physiological nerve damage and a self-perpetuating cycle of pain. Some static reflex inhibiting postures of the past may well have compromised the normal physiology of the nervous system by prolonged stretch in tension positions.

CONCLUSION

This chapter has touched only the 'tip of the iceberg'. There are not only many more considerations of neurodynamics applicable to neurological patients other than those following stroke but also many neurophysiology issues to be developed that could influence the rehabilitation of patients.

It is not suggested that treatment priorities with neurological patients should be rearranged to pursue normal neurodynamics to the detriment of tone. However, even an awareness can surely only improve treatment and ultimately the patient's outcome.

Acknowledgements

Thanks are extended to Jane Greening MSc MCSP MMACP and Louis Gifford MSc MCSP MMPAA for commenting on this chapter.

REFERENCES

Butler D S 1991 Mobilisation of the nervous system. Churchill Livingstone, Melbourne
Dhalin L B, McLean W G 1986 Effects of graded experimental compression on slow and fast axonal transport in rabbit vagus nerve. Journal of Neurological Sciences 72: 19–30
Elvey R L 1986 Treatment of arm pain associated with abnormal brachial plexus tension. Australian Journal of Physiotherapy 32: 225–230

Lundborg G, Myers R, Powell H C 1983 Nerve compression injury and increase in
    endoneurial fluid pressure. A miniature compartment syndrome. Journal of Neurology,
    Neurosurgery and Psychiatry 46: 1119–1124
Maitland G D 1979 Negative disc exploration; positive canal signs. Australian Journal of
    Physiotherapy 25: 129–134
Myers R, Powell H C 1981 Endoneurial fluid pressure in peripheral neuropathies. In:
    Hargens A (ed) Tissue fluid pressure and composition. Williams & Wilkins, Baltimore
Ogata K, Naito M 1986 Blood flow of peripheral nerve. Effects of dissection stretching and
    compression. Journal of Hand Surgery 11B: 10–14
Poulter N, Sever P, Thomas S 1993 Cardiovascular disease: practical issues for prevention.
    Caroline Black, St. Albans,
Powell H C, Myers R 1986 Pathology of experimental nerve compression. Laboratory
    Investigations 55: 91–100
Pullos J 1986 The upper limb tension test. Australian Journal of Physiotherapy 32: 258–259
Rubenach H 1985 The upper limb tension test: the effect of the position and movement of
    the contralateral arm. In: Proceedings, Manipulative Therapists Association of Australia,
    4th biennial conference, Brisbane
Rydevik B, Lundborg G, Bagge U 1981 Effects of graded compression on intraneural blood
    flow. Journal of Hand Surgery 6: 3–12
Sunderland S 1976 The nerve lesion in carpal tunnel syndrome. Journal of Neurology,
    Neurosurgery and Psychiatry 39: 615–626
Upton A R M, McComas A J 1973 The double crush in nerve entrapment syndromes.
    Lancet 2: 359–362

FURTHER READING

Lundborg G 1988 Nerve injury and repair. Churchill Livingstone, Edinburgh
Sunderland S 1978 Nerves and nerve injuries, 2nd edn. Churchill Livingstone, Edinburgh

11. How do physiotherapists view spasticity?

O. Gjelsvik

INTRODUCTION

For many years physiotherapists have tried to deal with the problem of spasticity. Considerable scientific research has been carried out in an attempt to explain the cause and complexity of the problem, and physiotherapists have tried to adapt their therapeutic approach accordingly. Their success in doing so has indeed been variable.

In the 1940s Berta Bobath and her husband Karel set up a practice in London. She was a physiotherapist widely known for her handling skills and he was a psychiatrist. Together they tried to postulate a scientific background to explain spasticity and why treatment worked. Some of their hypotheses have since been proven correct, while others have been proven incorrect.

Their work resulted in great interest among physiotherapists, as a result of which, the Bobaths' work has been passed on and is still being followed today. The Bobath concept is, now, widely known and highly respected in physiotherapy circles throughout the world.

In the 1980s neurophysiologists further widened the scope of knowledge and brought the understanding of neuromuscular tonus and activity to greater depths. Some neurophysiologists have also worked in close liaison with physiotherapists who treat hemiplegic patients on a daily basis. This has enabled the researchers and the clinical staff to create an atmosphere conducive to mutual learning.

So what is there to understand? What do physiotherapists have to take on board from this new knowledge? Obviously physiotherapists cannot, themselves, undertake the basic research down to the molecular level – this has to be done by scientists in laboratories. Yet what is much of this research worth if it is not applied in the daily treatment of the neurologically damaged person? Who else but physiotherapists treat patients using their handling skills in an effort to reaccess the potential which still lies within a damaged central neuromuscular system, and to enable movement that is as normal as possible. Physiotherapists can absorb new knowledge and make it work in daily treatments.

WHAT IS SPASTICITY?

Spasticity was much easier to deal with in the early days. It was believed to be caused by the release of primitive reflexes within the damaged central nervous system. Therefore, regardless of what one did, the spasticity would still be there to a greater or lesser degree.

Lance (1980) stated:

Spasticity may be defined as the result of plastic reorganisation of spinal cord reflexes released partially or wholly from brainstem or cerebro-cortical direction, i.e. the loss of inhibitory or modulatory control.

Asymmetry and associated reactions

Today spasticity is thought to be a developing process following damage to the central nervous system. It develops over time and is more a result of what the patients do or have done to them than a direct cause of the lesion. If a patient is allowed to move in a compensatory manner, – i.e. to use effort to get out of bed, to walk at an early stage with a walking aid and caliper, and to develop within him or herself a sense of being asymmetrical in all their activity – then they will become asymmetrical as a result.

If patients are told by the medical staff at an early stage to try as hard as they can to pull themselves into sitting by the use of their sound arm and hand, or to pull themselves into standing while trying to balance on one leg on their way from a chair to bed or vice versa, it is very likely that this undue effort will produce the first signs of associated reactions on the affected side. When associated reactions are repeated they become established, and once established they produce stereotyped patterns of movement, the result of which is spasticity.

Associated reactions may be defined (British Bobath Tutor's Association 1993) as:

... reactions or responses associated with a stimulus that goes beyond the patient's individual level of inhibitory control. They always produce an increase of tone and are always pathological. They are the observable feature of possible future spasticity.

This complex is illustrated in Figure 11.1. It shows that what the patient does or is allowed or encouraged to do following a neurological lesion is much more important in the development of spasticity than the lesion itself.

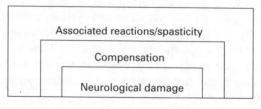

Fig. 11.1 Associated reactions in spasticity (Lynch 1990).

Plasticity

Geoffrey Kidd explains this differently and more on the molecular level with the term 'formfunction' (Kidd et al 1992). The form (the anatomy) has its function (physiology) and the function decides the form. This means that one becomes what one does. The neuromuscular system is adaptable to changes in its environment on both internal and external levels. This is called plasticity.

After damage to the central nervous system, cell death leads to axonal degeneration. This leads in turn to free synaptic spaces on cell bodies in neuronal sets at all levels in the system. Growth associated protein is released in large quantities and this protein acts as a magnet on sprouting axons. These new synaptic connections are 'unskilled' and will learn what they are taught; their function may be directed either towards pathology, as in development of spasticity, or back towards normality. Herein lies the joint therapeutic challenge.

The central nervous system responds to its environment 24 hours a day. It is constantly formed and reformed according to what it hears, thinks, feels, sees and does. It is proprioceptively controlled. This is still the case after damage. The main difference is that the central neuromuscular system does not possess the ability to regain its normal function, although the potential to do so continues to lie within the system. Whenever the patient tries to move, they are unsuccessful in terms of quality of movement because of the neurological deficit. Therefore the patient increases his or her effort in order to reach the goal and, to a small degree, is preoccupied with how the movement occurs. The quality of performance is reduced as a result, but as patients are goal-orientated they may not be aware that their movement has deviated from the normal. The following quotation may be applied, with reference to the plasticity (Kidd et al 1992):

The ability of the central nervous system to adapt its structure to suit the required function means that what goes in modifies the inside so that it can more easily give the same response in the future.
So abnormal movement in the short term will reinforce abnormal movement in the long term by making it easier for the central nervous system to respond to the same stimulus in the future.

Turning this statement on its head, this must mean that normal movement in the short term will reinforce normal movement in the long term.

Therefore, it is most important that the environment in which the patient interacts provides the right amount of physiological stress. This means that throughout the day the demands placed on the patient must correspond with what he or she is able to do at that moment in time. Later on the patient must be given the necessary aid and assistance in daily activities which cannot be performed to standard in order to regain the proprioceptive feedback that will provide the sensation of moving functionally and with a minimum of effort. This is called the 24-hour concept. Its prerequisite is a sound understanding by all parties responsible for the rehabilitation plan of the patient that spasticity can indeed be prevented.

Iris Musa (1986) presented the following hypotheses:

The manipulation of afferent input during the stage of spinal shock following a central nervous system damage can prevent spasticity from occuring.

and

The manipulation of afferent input from the periphery to the spinal cord can control spasticity in a limb and so facilitate normal movement.

The Bobath concept

Within the Bobath concept, it is a firm belief that spasticity can be prevented, although it is not always possible. Spasticity can be prevented to a certain extent, and many more different forms of abnormal movement with high neuromuscular tonus are seen today, but with a high degree of volitional control. So why has spastic man' as was seen on a regular basis 20 years ago changed into the far lesser 'spastic man' of today? Surely, looking at it from a medical point of view, the lesions are the same today as they were before. Does this mean that the joint treatment approach of today achieves more successful treatment results? If so, is it possible that deeper knowledge and better handling skills may improve the treatment results even further?

The Bobaths' answer was 'yes'. This author agrees and, furthermore, thinks that in working with neurologically damaged people one has to maintain an optimistic attitude.

Returning to Iris Musa's hypotheses and looking at the terms 'neuromuscular plasticity' and 'formfunction', an explanation as to how spasticity can be prevented is required, and if spasticity is established, can it then be treated successfully? It is appropriate here to present the definition of the Bobath concept (Lynch 1990):

The Bobath Concept is a holistic approach to the assessment and treatment of patients with damage within the central nervous system (brain, spinal cord, neuromuscular system) which causes a deviation from normal posture and movement.

It is based upon:

1. Analysis of normal movement.
2. Analysis of the deviation from normal movement
   a) main problem
   b) compensation.
3. Application of appropriate treatment techniques.

Uniform handling

The key to the successful treatment is uniform handling. Therein lies the application of the 24-hour concept. Physiotherapy creates the basis for the understanding of that particular patient's problem and the analysis forms the basis of the rehabilitation plan. Basically, this means that the regaining of postural control and activity against gravity will provide the patient with a basis for recovery of functional activity in arms and legs. The postural control will give back the sense of midline which further allows the patient to move and to alter position between symmetry and asymmetry. This is called balance. Balance means freedom to move and not having to cling on to the bed, a work surface or a walking aid.

In achieving this, it is believed that the routes to the already programmed areas of the brain and spinal cord have been reopened. Many of these areas are not directly affected by a cerebrovascular accident, but have been rendered inaccessible because entry to the 'programme' has been barred.

One hour of prescriptive physiotherapy per day may be sufficient to reopen the route, but it will not stay open unless the postural control, the symmetry and the alignment of the head, trunk and limbs are maintained throughout the day and night. This is the multidisciplinary responsibility.

For the patient with established spasticity, the potential for functional improvement is still present, but the challenge to accomplish this is far greater. This will be a patient who has compensated for functional loss and reached a plateau of self-sufficiency. This will be a situation that has developed itself over time and, due to the neuromuscular plasticity, the abnormal state has become normal to the patient. To change this state of spasticity takes a great deal of motivation and understanding on the part of the patient. The neuromuscular system possesses the ability to form itself into a wider scope of function. Again, one may refer to the term 'formfunction' (Kidd et al 1992).

Theoretically, it is possible; practically, it takes time and a motivated patient with a sound understanding of the functional gain. The therapeutic challenge is to show the patient in the treatment session that the treatment is successful. This can be achieved by proprioceptive control administered through handling skills.

Proprioceptive control

What are the proprioceptive controls? In treatment, the variety in choice of positions constitutes proprioceptive controls. The reason why the therapist will want to take a patient into standing instead of supine leads us to the next proprioceptive control, i.e. choice of motor goal. Standing is a position where the patient is able to maintain posture, while at the same time the arm is free from the body.

The standing position gives the patient the postural background of being able to transfer weight actively over one leg by a lateral tilt of the pelvis, thereby making it possible to take a step with the other leg. In this way, a motor goal can be broken up into its component parts.

Where the hands are placed and the pressure applied in treatment is a strong proprioceptive control. Through the hands the therapist can detect the patient's response to being moved and, by means of verbal and operational feedback, can give an indication of the direction, scope and speed of movement. The aim of this is to modulate the level of excitation and inhibition within the patient's central nervous system back towards normality by giving his/her the experience of:

- being up against gravity
- being able to move within the force of gravity.

As the controllers of proprioceptive information, therapists must decide what can be achieved in treatment through the facilitation of movement. Automatic responses can be utilized as opposed to conscious use of verbal commands, thereby calling upon volitional activity. The use of the voice in therapy will have variable effects. Expressions such as 'follow', 'come with me', 'grow tall', will have a more subtle effect than words such as 'pull', 'push' and 'stretch'. The latter will produce more volitional effort on the part of the patient and may cause an increase in muscular tonus far beyond the level required.

CONCLUSION

Physiotherapy is handling skills in combination with a sound theoretical knowledge. Therapists have to know and keep up with new scientific progress because only through research and the application in treatment of scientific results can an improvement in practical skills occur.

Berta Bobath was an artist with modulatory skill. She could mould spastic man back towards normality through her hands. Her science was up-to-date in its time, but obviously, greater knowledge has been acquired today through research.

There is, however, a scientific statement that was made in the 1920s that is still as sound today, and maybe this represents the bridge between the empirically based science and treatment approach of the earlier days and the more scientifically proven treatment methods of today, i.e. the shunting rule of Magus:

At any moment during a movement or postural change the central nervous system reflects faithfully the state of the body musculature.

At any moment during a movement or postural change the state of active elongation or contraction of the body musculature is faithfully mirrored within the central nervous system by the distribution of inhibitory or excitatory neurotransmission. The state of the body musculature can control the central nervous system.

Acknowledgement

Most of the ideas in this chapter have been communicated to me by my very good friend and colleague, Mary Lynch, to whom I am deeply and forever grateful.

REFERENCES

British Bobath Tutor's Association 1993 Personal communication
Kidd G, Lawes N, Musa I 1992 Understanding neuromuscular plasticity – a basis for clinical rehabilitation. Edward Arnold, London, chs 5–9
Lance J W 1980 Spasticity disordered motor control. In: Feldman R G, Young R R, Koella W P (eds) Spasticity: disordered motor control. Chicago, III, Year Book Medical Publishers, Inc., pp 185–205
Lynch 1990 Personal communication
Musa I 1986 The role of afferent input in the reduction of spasticity – an hypothesis. Physiotherapy 72(4): 179–182

Measurement and research

Measurement and research

12. Research in stroke rehabilitation

N. B. Lincoln

Research is a systematic enquiry to advance knowledge. Much of stroke rehabilitation is based on impressions and dogma with little scientific evidence for its accuracy. The aim must be to increase the knowledge base so that the most effective treatment possible can be provided for patients.

TYPES OF RESEARCH

There are different types of research which serve different purposes. Some questions may be answered in different ways. While one approach may be the optimum for answering a question, another may be more practical. Studies may be retrospective or prospective. In retrospective studies the researcher examines events that are past and analyses data that have been collected previously, whereas in prospective studies the data collected is planned in advance and information is gathered as it becomes available. The latter has the advantage that it is relatively easy and quick to do, but the disadvantage is that information may be missing, it may be necessary to rely on recall of information and not all that is needed may be available. Ideally, studies should be prospective, but useful preliminary information can be obtained from retrospective studies.

Studies may be descriptive or interventional. In descriptive studies events are observed as they occur in clinical practice. The role of the researcher is to provide an accurate report of events as they happen without changing them. In contrast, intervention studies will include a change in the pattern of clinical care, and the researcher records the effects of this change. Again, the former provides useful preliminary information but often, to answer the most important questions, intervention studies are required. Studies may be confined to an individual or may consider groups of patients. The former has the advantage that the information obtained is of relevance to the assessment and treatment of that individual, but it may not necessarily apply to others. Group studies provide information of general principles in the management of patients but do not necessarily apply to each individual in the group.

The most informative studies are generally prospective and interventional, but retrospective, descriptive studies provide useful background information from which a prospective intervention study may be planned. Therefore, there is a place for both in stroke rehabilitation research. The choice of study will often be based on practical constraints. The practical constraints of different types of study will be considered and illustrative examples given of some types of research in stroke rehabilitation.

DESCRIPTIVE STUDIES

Descriptive studies provide a record of events as they occur in clinical practice. For example, the detailed observation of reaching reported by van Vliet (Ch. 21) is a descriptive study. The aim is to learn general principles by detailed observation and recording of events as they happen. The development of assessment scales based on the pattern of recovery of stroke patients was based on descriptive studies. Adams (Ch.15) describes the systematic observations of different groups of patients using the Rivermead motor assessment to identify general rules about the pattern of recovery. The value of these studies depends to a large extent on the properties of the measurement scales used to record the observations. The requirements of such assessment procedures are described by Wade (1992). In addition there are practical constraints. Collecting systematic information takes time. It is not possible to draw general conclusions about stroke patients unless a representative cross-section of patients has been studied, which may mean large numbers of patients. If information is going to be collected in one centre, it may take several months.

An alternative approach is to involve several centres. For example, Partridge et al (1993) incorporated results from several centres in their study of recovery, but in this case the inter-observer reliability of the data collection method must be high, otherwise errors will occur due to observer variation. Studies by a single observer or a group of therapists working closely together will be less prone to this type of error but may take longer. The detailed analysis reported by van Vliet (Ch. 21) would be difficult to incorporate into routine clinical work, whereas the information reported by Partridge et al (1993) was collected as part of routine clinical practice.

Many therapists do not use standardized scoreable assessments in their clinical work (Sackley & Lincoln 1994). However, if they do, a wealth of research information immediately becomes available. The advantage of using such data is that the findings are of relevance to the therapist working in a general setting with a wide range of patients rather than, for example, in the specialist unit.

INTERVENTION STUDIES

The main purpose of intervention studies is to evaluate treatments or patterns of stroke care. These studies, at the same time, also provide a considerable amount of descriptive information. For example, some of the descriptive data reported by Adams were collected as part of an intervention study on domiciliary rehabilitation (Gladman et al 1993). Some intervention studies can be incorporated into routine clinical practice. This is perhaps most easily achieved using single case experimental designs.

SINGLE CASE EXPERIMENTAL DESIGNS

Single case experimental designs (SCED) are intervention studies which enable treatment of an individual patient to be evaluated. They differ from case reports in that they are prospective and are designed so that results can be interpreted objectively. There are some useful summaries of the application of single case experimental designs in neurological rehabilitation (Riddoch 1991, Riddoch & Lennon 1991, Sunderland 1990, Wilson 1987). Two examples will be given to illustrate the practical constraints of SCED.

Sackley & Baguley (1993) describe the application of SCED to evaluate treatment with a balance performance monitor. The design used was an ABAB design. During the A phase, baseline recordings are taken while the patient receives routine treatment. These baseline recordings demonstrate the pattern of change over time. If there is no significant change during the baseline period it can be assumed that the treatment being applied at this time is not having a significant effect on the outcome being assessed. During the B phase, a specific treatment is introduced and the effect is recorded over time. If there is a significant change of level or slope of the assessment over time during the B phase then it could be because the treatment is having an effect or because, by chance, the patient has started to improve at that time. The second baseline phase helps to identify which of these possibilities is the more likely. If improvement continues during the second baseline phase, as during the B phase, then the observed change may have been due to chance. However, if the patient's improvement stabilises or declines during the second A phase then it is likely that the observed change was due to the treatment being given.

It is possible to include various forms of control phases in the basic ABA design. For example, De Weerdt et al (1989) designed their SCED to differentiate between the general effects of a new therapist and impressive equipment, and the specific effects of a balance performance monitor. Two baselines were included, one with no treatment and the other with the new therapist and some equipment, but not the specific treatment that was to be evaluated.

Advantages

The advantages of SCED are that they do not require large numbers of patients. They are appropriate for the rare or exceptional patient. This may be particularly important for those working with elderly stroke patients with multiple causes of disability. For example, most stroke patients who also had an amputation would be excluded from group studies of stroke rehabilitation. Therefore, there is little information on the effectiveness of treatment strategies with these patients. However, an SCED would evaluate treatment for that individual. Apart from planning, these studies need little additional work and can therefore easily be incorporated into routine clinical practice. To do this, however, it is important that the assessments used to monitor the treatment are very quick to perform. De Weerdt et al (1989) used a balance coefficient reading at the beginning of each session which took only about 30 seconds to obtain. The requirements for such measurements are the same as the longer scales described by Wade, but some of the more general scales are not appropriate for SCED. The measures need to be very specific to the ability being treated and sensitive to small changes.

Another advantage of SCED is that the design can be modified according to the progress of the patient. If, for example, De Weerdt et al (1989) had observed a marked shift in baseline in response to a new therapist and equipment, it might have been necessary to modify the design at this stage to extend the baseline for a further week to determine if the base line stabilized, or to incorporate a phase with a new therapist but no special equipment, to assess whether it was the therapist or the equipment that produced the observed change in ability. Studies employing SCEDs have provided a useful means of evaluating new treatment techniques (Lennon 1991), or determining whether there is sufficient evidence to justify a larger scale study (Wagenaar et al 1990).

A series of SCED studies will give an indication whether the effects observed are specific to the one patient or whether they also apply to other patients. However, to obtain an overall indication of the general applicability it is necessary to do a group study.

GROUP STUDIES

Group studies provide a means of evaluating treatments with a wide range of patients. They provide general principles about the effectiveness of a treatment procedure, which may not necessarily apply to each individual in that group. For example, on the basis of the SCED studies reported by De Weerdt et al (1989), Sackley (1992) evaluated the same procedure in a group study. Patients were randomly allocated to either a visual feedback group or a control group in which the same activities were used but without visual feedback of weight distribution.

The significant differences between the specific feedback technique used and the placebo treatment indicated that the treatment had a specific effect which was generally applicable to the patients included in the study. However, it was not necessarily applicable to patients not included, such as those with severe communication problems. Although less easy to conduct as part of routine clinical practice, it is still feasible. The patients were all being treated as would occur in routine clinical practice. The content of the treatment differed according to the group allocation, but this too occurs in clinical work. One therapist may rely heavily on one technique and another on a different one. Assessment of outcome should be conducted by an independent observer who is not aware of the treatment being given. This may be achieved by an exchange arrangement between two therapists with each acting as the independent assessor for the other. Alternatively, automatic recording systems which can be transferred directly for computer analysis save the therapist from knowing the results of the assessment without the need for a separate individual.

Although evaluations of general stroke management procedures such as domiciliary treatment, or intensive treatment as compared with standard treatment, require large numbers of patients, this is not necessarily the case if specific components of treatment are being evaluated. Studies with smaller numbers, such as evaluations of EMG biofeedback for arm function (Crow et al 1989) and ice in the management of painful shoulder (Partridge et al 1990) have yielded useful results of clinical relevance.

FUTURE RESEARCH IN STROKE REHABILITATION

There are many questions about physiotherapy in stroke rehabilitation to be answered. Large scale trials have indicated some general findings. There is evidence to suggest that more treatment is better than less (Sivenius et al 1985, Smith et al 1981, Sunderland et al 1992, Wade & Collen 1992). Co-ordinated multidisciplinary care is better than more fragmented services (Langhorne et al 1993, Kalra et al 1993, Juby et al 1994) and domiciliary physiotherapy has advantages for selected groups of patients over outpatient hospital services (Gladman et al 1993, Young & Forster 1992).

However, there is relatively little information on the content of these treatment packages. Which components of physiotherapy are essential and which are not is still open to debate. A review of physiotherapy for stroke patients (Ernst 1990) concluded that there was evidence to suggest that stroke patients benefit from rehabilitation but that there was no evidence to indicate that it mattered which treatment was chosen.

Since this review in 1990, some progress has been made. Some techniques, such as biofeedback, have been relatively well evaluated (Lincoln & Sackley 1992) but are little used in routine clinical practice. Other widely used practices, such as the use of inflatable splints, strapping and trunk mobilizations, have not been evaluated. The most likely means of achieving this is by incorporating research into routine clinical practice. If clinicians are conducting research as part of their clinical management of the patients, then the questions that are important to clinicians will be answered and stroke rehabilitation will have a sound scientific basis. Patients deserve to receive treatments of proven effectiveness and not just those that are the fashion of the decade.

REFERENCES

Crow J L, Lincoln N B, Nouri F M, De Weerdt W G 1989 The effectiveness of EMG biofeedback in the treatment of arm function after stroke. International Disability Studies 11: 155–160

De Weerdt W G, Crossley S M, Lincoln N B, Harrison M A 1989 Restoration of balance in stroke patients: a single case study design. Clinical Rehabilitation 3: 139–147

Ernst E 1990 A review of stroke rehabilitation and physiotherapy. Stroke 21: 1081–1085

Gladman J R F, Lincoln N B, Barer D H 1993 A randomised control trial of domiciliary and hospital based rehabilitation for stroke patients after discharge from hospital. Journal of Neurology, Neurosurgery and Psychiatry 56: 960–966

Juby L C, Lincoln N B, Berman P 1994 A randomised control trial to evaluate the effect of rehabilitation in a stroke unit on functional outcome. Submitted for publication

Kalra L, Dale P, Crome P 1993 Improving stroke rehabilitation: a controlled study. Stroke 24: 1462–1467

Langhorne P, Williams B O, Gilchrist W, Howie K 1993 Do stroke units save lives? Lancet 342: 395–398

Lennon S 1991 Wheelchair transfer training in a stroke patient with neglect: a single case study design. Physiotherapy Theory and Practice 7: 51–55

Lincoln N B, Sackley C M 1992 Biofeedback in stroke rehabilitation. Critical Reviews in Physical and Rehabilitation Medicine 4: 37–47

Partridge C J, Edwards S M, Mee R, van Langenberghe H V K 1990 Hemiplegic shoulder pain: a study of two methods of physiotherapy treatment. Clinical Rehabilitation 4: 43–50

Partridge C J, Morris L W, Edwards S M 1993 Recovery from physical disability after stroke: profiles for different levels of starting severity. Clinical Rehabilitation 7: 210–217

Riddoch J 1991 Evaluation of pratice. Physiotherapy 77: 439–444

Riddoch J, Lennon S 1991 Evaluation of practice: the single case study approach. Physiotherapy Theory and Practice 7: 3–11

Sackley C M 1992 A randomised controlled trial of visual feedback after stroke. Proceedings of World Congress of Physiotherapy, London, pp 475–477

Sackley C M, Baguley B I 1993 Visual feedback after stroke with the balance performance monitor: two single case studies. Clinical Rehabilitation 7: 189–195

Sackley C M, Lincoln N B 1994 A survey of rehabilitation practice for stroke patients. In preparation

Sivenius J, Pyorala K, Heinonen O P, Salonen J T, Riekkinen P 1985 The significance of intensity of rehabilitation of stroke – a controlled trial. Stroke 16: 928–931

Smith D S, Goldenberg E, Ashburn A et al 1981 Remedial therapy after stroke: a randomised controlled trial. British Medical Journal 282: 517–518

Sunderland A 1990 Single case experiments in neurological rehabilitation. Clinical Rehabilitation 4: 181–192

Sunderland A, Tinson D J, Bradley E L, Fletcher D, Langton-Hewer R, Wade D T 1992 Enhanced physical therapy improves recovery of arm function after stroke: a randomised controlled trial. Journal of Neurology, Neurosurgery and Psychiatry 52: 530–535

Wade D T 1992 Measurement in neurological rehabilitation. Oxford University Press, Oxford

Wade D T, Collen F M, Robb G F, Warlow C P 1992 Physiotherapy intervention late after stroke. British Medical Journal 405: 609–613

Wagenaar R, Meijer O G, van Wieringen P C W et al 1990 The functional recovery of
stroke: a comparison between neurodevelopmental treatment and the Brunnstrom
method. Scandinavian Journal of Rehabilitation Medicine 22: 1–8

Wilson B A 1987 Single case experimental designs in neurological rehabilitation. Journal of
Clinical Experimental Neuropsychology 9: 527–544

Young J B, Forster A 1992 The Bradford community stroke trial: results at 6 months.
British Medical Journal 304: 1085–1089

13. The role of the physiotherapist in research

B. Bergman

INTRODUCTION

The professionalization of physiotherapy as an occupation is much discussed and has attracted considerable interest in recent decades (Hislop 1975, Jensen 1988, Raz et al 1991, Miles-Tapping et al 1992, Soderberg 1993). It is mostly a discussion concerning expansion of the specific and theoretical body of knowledge in physiotherapy and remodelling of the professional role in order to define occupational practice. Research is identified as an area of concern for physiotherapists. Time–budget studies show, however, that practising physiotherapists devote very little of their worktime to developmental work and research (Allen 1983, Bergman 1988). Although research could be included in the professional role of physiotherapists, the research arena is not entered easily by the average physiotherapist. Indeed, the research physiotherapist is a rarity about whom very little is written, even though the topic is ardently discussed among physiotherapists themselves.

This chapter discusses the role of the physiotherapist, with the focus on research, setting out from a series of studies undertaken in Sweden in the 1980s (Bergman 1989).

HOW PHYSIOTHERAPISTS UTILIZE THEIR WORKING HOURS

In a time–budget study it was shown that the treatment of patients occupied on average 33% of the physiotherapists' gross working time. Continuing education and developmental work amounted to 6% and the remaining occupational tasks totalled 38% (Bergman 1988). A similar utilization of working hours is reported in unpublished replications of the study in Sweden and by Allen (1983). Therefore, the results of time–budget studies show that practising physiotherapists use very little of their working day for developmental work and research. Such work appears not to form part of the average physiotherapist's duties.

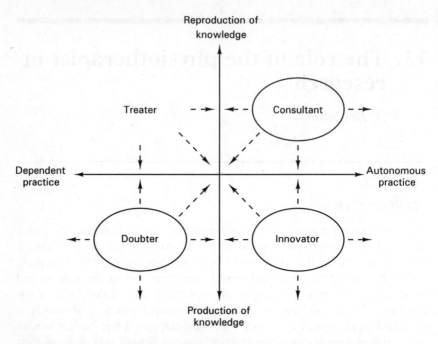

Fig. 13.1   An interpretation of the approaches and wishes of the four ideal types to professional knowledge and autonomy, with the arrows suggesting various possible future prospects. (Adapted with permission from Sjukgymnasten, Vetenskapligt supplement 1991.)

VOCATIONAL STRATEGIES AMONG PHYSIOTHERAPISTS

To gain an understanding of the ideas and beliefs underlying the way physiotherapists work, an interview study was conducted. Data were analysed qualitatively and presented in the form of four ideal types (Fig.13.1): the treater, the consultant, the doubter and the innovator (Bergman 1991).

The treater was characterized as giving priority to patient treatment, taking the view that he/she is responsible for providing care and service in the form of physiotherapy, but also keeping their own interests in mind.

The consultant was characterized by an intention to work as an adviser and expert on physiotherapy, rather than on patient treatment.

The doubter gave priority to patient treatment, even when suspecting that combining treatment with research would promote professional knowledge as well as benefiting clinical work.

The innovator was characterized by a deliberate desire to work with management and research as well as with patient treatment, in order to promote both the latter and professional autonomy.

These ideal types can all be perceived to emanate from and be related to the conceptions the physiotherapist held about professional *responsibility*, professional *autonomy* and professional *knowledge*.

PATIENT PRIMACY – THIS NARROW CONCEPT OF PROFESSIONAL RESPONSIBILITY

The physiotherapy profession was seen to have twin objectives: care and service in general and the provision of physiotherapy in particular, both equally important. Care-giving, service and availability were ideas central to the physiotherapist's role. Preventive work, management, and research were not looked upon as routine matters for the average physiotherapist. The systematic assessment of work outcome, being regarded as research, was also not included in the duties of the average physiotherapist.

Physiotherapists are socialized in certain health professional behaviours, one of which is 'patient primacy' (Shepard & Jensen 1990). This is the belief that the patient comes first, above all other activities in which a therapist may be involved, such as engagement in research. The professional culture – the ideas about and values enshrined in the purposes and practices of work – as described in physiotherapy practice, is assumed to emanate from the physiotherapist as a treater or 'doer'; what Purtilo (1986) calls 'this narrow concept' of professional responsibility. Such a concept was, however, questioned by the *doubter* and the *innovator*, chiefly from an experienced need to be able to verbalize about and give reasons for treatment methods and results. This in turn was described as being linked with an extended professional autonomy, with the possibility of actively participating in devising overall work objectives and routines, and with developing relationships and collaboration with other medical profes-sions.

AUTONOMY AND PROFESSIONAL KNOWLEDGE

According to Abbot (1988), full professional status implies the unrestricted right to use, control, and structure both practical know-how and abstract theory of physiotherapy. Responsibility for the outcome of one's work is closely connected with autonomy. Swedish physiotherapists were seen to be in firm control of their treatment methods, but their freedom to decide who to treat, and when to terminate treatment was somewhat limited (Bergman 1990). They seemed to have 'powerless discretion' rather than 'discretion-ary power'. They were not completely in sole control. Consequently, they were not always able to see their work through from start to finish or to demonstrate manifest and measurable results. Nor did they always regard themselves as those ultimately responsible for the results or evaluation of their efforts. This must have hampered their ability to give their patients optimal treatment.

Research is a means with which to improve the quality of physiotherapy. Few systematically evaluated their treatments and methods, and hence few obtained any objective feedback from their work. Consequently, few could evolve physiotherapeutic methods and knowledge. Professional autonomy appears to be a prerequisite for the evolution of the role of the physiotherapist in research.

THE ROLE OF THE PHYSIOTHERAPIST IN RESEARCH

In 1977, education for and training in the profession of physiotherapy in Sweden was accorded university status. This enabled physiotherapists to enrol in courses leading to a postgraduate degree. Since then, 40 physiotherapists have gained doctorates, but only one of these has undertaken research on stroke (Lindmark 1988). This is illustrative of the marvellous progress made, but also of the loneliness of the individual physiotherapy researcher. This particular physiotherapist studying physio-therapy and stroke must have had very few, if any, physiotherapy researchers with whom to plan and discuss the actual work.

Furthermore, there are very few professional archetypes or models for the role of physiotherapists in research. Moreover, in Sweden there is only one department of physiotherapy with a chair in the discipline. Thus, most physiotherapists are associated with university departments other than physiotherapy per se. Consequently, the focus of the research questions often differs from what would be asked by physiotherapists.

The twin roles of clinical and research physiotherapist have much in common. Progress is often the result of a shift in perspective – to look at a problem from another angle. In this way, hidden secrets are revealed.

To sum up, the development of the role of the physiotherapist in research appears to be bound up with an extended professional autonomy and with a widening of the concept of professional responsibility. It is also a question of redesigning the organization of work, and of the evolution of professional models and creative research environments.

REFERENCES

Abbot A 1988 The system of professions. An essay on the division of expert labour. University of Chicago Press, Chicago

Allen J M 1983 Work sampling: a means of determining physiotherapy activities and reviewing caseloads. Physiotherapy Canada 35: 31–35

Bergman B 1988 Work sampling: the way in which physiotherapists utilise their working hours. Scandinavian Journal of Caring Sciences 2: 155–162

Bergman B 1989 Being a physiotherapist: professional role, utilization of time, and vocational strategies. Medical dissertation, new series no. 251. University of Umeå, Sweden

Bergman B 1990 Professional role and autonomy in physiotherapy. A study of Swedish physiotherapists. Scandinavian Journal of Rehabilitation Medicine 22: 79–84

Bergman B 1991 Vocational strategies among physiotherapists: a qualitative study. Sjukgymnasten, Vetenskapligt supplement 2: 20–25

Hislop H J 1975 The not-so-impossible dream. Physical Therapy 55: 1069–1080

Jensen G M 1988 The work of accreditation on-site evaluators: enhancing the development of a profession. Phys Ther 68: 1517–1525

Lindmark B 1988 Evaluation of functional capacity after stroke with special emphasis on motor function and activities of daily living. Medical dissertation, Uppsala University, Sweden

Miles-Tapping C, Rennie G A, Duffy M, Rooke L, Holstein S 1992 Canadian physiotherapists' professional identity: an exploratory survey. Physiotherapy Canada 44: 31–35

Purtilo R 1986 Professional responsibility in physiotherapy: old dimensions and new directions. Physiotherapy 72: 579–583

Raz P, Jensen G M, Walter J, Drake L M 1991 Perspective on gender and professional issues among female physical therapists. Physical Therapy 71: 530–540

Shepard K F, Jensen G M 1990 Physical therapist curricula for the 1990s: educating the reflective practitioner. Physical Therapy 70: 566–573

Soderberg G L 1993 On passing from ignorance to knowledge. Physical Therapy 73: 796–807

14. The Sødring motor evaluation of stroke patients

K. M. Sødring

INTRODUCTION

Management of stroke rehabilitation is based upon appropriate assessments used by different members of the rehabilitation team. To obtain a thorough picture of the patient's functional level, various aspects of function must be assessed by separate and clinically relevant assessment methods. Many tests for assessing motor function have been developed, but there is a lack of instruments which fulfil the requirements necessary for scientific use (Wagenaar & Mejier 1991). Basic demands are reliability and validity.

RELIABILITY

Reliability concerns the extent to which a test is consistent on repeated trials. In any measurement situation there are certain factors which may influence the results. Reliability is closely linked to the extent of random error, while validity depends mainly on the extent of non-random error in the measurement procedure (Carmines & Zeller 1979). Random error is all those factors which obscure the results in an unpredictable way, e.g. variations in motivation, daily fitness or the interpretation of the evaluator. The effects are unsystematic in character, and may vary from one measurement to the next. A reliable indicator of an assessment is therefore one that leads to consistent results on repeated measurements because it does not fluctuate greatly due to random error (Carmines & Zeller 1979).

Standardizing the procedures of the assessment and writing exact instructions in a manual improves the reliability, ruling out some of the sources of random variation in the assessment situation.

VALIDITY

Validity is defined as the extent to which an assessment measures what it is intended to measure, but as Keith (1984) states: 'An assessment measure itself is not validated, but only the particular uses to which it is put'. Types

119

of validity appropriate for judging functional assessments are criterion-related validity and construct validity.

Criterion-related validity

Criterion-related validity comprises two factors: concurrent validity and predictive validity.

Concurrent validity

This is assessed by correlating a test and the criterion or reference method at the same point in time.

Predictive validity

This concerns a future criterion which is correlated with the relevant test. In this respect, the predictive validity is by far the most interesting and important question. However, the scientific and practical utility of criterion validation depends as much on the measurement of criterion as it does on the quality of the measuring instrument itself (Carmines & Zeller 1979).

Construct validity

Perhaps the most important measure of validation in the development of an assessment method is *construct validity*. If this is not good, neither the reliability nor the validity can possibly be acceptable.

Construct validity is related to the theory behind what is being measured. In this context, it means that the assessment must have a logical structure, where the scores on the scale give adequate information about the motor function of the patient. Within the wide area of motor function, there must be a clear definition of what is clinically relevant to measure. Thus the *selection of test items* is an essential part of the construction of the scale.

The test items must intercorrelate to form an internally consistent instrument. Internal consistency implies that the items have a common construct. Within a construct, items should be ordered in difficulty according to clinical experience. The validity is ensured by the registration of a unidimensional phenomenon at different levels.

THE RATING SCALE

A rating scale of each item is intended to describe the patient's performance. Thus the scores must be placed in a clinical context. Which aspects of performance are relevant? How do physiotherapists evaluate motor function in a stroke patient? There ought to be a close connection between the professional way of analysing motor function in a stroke patient, and the way it is recorded in an assessment chart. The scores should be clear and discrete; in this way they are also easy to understand. Most frequently a numerical, ordinal scale is used. The numerical scores are applicable in research, whereas descriptive details are not. Likewise, the scores may be better than a long description for enabling other members of the rehabilitation team to visualize a functional level.

SENSITIVITY/RESPONSIVENESS

In the literature, sensitivity and responsiveness are often used to designate the same phenomenon. It means that the scale has the ability to detect small changes in improvement or deterioration. This is an extremely important property of functional assessments and is not easy to obtain.

A rating scale with more score levels will be more adequate than one which is dichotomous. On the other hand, this may cause a reduced reliability due to an expected increase in random error. Obviously this matter creates an extra challenge in the developmental process of an assessment method.

SUMMATION OF ORDINAL DATA

Logically speaking, only variables at interval level should be added to a sumscore. Nevertheless, summation of ordinal data is a common procedure in functional assessment instruments, often without documentation to justify it. The use of an ordinal scale has its limitations, as it gives a relative, not a definite, measure. In the author's opinion there are at least three requirements which, if they are fulfilled, may support the adequacy of summation. These are:

- unidimensionality
- uniformly high factor loadings which indicate that the items are approximately the same weight
- an acceptable ordinality of the rating scale.

Basic principles as applied to the Sødring Scale

In the Sødring Scale (SS), the construct validity concentrates on two main issues:

- the design of an item pool with a common construct
- the adequacy of adding ordinal data.

The items were subjected to exploratory factor analysis in order to study the dimensionality of the assessment and the extent to which the items intercorrelated. The internal consistency of the factors was measured by calculating the Cronbach's alpha coefficient.

Depending on the function assessed, the scoring of the items of the Sødring Scale is ordinal with three or five levels. The addition of the scorings to a sumscore requires that the ordinal scaling on each item functions well. This was examined by means of linear regression analyses. The scoring of each item, with N (three or five) scoring levels, was described by means of N-1 dummy variables, using the lowest scoring level as the reference level. The dummy variables were introduced as explanatory variables for the sumscore on the factor to which the item was allocated (Hosmer & Lemeshow 1989). A well-functioning ordinal scaling requires a reasonably monotonous linear increase in the regression coefficients for the dummy variables describing each scoring level.

The rating of each item in the SS reflects quantity as well as quality in the unassisted motor performance of the patient. Quality is defined in relation to the degree of normality in the performance of movement patterns. As it is possible to observe different levels of normality during performance, it seems logical to describe these levels from a clinical point of view. In order to operationalize the clinical observations in the SS, the author has described all scores for each variable. From this interpretation, certain categories emerged. These were marked numerically 1-2-3-4-5 with level 5 as the 'normal performance' category.

The introduction of a rating of quality in movement is in accordance with the clinical concept of motor control being the main issue in stroke rehabilitation.

EVALUATION OF UNASSISTED PERFORMANCE

Common to functional assessments used in the evaluation of motor function in the stroke patient, is the registration of the quantity of the patient's performance. Another characteristic is the assistance that the patient receives during the test situation, i.e. in getting into the starting positions. The author believes that the rating of the unassisted performance of the patient's motor activity is crucial; first, because it is the unassisted performance that gives a realistic level of the patient's functional ability; second, because this may contribute to a more systematic, valid and reliable recording from one assessment point to the other.

PRACTICALITY IN CLINICAL WORK

Finally, it is essential that an assessment is reasonably simple to use for both the therapist and the patient. This also implies that the test must not be too time-consuming. In the SS, these criteria are met for therapists who are familiar with the problems of the stroke patient. The test items are movements used in functional activities, and are thus convenient for the patients as well. The assessment is carried out over 5–25 minutes, depending on the condition of the patient and the experience of the evaluator.

Modern times, with their demands for health services to be acutely cost-effective, make it necessary to substantiate the profession of physiotherapy. It is essential that physiotherapists are critical of the instruments that are used in clinical work. It should not be acceptable any longer to use assessment instruments which do not possess the basic requirements and qualifications. These form the basis on which physiotherapists can evaluate different treatment methods in the most professional way.

REFERENCES

Carmines E, Zeller R 1979 Reliablity and validity assessment. Quantitative Applications in the Social Sciences 17, Sage, Newbury Park
Hosmer D W Lemeshow S 1989 Applied logistic regression. John Wiley, New York
Keith R A 1984 Functional assessments measures in medical rehabilitation: current status. Archives of Physical Medicine and Rehabilitation 65: 74–78
Wagenaar R C, Meijer O G 1991 Effects of stroke rehabilitation (1). Journal of Rehabilitation Sciences 4(3): 61–73

15. The Rivermead motor assessment

S. A. Adams

INTRODUCTION

The aim of this chapter is to present a published motor assessment for use after stroke, and to discuss its reliability and validity. Results of a literature review are also presented.

There is no one assessment of motor function after stroke that is used extensively throughout the United Kingdom, which makes service comparisons between districts, units, or even within the same department, impossible. The needs of the stroke patient must be identified at every stage of recovery, so that appropriate intervention may be given. There is also an increasing requirement to audit services and to evaluate the effectiveness of treatment modalities and therapy input. There is a need for a short, simple motor assessment that is clinically appropriate, can be performed repeatedly, and which can be used both to monitor patients' progress, and as a research tool.

THE RIVERMEAD MOTOR ASSESSMENT FOR STROKE

In 1979, Lincoln & Leadbitter published the Rivermead assessment of motor function in stroke patients (RMA). The RMA was developed because of the lack of short, reliable, valid, and scorable assessments of motor function. It was designed for both clinical and research use, based on the assumption that stroke patients follow a consistent pattern of recovery. Items in the assessment were chosen to reflect the abilities of stroke patients in all stages of recovery. The emphasis of the design was on a standardised procedure, scorable results (so that statistical analysis of data would be feasible if it were to be used in research projects), reliability and validity.

Structive of the RMA

The RMA is divided into three sections: gross function, leg and trunk function, and arm function. Within these three subsections, test items are ordered according to their difficulty. The easiest items are tested first. The scoring system is dichotomous, so that a patient passes or fails each item of each section. The summed total number of items passed in each section is recorded. The score obtained for each section of the RMA relates to the patient's level of ability. The assessment mixes impairments (arm and leg and trunk sections) with disabilities (gross function). The leg and trunk and arm sections test qualitative aspects of motor function. (See Appendices I and II, pp. 134–138, for a copy of the assessment form and detailed instructions for use.)

Gross function section

The first section of the RMA concerns gross function, and comprises 13 test items. The easiest item in this section is sitting without support for 10 seconds. The most difficult item is hopping five times on the affected leg.

Leg and trunk section

The second section concerns the leg and trunk, and comprises 10 items, six of which are tested on a bed, the other four being tested in standing. This section starts with rolling to the affected side. Item six involves standing without support, balancing on the affected leg, and stepping the unaffected leg on and off a 9 cm block or step.

Arm section

This section contains 15 items, including picking up a ball with two hands, or picking up a small ball, or a pencil, or a piece of paper with the affected hand. The patient is also asked to cut up modelling clay with a knife and fork.

Equipment

Test equipment is needed for some activities. This comprises a large ball, a small ball, a beanbag, a pencil, a piece of paper, a knife, fork, plate and modelling clay, a piece of string (100 cm long), and a step or block (9 cm high; 30 cm × 25 cm surface). A table, chair and bed are also used, for items such as transfers and rolling.

Validity

The validity of each section of the RMA as a Guttman scale was established by calculations of coefficients of scalability and reproducibility (Menzel 1953) on data from patient assessments. A Guttman scale is a set of individual items that are ranked to form a hierarchy of severity such that items are passed in the same order by all patients. When high scalability has been obtained, the number of items passed (until the first 'fail') is expected to produce a score equivalent to that which would have been obtained if all items had been tested. The assessor does not have to test every item in each section of the assessment, and testing can be stopped after an item has been failed. This speeds up the assessment procedure. The patient is less prone to fatigue, thus reducing the risk of an incomplete assessment and lost data. The summed score for each section provides information on what a patient can do, not purely on how many items have been passed.

The RMA was standardised on a group of 51 young non-acute stroke patients (aged 17–65 years). These patients had either a right or left hemiplegia, and no additional disabilities. The results indicated that each of the three sections of the RMA formed a valid Guttman scale. The scale ordering was imposed on the RMA data obtained from a further 40 hemiplegic stroke patients, the results further validating the scale.

Reliability

Inter-rater reliability, over a 4-week period, was established using videotaped assessments. Correlation coefficients for test–retest assessments on 10 young non-acute stroke patients indicated that the RMA had adequate test–retest reliability to be used as a measure of change in motor function with this patient group.

Reliability was not checked with centres other than Rivermead in Oxford. The scalability and reliability of the RMA were not established with acute stroke patients, nor with stroke patients over the age of 65. As the risk of stroke for those aged 75 or over is 15–30 times higher than for those aged under 65 (Barer 1991), these restrictions limit the clinical usefulness of the RMA, as well as its value as a research tool.

CITATIONS OF THE RMA

The scalability and reliability of the RMA have been acknowledged by several authors (Cote et al 1986, Lindmark & Hamrin 1988, Loewen & Anderson 1988, Goldie et al 1990, Mawson 1993). All rejected the RMA for measures more suited to their specific requirements.

Partridge et al (1987) cited the RMA as including items similar to those chosen when they established recovery curves in acute stroke.

REPORTED USE OF THE RMA IN CLINICAL RESEARCH

The usefulness and relevance of the RMA, both in clinical practice and in research, have been examined by a review of published studies. The

Table 15.1 Studies that have used the RMA

Authors	Number of subjects	Age range mean; SD	Time since stroke
Blake 1991	7	–	–
Collen et al 1990	25	48–82 72; –	2–6 yrs
Collin & Archdeacon 1989	20	–	6 weeks +
Collin & Wade 1990	12 female	45–69 59.9; –	6 weeks +
	24 male	15–77 56.1; –	
De Weerdt et al 1989	2	60	15 months
		61	6 months
Gladman et al 1993	327	44–101	6 months +
Lincoln et al 1989	70	36–88 62.8; 10.6	1–13 weeks
Lincoln et al 1990	60	21–83 63.7; 10.3	–
Sackley 1990	52 right hemiplegia	21–87; 63.4; –	6–26 weeks
	38 left hemiplegia	33–86; 63.2; –	
Sackley & Lincoln 1990	49	–	6 months
Taylor et al 1994	38	49–86 72; –	1 week
Wade et al 1992	49 early intervention	–72.3; 9.7	–
	45 late intervention	–72.0; 10.6	
Walker & Lincoln 1991	60	21–79 62.4; 9.5	2–12 weeks

Note – indicates information not available.

following studies all involved the use of the RMA as an assessment of motor function. Table 15.1 summarises the number of subjects in each study, their ages, and time since onset of stroke. It is of interest to note that almost all studies included patients over the age of 65. Also, while the subjects in some studies were 6 months or more poststroke (non-acute), other studies assessed patients as early as 1 week after onset of stroke.

The use of the RMA is assumed to be satisfactory, as none of the authors reported problems, either with administration or with sequential use. The following accounts report on these studies. Many authors did not comment on why the RMA was chosen for use in their study.

Two studies in 1990 (Sackley & Lincoln 1990, Collen et al 1990) demonstrated that the gross function section of the RMA is a valid and reliable assessment when patients are questioned rather than physically assessed. It is unlikely that the leg and trunk or arm sections could be assessed by self-report as they require the skilled observation of a trained physiotherapist (Collen et al 1990). Items in these two sections have very specific instructions as to what is required for a patient to 'pass' each item.

It is assumed that the detail of the instructions is intended to confer a degree of quality on the performance of the item. A poor performance (one that does not reach the standard of the instructions) constitutes a 'fail' (see Appendix II, p.136).

The summed score of the gross function section of the RMA has also been used in a predictive equation (generated in Lincoln et al 1989) to demonstrate that motor function is one of the important determinants of outcome for patients on the Stroke Unit at Nottingham, UK (Lincoln et al 1990). Patients were admitted to the stroke unit only when they had 'recovered from the acute stage and were in need of rehabilitation'. In this study, patients were admitted at 1–13 weeks after onset of stroke (mean 3.6 weeks). Many patients (73%) were admitted to the stroke unit within a month of their stroke. The initial assessment took place during the first week of admission to the stroke unit.

All three sections of the RMA were used in a study to investigate the relationship between dressing abilities and cognitive and physical problems (Walker & Lincoln 1991). Dressing as a global skill was demonstrated to be heavily dependent on the physical abilities of stroke patients, particularly patients who have difficulty putting garments on the lower half of their body. It was concluded that the ability of stroke patients to dress is heavily overshadowed by their physical abilities. The authors commented that standardised assessments were used when available, but, as with many studies, they made no other comment as to why the RMA was chosen, and no problems or difficulties with the RMA were reported.

The RMA has also been used as an outcome measure in studies of the use of visual biofeedback during the re-education of balance and weight transference after stroke (De Weerdt et al 1989, Sackley 1990). De Weerdt used single case designs to assess two subjects. The authors used the RMA to document recovery over time, and did not raise any problems with its use.

The gross function section of the RMA was used as an outcome measure in a randomised crossover design study to determine whether the intervention of a physiotherapist improved mobility in patients seen more than 1 year after stroke (Wade et al 1992). There was no significant change in RMA gross function scores.

Wade (1989) cites the RMA as an example of a motor assessment for use predominantly by physiotherapists in planning treatment which includes specific parts relating to the arm, but gives it no further attention. The arm function section of the RMA has been used in a small study of seven stroke patients (Blake 1991) to compare the relationships between motor function and spontaneous use and observed use of the hemiplegic arm. The best agreement was between motor function and spontaneous use, although the effects of such variables as dominance of hand, sensation and neuropsychological factors on outcome could not be identified from such a small sample. The ages of the subjects, and the time since stroke, are not known.

The RMA has been used in a study to investigate the validity of the motricity index (MI) and the trunk control test (TCT) (Collin & Archdeacon 1989, Collin & Wade 1990). All three sections of the RMA appeared to be as sensitive in detecting change as the MI arm and leg sections and the TCT, when assessed at paired assessments, 6 weeks apart. Results showed strong correlations between the RMA and the two shorter tests of motor function, especially between the leg and trunk section of the RMA and the leg section of the MI for mild motor impairment. Concern was expressed that the RMA was insensitive for more severe levels of motor impairment, which could be regarded as a floor effect. (Patients with severe motor deficit were failing to score, when the other two assessments were able to differentiate between different levels of disability.) Patients with very poor function have been excluded from other studies (e.g. Sackley & Lincoln 1990) as the gross function scale was said to be insensitive below this level of ability. Collin & Wade (1990) acknowledged that the RMA looks at type and quality of movement, rather than simply gross change, but this study did not find the RMA any more sensitive to minor changes than the two simpler tests (MI and TCT).

The RMA gross function section has recently been used to develop the Rivermead mobility index (RMI), a measure of mobility disability which concentrates on body mobility, for use with neurologically impaired patients (Collen et al 1991). The RMI comprises 14 questions and one direct observation, including nine items from the gross function section of the RMA. It has been tested not only on patients who have suffered a stroke, but also those with head injuries. The RMI is not specifically designed for use with stroke patients and is limited to the assessment of mobility. It does not assess leg, trunk, or arm function, nor does it assess quality of movement.

Taylor et al (1994) used the RMA as a measure of motor recovery in a study to determine whether asymmetrical sitting posture (to the affected side) and motor function following hemispheric stroke were related to the side of lesion or the presence of unilateral neglect. The subjects who sat with their trunk leaning to their affected side, and who tended to have unilateral neglect, had significantly worse gross function scores at 3 and 6 weeks than those who sat with their trunk in midline or towards their unaffected side. There were no differences in leg and trunk or arm function scores.

Recent studies (Adams 1993a, b) investigated the scaling properties of the RMA with groups other than the young non-acute stroke patients on whom it was originally standardised. To test the scalability of the RMA with acute strokes, data from 51 stroke patients (including those over 65), assessed at 1, 3 and 6 weeks poststroke, were used to calculate the coefficients of reproducibility and scalability (CS and CR) (Menzel 1953) for each section of the RMA, at each of the three assessments. The results indicated that only the gross function and arm sections met Guttman scale criteria (CS > 0.6; CR > 0.9) when used with acute strokes. The gross function and arm sections demonstrated recovery following a hierarchical pattern, whereas the leg and trunk section demonstrated a more uneven pattern of recovery, which did not correspond to the hierarchical listing of the items in the assessment. Items which required a patient to be able to stand were those most likely to break the scale order. The leg and trunk section cannot be assumed to scale with acute stroke patients, and should only be used as a checklist with this group.

Test–retest reliability was also calculated for 24 of these acute subjects. The RMA was shown to be a very reliable assessment when used by the same therapist with selected acute stroke patients (Adams 1992).

A study to assess the scalability of the RMA with non-acute stroke patients over 65 years of age (Adams 1993b) used data from subjects who were in the DOMINO study (Gladman et al 1993). Patients were assessed with the RMA at 6 and 12 months after discharge from hospital. The results indicated that the gross function section met Guttman scale criteria when used with non-acute strokes in patients over 65 years old. The leg and trunk and arm function sections did not meet Guttman scale criteria with these subjects. More items in the leg and trunk section were passed in reverse order than in scale order.

Only the gross function section retains the properties of a Guttman scale with all groups of stroke patients. As there is most need for an assessment with acute patients, and as the majority of stroke survivors are aged 65 or over, the usefulness of the RMA, both in clinical practice and as a research tool, may be limited.

CONCLUSION

The Rivermead motor assessment (RMA) is based on the assumption of a consistent pattern of recovery following stroke. The three sections of the RMA have good test–retest reliability, and have been shown to demonstrate the properties of Guttman scales when used with non-acute stroke patients under the age of 65.

The RMA has been used in studies of motor function as a predictor of outcome and in studies to investigate a variety of aspects of recovery from stroke. It has been used to investigate the validity of simpler measures of motor function, and to develop a new measure of mobility. It has also been used in a study which investigated unilateral neglect and midline position. When cited, the reliability of the RMA has not been questioned and no direct criticisms have been made of it as an instrument for measuring motor impairment.

Studies to test the scaling properties of the RMA with acute stroke patients and with older non-acute stroke patients, suggest that only the gross function section can be used as an hierarchical Guttman scale with a final, meaningful score, for all stroke patients. These restrictions limit the clinical usefulness of the RMA, as well as its value as a research tool.

Acknowledgement

The financial support for this work was received from the Department of Health (United Kingdom) through a Department of Health Research Training Award for Therapists.

REFERENCES

Adams S A 1992 A study to test the scalability and reliability of the Rivermead motor assessment with acute stroke patients, and the scalability with non-acute stroke patients over the age of sixty five. Dissertation for MSc in Rehabilitation Studies, University of Southampton

Adams S A 1993a A study to test the scalability of the Rivermead motor assessment with acute stroke patients. Physiotherapy 79: 506 (abstract)

Adams S A 1993b A study to test the scalability of the Rivermead motor assessment with non-acute strokes over 65. Clinical Rehabilitation 7: 358 (abstract)

Barer D H 1991 Stroke in Nottingham: provision of nursing care and possible implications for the future. Clinical Rehabilitation 5: 103–110

Blake P F 1991 Is movement of the upper extremity after stroke always translated into useful function? Proceedings of the World Confederation for Physical Therapy 11th International Congress, London, Book 1: 502–504

Collen F M, Wade D T, Bradshaw C M 1990 Mobility after stroke: reliability of measures of impairment and disability. International Disability Studies 12: 6–9

Collen F M, Wade D T, Robb G F, Bradshaw C M 1991 The Rivermead mobility index: a further development of the Rivermead motor assessment. International Disability Studies 13: 50–54

Collin C, Archdeacon L 1989 Motor assessment study. Clinical Rehabilitation 3: 81 (abstract)

Collin C, Wade D 1990 Assessing motor impairment after stroke: a pilot reliability study. Journal of Neurology, Neurosurgery and Psychiatry 53: 576–579

Cote R, Hachinski V C, Shurvell B L, Norris J W, Wolfson C 1986 The Canadian neurological scale: a preliminary study in acute stroke. Stroke 17: 731–737

De Weerdt W, Crossley S M, Lincoln N B, Harrison M A 1989 Restoration of balance in stroke patients: a single case design study. Clinical Rehabilitation 3: 139–147

Gladman J R F, Lincoln N B, Barer D H 1993 A randomized controlled trial of domiciliary and hospital-based rehabilitation for stroke patients after discharge from hospital. Journal of Neurology, Neurosurgery and Psychiatry 56: 960–966

Goldie P A, Matyas T A, Spencer K I, McGinley R B 1990 Postural control in standing following stroke: test–retest reliability of some quantitative clinical tests. Physical Therapy 70(4): 234–243

Lincoln N B, Leadbitter D 1979 Assessment of motor function in stroke patients. Physiotherapy 65(2): 48–51

Lincoln N B, Blackburn M, Ellis S, Jackson J, Edmans J A, Nouri F M, Walker M F, Haworth H 1989 An investigation of factors affecting progress of patients on a stroke unit. Journal of Neurology, Neurosurgery and Psychiatry. 52: 493–496

Lincoln N B, Jackson J M, Edmans J E, Walker M F, Farrow V M, Latham A, Coombes K 1990 The accuracy of predictions about progress of patients on a stroke unit. Journal of Neurology, Neurosurgery and Psychiatry 53: 972–975

Lindmark B, Hamrin E 1988 Evaluation of functional capacity after stroke as a basis for active intervention. Scandinavian Journal of Rehabilitation Medicine 20(3): 103–109

Loewen S C, Anderson B A 1988 Reliabilty of the modified motor assessment scale and the Barthel index. Physical Therapy 68(7): 1077–1081

Mawson S J 1993 Measuring physiotherapy outcome in stroke rehabilitation. Physiotherapy 79(11): 762–765

Menzel H 1953 A new coefficient of scalogram analysis. Public Opinion Quarterly 17: 268–280

Partridge C J, Johnstone M, Edwards S 1987 Recovery from physical disability after stroke: normal patterns as a basis for evaluation. Lancet 1: 373–375

Sackley C M 1990 The relationship between weight-bearing asymmetry after stroke, motor function and activities of daily living. Physiotherapy Theory and Practice 6: 179–185

Sackley C M, Lincoln N B 1990 The verbal administration of the gross function scale of the Rivermead motor assessment. Clinical Rehabilitation 4: 301–303

Taylor D, Ashburn A, Ward C D 1994 Asymmetrical trunk posture, unilateral neglect and motor performance following stroke. Clinical Rehabilitation 8: 48–53

Wade D T 1989 Measuring arm impairment and disability after stroke. International Disability Studies 11(2): 89–92

Wade D T, Collen F M, Robb G F, Warlow C P 1992 Physiotherapy intervention late after stroke and mobility. British Medical Journal 304: 609–613

Walker M F, Lincoln N B 1991 Factors influencing dressing performance after stroke. Journal of Neurology, Neurosurgery and Psychiatry 54: 699–701

APPENDIX I

RIVERMEAD ASSESSMENT OF MOTOR FUNCTION IN STROKE PATIENTS (Lincoln & Leadbitter 1979)

Gross function
Score 1 or 0

1. Sit; feet unsupported (10 secs) ____
2. Lying to sitting on side of bed ____
3. Sit to stand, in 15 secs for 15 secs ____
4. Transfer from chair to chair towards unaffected side ____
5. Transfer from chair to chair towards affected side ____
6. Walk 10 metres independently with an aid ____
7. Climb stairs; may use banister ____
8. Walk 10 metres without an aid ____
9. Walk 5 metres, pick up beanbag from floor and return ____
10. Walk outside 40 metres (aid if needed) ____
11. Walk up and down four steps (no banister or wall support) ____
12. Run 10 metres (4 secs) ____
13. Hop on affected leg five times on the spot ____

Total ____

Leg and trunk

1. Roll to affected side (supine to side lying) ____
2. Roll to unaffected side (supine to side lying) ____
3. Half bridging ____
4. Sit to stand, hips 90° flexion, weight through both feet ____
5. Half crook lying; affected leg over side of bed and return ____
6. Standing; step with unaffected leg on and off block ____
7. Standing; tap ground lightly with unaffected foot five times ____
8. Lying; dorsiflex affected ankle with leg flexed ____
9. Lying; dorsiflex affected ankle with leg extended ____
10. Standing with affected hip in neutral, flex affected knee ____

Total ____

Arm

1. Lying; protract shoulder girdle with arm in elevation ____
2. Lying; hold extended arm in elevation, with external rotation ____
3. Flex and extend elbow with arms as in point 2 ____
4. Sitting; elbow into side of body, pronate and supinate ____
5. Reach forwards, pick up large ball with both hands ____
6. Pick up tennis ball, release on midthigh × 5 ____
7. As point 6 with pencil × 5 ____
8. Pick up piece of paper from table and release × 5 ____

9. Cut up putty with knife and fork and put in container (mat)   ____
10. Stand; pat large ball on floor with palm of hand × 5   ____
11. Continuous opposition thumb and fingers × 14 in 10 secs   ____
12. Pronation and supination onto palm of unaffected   ____
    hand × 20 in 10 secs
13. Stand; hand on wall, shoulders 90° flexion, elbow extended,   ____
    walk round arm
14. Tie string in a bow behind head (use both hands)   ____
15. 'Pat a cake' × 7 in 15 secs   ____

                                                    Total ____

APPENDIX II

INSTRUCTIONS FOR THE USE OF THE RIVERMEAD MOTOR ASSESSMENT FOR STROKE (Lincoln & Leadbitter 1979)

General instructions

Go through items in order of difficulty. Score 1 if patient can perform activity, 0 if patient cannot. Three tries are allowed; after three consecutive failures stop that section and proceed to next.

Give no feedback of whether correct or incorrect but just general encouragement.

Repeat instructions and demonstrate to patient if necessary.

All exercises to be carried out independently unless otherwise stated.

All arm tests refer to affected arm unless otherwise stated.

Gross function

1. Sit; feet unsupported (10 seconds). Without holding on, on edge of bed.
2. Lying to sitting on side of bed. Using any method.
3. Sit to stand, in 15 seconds for 15 seconds. May use hands to push up. May stand with an aid if necessary.
4. Transfer from chair to chair towards unaffected side. May use hands.
5. Transfer from chair to chair towards affected side. May use hands.
6. Walk 10 metres independently with an aid. Any walking aid. No stand-by help.
7. Climb stairs; may use banister. Any method. May use a walking aid. Must be a full flight of stairs.
8. Walk 10 metres without an aid. No stand-by help. No caliper, splint or walking aid.
9. Walk 5 metres, pick up beanbag from floor and return. Bend down any way. May use aid to walk if necessary. No stand-by help. May use either hand to pick up beanbag.
10. Walk outside 40 metres. May use walking aid, caliper or splint. No stand-by help.
11. Walk up and down four steps (no banister or wall support). May use an aid if one is normally used, but may not hold on to a rail. This is included to test ability to negotiate kerb or stairs without a rail.
12. Run 10 metres (4 seconds). Must be symmetrical.
13. Hop on affected leg five times on the spot. Must hop on ball of foot without stopping to regain balance. No help with arms.

Leg and trunk

1. Roll to affected side (supine to side lying). No abnormal movement patterns. Starting position should be lying, not crook lying. May not use hands.

2. Roll to unaffected side. Same conditions as point 1.

3. Half bridging. Starting position – half crook lying. Patient must put some weight through affected leg to lift hip on affected side. Physiotherapist may position leg, but patient must maintain position even after movement is completed.

4. Sit to stand, hips 90° flexion and, in standing, weight through both feet. May not use arms. Feet must be flat on the floor. Must put weight through both feet.

5. Half crook lying, unaffected leg over side of bed and return to same position. Affected leg in half crook position. Lift leg off bed on to support (e.g. box, stool, floor) so that hip is in neutral and knee at 90° while resting on support. Must keep affected knee flexed throughout the movement. Do not allow external rotation at hip. This tests control of knee and hip.

6. Standing; step with unaffected leg on and off 9 cm high block. Without retraction of pelvis or hyperextension of knee. This tests hip and knee control while weight-bearing through the affected leg.

7. Standing; tap ground lightly five times with unaffected foot. Without retraction of pelvis or hyperextension of knee. Weight must stay on affected leg. This again tests hip and knee control while weight bearing through the affected leg, but is more difficult than point 6.

8. Lying; dorsiflex affected ankle with leg flexed. Physiotherapist may hold affected leg in position, knee at 90°. Do not allow inversion. Must have half range of movement of unaffected foot.

9. Lying; dorsiflex affected ankle with leg extended. Same conditions as point 8, with leg extended. Do not allow inversion or knee flexion. Foot must reach plantigrade (90°).

10. Stand with affected hip in neutral, flex knee (45°+). Physiotherapist may not position leg. This is extremely difficult for most hemiplegic patients, but is included to assess minimal dysfunction.

Arm function

1. Lying; protract shoulder girdle with arm in elevation (arm may be supported).

2. Lying; hold extended arm in elevation, some external rotation, for at least 2 seconds. Physiotherapist should place arm in position and patient must maintain position with some external rotation. Do not allow pronation. Elbow must be held within 30° of full extension.

3. Flexion and extension of elbow with arm as in point 2. Elbow must extend to at least 20° of full extension. Palm should not face outwards during any part of the movement.

4. Sitting; elbow into side body, pronation and supination. Three-quarters range is acceptable, with elbow unsupported and at right angles.

5. Reach forward, pick up large ball with both hands and put down again. Ball should be on table so far in front of patient that he has to extend arms fully to reach it. Shoulders must be protracted, elbows extended, wrists neutral or extended, and fingers extended throughout movement. Palms should be kept in contact with the ball.

6. Stretch arm forward, pick up a tennis ball from table, release on midthigh on affected side, return to table, then release again on table. Repeat five times. Shoulder must be protracted, elbow extended and wrist extended or in neutral during each phase.

7. As point 6, with a pencil × 5. Patient must use thumb and fingers to grip.

8. Pick up piece of paper from table in front and release × 5. Patient must use thumb and fingers to pick up paper, not pull to edge of table. Arm position as in point 6.

9. Cut putty with knife and fork on plate with non-slip mat and put pieces into a container at side of plate. Bite-size pieces.

10. Stand on spot, maintain upright position, pat a large ball on floor with palm of hand for five continuous bounces.

11. Continuous opposition of thumb and each finger more than 14 times in 10 seconds (tap = 1). Must do movements in consistent sequence. Do not allow thumb to slide from one finger to the other.

12. Supination and pronation on to palm of unaffected hand (tap = 1) 20 times in 10 seconds. Arm must be away from body, palm and dorsum of hand must touch palm of good hand. This is similar to point 4 but introduces speed.

13. Standing, with affected arm abducted to 90° with palm flat against wall. Maintain arm in position. Turn body towards wall and as far as possible towards arm, i.e. rotate body beyond 90°. Do not allow flexion at elbow, and wrist must be extended with palm of hand fully in contact with wall.

14. Place string (100 cm long) around head, tie bow at back. Do not allow neck to flex. Affected hand must be used for more than just supporting string. This tests function of hand without help of sight.

15. 'Pat-a-cake' seven times in 15 seconds. Mark crosses on wall at shoulder level (or assessor can hold hands up in position). Clap both hands together – both hands touch crosses; clap – one hand touches opposite cross; clap – other hand touches opposite cross. Must be in correct order. Palms must touch. Each sequence counts as one. Allow patient three attempts. This is a complex pattern which involves coordination, speed and memory as well as good arm function.

16. Functional independence measure scale on stroke patients

T. Glott

INTRODUCTION

One of the most important aspects of rehabilitation is for the individual to become as independent from assistance as possible. The more the need for assistance, the more likely is discharge to a permanent institution after rehabilitation. Being independent from assistance is also important for life satisfaction. Rehabilitation of the individual should always include detailed documentation about what the subject is able to do independently. One of the major problems has been to standardize and scale an instrument suitable for rehabilitation of different groups. Such an instrument must include activities performed frequently by most individuals, i.e. activities of daily living. It is also important to detect progress during rehabilitation, and to make the instrument adequately sensitive.

OUTLINE OF FUNCTIONAL INDEPENDENCE MEASURE

At the Sunnaas Rehabilitation Hospital in Norway there was a desire to test the functional independence measure (FIM) on stroke patients to obtain first-hand experience of one of the major instruments in rehabilitation. The FIM was initiated by the American Congress of Rehabilitation Medicine and the American Academy of Physical Medicine and Rehabilitation. The aim in 1986, was to develop a National Uniform Data System for medical rehabilitation. It is based on the well-known Barthel index. Approximately 50% of all rehabilitation hospitals in the United States of America are now subscribing to the Uniform Data System and are using the FIM. The national data collection now contains about 100 000 FIM ratings of which tens of thousands are ratings from stroke patients. Outside the United States it is currently used in several countries around the world. The FIM was introduced to the author and team by Professor Gunnar Grimby of Sahlgrenska hospital in Gothenburg, Sweden.

The FIM consists of 18 items (Table 16.1) and is intended to include a minimum number of items. It is not expected to include all activities that might need to be measured in the rehabilitation phase. It may be extended with other instruments in areas other than those covered by the FIM. The

Table 16.1 Summary of items (this is not the complete definition of each item)

Self-care activities

- feeding – includes eating and drinking once meal is properly prepared
- grooming – includes oral care, hair grooming, washing hands and face and, depending on the individual, either shaving or applying make-up
- bathing – includes bathing the body from neck and down in bath, shower or bed-bath
- dressing upper body – includes dressing and undressing above the waist
- dressing lower body – includes dressing and undressing below the waist
- toileting – includes maintaining perineal hygiene and adjusting clothing after toileting.

Sphincter control

- bladder management – includes complete intentional control of urinary bladder and use of equipment or agents necessary for bladder control
- bowel management – includes complete intentional control of bowel movement and use of equipment or agents necessary for bowel control.

Transfers

- from bed to chair – includes all aspects of transferring to and from bed, chair or wheelchair, or coming to a standing position if walking is the typical mode of locomotion
- to toilet – includes getting on and off a toilet
- to bath or shower – includes getting into and out of a bath or shower.

Locomotion

- includes walking once in a standing position, or using a wheelchair once in a seated position, indoors; depending on most frequent mode of locomotion
- stairs – includes going up 12–14 stairs indoors.

Communication

- comprehension by auditory or visual means – understanding linguistic information by spoken or written word
- expression – includes expression of verbal or non-verbal language.

Social cognition

- social interaction – includes skills related to getting along and participating with others in therapeutic and social situations
- problem-solving – includes skills related to solving problems of daily living
- memory – includes skills related to awareness in performing daily activities in an institutional or community setting.

functional assessment scale (FAM) is such a supplementary instrument useful in patients with traumatic brain injury.

Each item is rated on seven different levels. It is important to observe what the patient actually does and how much help is needed. The general desciption of each level is:

7. complete independence – every part of the item done safely and on time
6. modified independence – the subject uses an assistive device
5. modified dependence – supervision or setup is required
4. minimal assistance – the subject performs more than 75%
3. moderate assistance – the subject performs 50–75%

2. maximal assistance – the subject performs 25–50%
1. total assistance – the subject performs less than 25%.

In addition to rating these items, background information on the patients is recorded on a data set. This includes specific impairments such as paresis, the presence of spasticity, pain and neuropsychological impairment. Information such as marital status, ICD-9 diagnosis, living arrangements at discharge and length of stay are also recorded.

SUNNAAS REHABILITATION HOSPITAL STUDY

The FIM is discipline-free and can be used by any trained clinician. The physiotherapist is often responsible for rating transfer, locomotion and stairs. In the study discussed, the rating was carried out in a multidisciplinary conference with a nurse, an occupational therapist, a physiotherapist and a medical doctor present. A 3-hour introductory course was given to the participating staff. A flowchart was drawn up to describe each level on every item, avoiding the use of percentages.

Experience demonstrated that there was a great variation in time needed to rate each patient from a minimum of 5 minutes to a maximum of 20 minutes. 30 consecutive stroke patients admitted for rehabilitation were included. All had a recent lesion from cerebrovascular disease, and time between acute stroke and admission to rehabilitation was 33 day ± 14 days. An FIM rating was performed during week 1, week 3 and weeks 6–8 after admission.

The scores were not available to the doctors responsible for the patients.

- 23 patients were discharged home
- 5 patients were discharged to a permanent institution
- 2 patients had a transitional place to live after discharge.

FIM scores

The FIM score at admission seems to have a predictive value. A score of higher than 60 (average score > 3.3) at admission predicted discharge home in 25 of 28 patients. A score of higher than 90 (average score > 5.0) at admission, coupled with being married, predicted discharge home without assistance in 16 of 17 patients.

An FIM score at discharge of higher than 80 (average score < 4.4) was previously reported to indicate discharge home. This was also the case in this study in 26 out of 28 patients.

In patients with a score of higher than 110 (average score > 6.1) at discharge, coupled with being married, predicted discharge home without assistance occurred in 14 out of 17 patients.

An FIM score after 3 weeks did not give any additional information on discharge score; neither did progress between first and second scores.

In predicting hours of care needed, the FIM was compared with a classification method developed at the RUSH hospital in Chicago. Several common nursing tasks are not included in the FIM, e.g. administration of medication, social activities with patients, and giving information to relatives and patients. However, in patients with a lower FIM score (< 100) the burden of care seems to be dominated by activities included in the FIM. Looking at this group, it was found that the time needed was 5.50 ± 0.96 minutes per FIM score below maximum. This is close to other studies, which indicate 3–5 minutes per FIM score.

Using a mathematical tool – Rasch analysis – it is possible to transform these ratings to an interval scale on which the intervals between units of the scale have equal values.

All FIM items are recorded on an ordinal scale from complete independence to total assistance. However, it is easier to achieve independence in feeding than in climbing stairs. Thus there is a difference between gaining an improvement from 4 to 7 in feeding and gaining an improvement from 4 to 7 in climbing stairs.

Figure 16.1 illustrates the Sunnaas Rehabilitation Hospital results. The x-axis shows the items and the y-axis demonstrates the relative measure of difficulty. Bowel management is the easiest item and climbing stairs is the most difficult non-cognitive item. Rasch analysis of a patient group can be used as a model where improvement in the FIM score follows a curve during rehabilitation. The patients' FIM score will be transformed to a single number describing the location along this curve.

The change in score will give a linear measure of improvement in the FIM score. Thus it is possible to use non-parametric statistics to compare, for example, treatment programmes or different hospitals. The existence of powerful computer software and the large collection of data worldwide make the FIM a valuable research instrument.

EVALUATION AND APPLICATION

Evaluation of different treatment programmes should always include a measure of independence in daily activities. A physiotherapist might make efforts to improve patients on the level of impairment, e.g. to reduce spasticity or to increase muscle strength. The outcome must be evaluated from what the patient is able to do in daily activities and not only on the performance in a test situation. Many of the widely used treatment programmes today lack such documentation.

According to this experience with the FIM rating on stroke patients, the instrument is a convenient method for clinical use and research within a rehabilitation hospital. There is no apparent 'ceiling' or 'floor' effect in hospitalized stroke patients. Correct use of the manual is important. The user must know the definition of each item. Because of its widespread use,

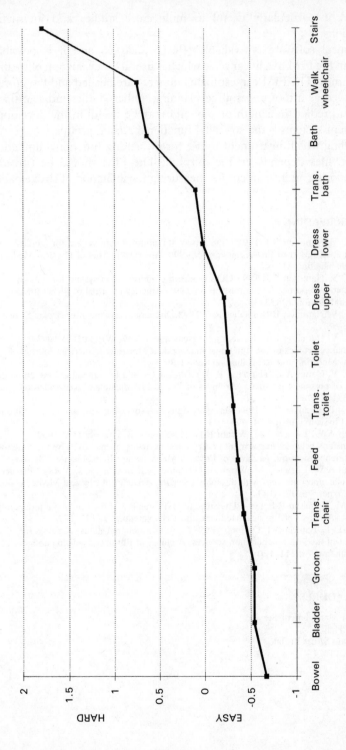

Fig. 16.1   Sunnaas Rehabilitation Hospital FIM results.

the FIM is particularly useful in multicentre studies and international publications.

Statistical software is available (Rasch analysis) and it is possible to transform the FIM to a linear scale which is useful for evaluation of treatment programmes. The FIM can estimate hours of care needed and therefore can be included as a tool in resource planning. Other studies indicate that the FIM can predict the length of stay and may be useful in the development of payment systems – the so-called functional related groups.

Deciding which instrument to use for measuring functional limitation in daily activities depends on the purpose. The FIM should be considered when choosing an instrument for measuring rehabilitation of stroke patients.

FURTHER READING

Granger C V, Hamilton B B 1992 UDS report: the uniform data system for medical rehabilitation report of first admission for 1990. Americal Journal of Physical Medicine and Rehabilitation 71: 108–113

Granger C V, Hamilton B B 1993 UDS report: the uniform data system for medical rehabilitation report of first admission for 1991. American Journal of Physical Medicine and Rehabilitation 72: 33–38

Granger C V, Hamilton B B, Fiedler R C 1992 Discharge outcome after stroke. Stroke 23: 978–982

Granger C V, Hamilton B B, Linacre J M, Heinemann A W, Wright B D 1993 Performance profiles of the functional independence measure. American Journal of Physical Medicine and Rehabilitation 72: 84–89

Granger C V, Cotter A C, Hamilton B B, Fiedler R C 1993 Functional assessment scales: a study of persons after stroke. Archives of Physical Medicine and Rehabilitation 74: 133–138

Hamilton B B, Granger C V 1994 Disability outcomes following inpatient rehabilitation for stroke. Physical Therapy 74: 494–503

Heinemann A W, Linacre J M, Wright B D, Hamilton B B, Granger C V 1993 Relationships between impairment and physical disability as measured by the functional independence measure. Archives of Physical Medicine and Rehabilitation 74: 566–573

Heinemann A W, Linacre J M, Wright B D, Hamilton B B, Granger C V 1994 Prediction of rehabilitation outcomes with disability measure. Archives of Physical Medicine and Rehabilitation 75: 133–143

Linacre J M, Hamilton B B 1994 The structure and stability of the functional independence measure. Archives of Physical Medicine and Rehabilitation 75: 127–132

Wilkerson D L, Batavia A I, De Jong G 1992 Use of functional status measures for payment of medical rehabilitation services. Archives of Physical Medicine and Rehabilitation 73: 111–120

USEFUL ADDRESS

UDS Data Management Service
82 Farber Hall
SUNY Main Street Buffalo
New York 14214
USA

17. TELER: the way forward in stroke outcome audit

S. J. Mawson,   M. J. McCreadie

INTRODUCTION

Recent changes within the National Health Service have resulted in an increasing need for physiotherapists to quantify the outcome of their therapeutic interventions. Only by developing a system for measuring outcome can the profession undertake a purposeful and valuable clinical audit that will promote and develop high standards of patient care.

In its document *The Health of the Nation* (DoH 1990) the British Government highlighted the need to develop effective measures of outcome from health care. As many clinicians had expected, the document specifically identified rehabilitation services for an evaluation. Since the implementation of resource management, physiotherapy managers, clinicians and researchers have endeavoured to quantify outcome and provide the hard data essential to back any case for resources in a now competitive market place (DoH 1990). The need for information about health gains from physiotherapy was reinforced by Tallis (1989) who quoted evidence submitted to the King's Fund Consensus Forum on Stroke Management:

Rehabilitation varies widely, mainly reflecting differences in resources but also reflecting different beliefs. There is no absolute proof that individuals or collective services benefit patients. Should rehabilitation be abandoned?

Although an overstatement of the case, it demonstrates the need to identify measurable outcomes and reinforces the importance of both research and clinical audit. The Government White Paper *Working for Patients* (DoH 1989) proposed that all doctors should be actively involved in formal audit of their work. More recently, the requirement for audit has been extended to all health care professionals and is termed 'clinical audit'

By definition, audit requires review, commonly by comparison with a set standard. The term 'medical audit' refers to the work of doctors, whereas clinical audit refers to the work of all health care professions, which may or may not include doctors.

The Department of Health (1989) defined audit as:

...the systematic critical analysis of the quality of (medical) care, including the procedures used for diagnosis and treatment, the use of resources and the resulting outcome and quality of life for the patient.

More recently, 'audit/quality assurance' has been defined (DoH 1993a) as:

...monitoring of current practice and set standards, preferably employing criteria derived from research findings on best practice as well as professional, management judgements and consumer preferences.

Consequently, 'clinical audit' is used as a generic term in this chapter.

CLINICAL AUDIT

Aims

The aims of clinical audit have been defined as follows (Joint Council for Education in Medicine 1992):

- to identify ways of improving and maintaining the quality of care for patients
- to assist in the training and education of health care professionals
- to make the most of resources available for health services.

These aims can be achieved via the audit cycle.

The audit cycle

Stage 1

The first stage of any audit cycle is the requirement to *select a topic* for audit. Various frameworks have been used to identify and structure topics for audit. For example, Donabedian (1966) described a framework where health care is considered in terms of its structure, process and outcome.

Structure is concerned with the amount and type of resources, asking where the service is provided, with what facilities and by whom.

Process relates to the amount and type of health care activities, asking what is done and how it is done. Process is normally more relevant to health care professionals than structure and may be the most appropriate area to begin audit.

Outcome describes what has been done, how appropriate it was and what the effect was. Donabedian (1966) defined outcome as:

...the change in the patient's current or future health that can be attributed to medical intervention or any other type of antecedent care.

Stage 2

The second stage of the audit cycle is *observation of current practice*. Information can be gathered using various audit tools, and will fall into the categories described by the Donabedian framework above.

Stage 3

The essence of audit is found in the third stage of the audit cycle where *current practice is compared with an agreed standard*, which should have been set at an early point in the audit cycle.

Standards are explicit statements about quantifiable aspects of care. They should be precisely defined, capable of being measured objectively, appropriate to the topic chosen and applicable to that area of practice. Standards can be set in two ways, either as a percentage to be achieved overall, i.e. this standard will be achieved in 90% of cases or as 100% compliance (or possibly 0% depending on the wording) with certain defined exceptions. Standards may be generated and agreed through observation of current clinical practice or by adapting existing standards which may come from various sources, such as national guidelines, Royal Colleges or literature reviews.

Stage 4

Following the comparison stage of the audit cycle it may be necessary to move on to the fourth stage of *implementing change*. During this phase appropriate and agreed changes in practice are implemented to 'close the gap' between the observed current practice and the agreed standards.

Stage 5

The final stage of the audit cycle is *re-audit* where the topic is audited for a second time after an appropriate interval using the same standards. This is to ascertain whether the change implemented actually resulted in an improvement in the quality of patient care.

OUTCOME MEASURES

At the Northern General Hospital Sheffield, UK (NGH) the Physiotherapy service had a commitment to the audit of clinical practice. However, the clinicians within the area of neurological rehabilitation had considerable reservations regarding the outcome measures used within the Donabedian framework, which had been implemented within the hospital.

This problem of identifying measurable outcomes has had two effects on the development of rehabilitation, both regionally and nationally. Research undertaken over the past two decades has failed to provide conclusive evidence of the effects of treatment or to contribute knowledge regarding the identification of specific theoretical models underpinning treatment approaches. This evidence, as previously discussed, has become essential in the purchaser–provider environment of the newly developed National Health Service; without it contracts could be lost and stroke units closed. The second effect of the lack of outcome measures, was that clinicians had become increasingly reticent about participating in audit or research when the measures used did not reflect the conceptual framework of the treatment model implemented.

NGH study

This anxiety together with the urgent need to be proactive in the area of stroke rehabilitation outcome audit resulted in the funding of a long-term research project. This initially involved the NGH stroke unit and four other regional units, and ultimately involved the cooperation and enthusiasm of the British Bobath Tutors Group, in the validation of a measure that did fulfil the specifications required by the specialist profession, patients and service managers.

The purpose of the investigation, was to develop a theory of recovery during physiotherapy intervention in the rehabilitation of patients following acute cerebral infarction, as a basis for effective clinical audit. Prior to the implementation of the study, a review of existing outcome measures deemed to be reliable and valid was undertaken to identify an appropriate measure.

During the literature search a number of well documented, reliable and valid measures of function and activities of daily living (ADL) status were identified including the Barthel index (Mahoney & Barthel 1965), and the Rivermead assessment (Lincoln & Leadbitter 1979).

It became apparent that when choosing or modifying a measure of outcome to be used in this study, it was required to fulfil the needs of the conceptual framework which was being evaluated. These needs can only be defined when the assumptions on which the conceptual model is based have been identified.

Conceptual model

The conceptual model being evaluated in the stroke outcome audit was that of the Bobath normal movement concept (Bobath 1990), where the emphasis is a non-prescriptive, patient-specific, treatment evaluation approach. It was these principles that had to be reflected in any outcome measure used, so that appropriate information was collected and subsequently analysed.

Criteria

Analysis of the qualitative data produced by the preliminary study resulted in the identification of criteria for a measure of outcome in rehabilitation. Those needs which were identified by health care professionals were then synthesised into a list of specifications to be fulfilled by any measuring system to be used for both research and clinical audit within the hospital.

The first criteria identified for any measuring system is *feasibility*, i.e. rapid and easy administration. Secondly the system requires *focus*, allowing for a choice and definition of items specific to individual patients' needs, and facilitating the definition and measurement of patient orientated goals. *Precision* is also required so that clinically significant changes in the patients' health status may be recorded. *Attribution* is necessary to provide statistically significant data to show that the outcome is the result of intervention and not of spontaneous recovery.

The system should provide *auditable* data including the measurement of change in health status and the documentation of all intervention including its timing and frequency.

Finally, the system should have the potential for *multidisciplinary* use and the ability to be incorporated in multidisciplinary audit.

Deficiencies

When the standardised measures revealed by the literature search were compared to the list of required specifications it became apparent that they were deficient in a number of areas. Standardised measures cover many aspects of patient care, e.g. basic self-care skills, functional independence, social activities, mental and psychological status and perceptual skills. Some were designed specifically for institutional care, others for community care, and the scales of measurement and their weightings vary accordingly (Murdock 1992). Rehabilitation outcomes are, however, multifarious and to achieve an accurate reflection of combinations of measures would be required, thereby reducing the feasibility of the system.

Clinicians have commented on the lack of sensitivity of standardised measures such as the Barthel index (Murdock 1992) to record clinically significant changes in health status, particularly when apparently measuring function or motor tasks. Standardised measures may fail to achieve precision as defined in the specification.

A number of the measures which emerged from the literature search are recommended for use as outcome audit tools (Nuffield Institute of Health 1993). However, these stand-alone measures are deficient as facilitators of clinical audit as they do not provide information that would allow the correlation of the relationship between changes in health status, treatment input, timing, frequency and staff mix (Mawson & McCreadie 1993).

THE TELER SYSTEM

Only one of the measurement systems appeared to fulfil all the specifications stated. This was the TELER system (Le Roux 1993), a system which was not previously documented but was used in a number of health authorities within the Trent Regional Health Authority.

Principles

The TELER system is a simple and effective method for evaluating the treatment of individual patients and is capable of the following:

1. Providing a simple and effective record of patient treatment.
2. Establishing an ordinal scale for recording response to treatment, the TELER indicator.
3. Providing a visual display of a patients' response to treatment.
4. Providing an easy to follow display of the relationship between response to and delivery of patient treatment.
5. Recording clinically significant changes in functional status.

A TELER indicator is an ordinal measuring scale for tracing changes in the ability to perform a named function. It provides six reference points coded 0 to 5. The title of the indicator denotes a negotiated rather than an imposed goal to be achieved as a result of intervention. There are a number of types of indicator, several of which may be used in stroke outcome audit, e.g. motor task or component indicators, and environmental or quiz style indicators.

Following on from this pilot study a catalogue of normal movement

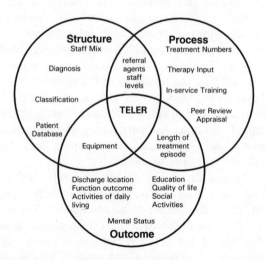

Fig. 17.1   Information provided by the TELER system.

TELER indicators is being developed and validated in conjunction with the UK National Bobath Tutors Group. This will ultimately enable evaluation of the Bobath principles (Bobath 1990) and determine both the effect and efficacy of treatment.

As previously stated, the TELER system appears to fulfil all the specifications required of a measuring system. TELER can incorporate any aspect of outcome covering all the domains which have been previously defined and therefore achieves a feasibility not reached by combining standardised measures. Clinical significance is an integral and essential component of the TELER outcome indicator (Le Roux 1993) enabling the achievement of precision as defined in the specifications. TELER facilitates clinical audit as it can be modified to provide a variety of information. The system enables both clinicians and managers to obtain information pertinent to the structure, process and outcome of their service, thus providing the previously missing link between the aspects of health care defined by Donabedian (1966) (Fig. 17.1).

Variables

Another failure of standardised measures of outcome is their inability to identify *variables* which could affect the eventual outcome of any intervention. Ideally, all variables should be identified at the beginning of a treatment programme. However, as clinical treatment is a dynamic situation, some variables may be identified during the process stage.

Obvious variables which exist in stroke rehabilitation practice include the severity of initial impairment and emotional or psychosocial well-being. These must be identified together with emerging variables such as 'staff mix', in-service training and therapeutic interaction. Change should not be implemented as a result of outcome audit until all the appropriate variables have been identified (Mawson & McCreadie 1993).

The TELER system is able to account for all variables within the structure and process of treatment that may have resulted in or influenced the outcome achieved. It can also be modified and adapted to provide a variety of management- and client-based information. Inclusion of a standardised scale of impairment will provide valuable information regarding the severity of specific areas of impairment such as visual, language or perceptual deficits (Brott et al 1989). This will allow the identification and analysis of relationships which may exist between treatment input, achieved outcome and initial severity.

An example of such a relationship would be the effect that global aphasia has on the ultimate outcome of therapeutic input. Figure 17.2 is a graphical representation of functional goal achievement in a patient with stroke who has a receptive and expressive aphasia. The fluctuating progress with repeated 'fall-backs' in achievement can be seen quite clearly and could be used by clinicians in both peer audit and future research.

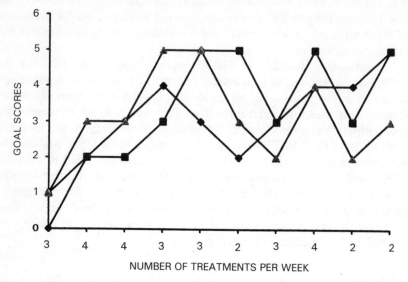

Fig. 17.2   Physiotherapy stroke outcome audit: pattern of recovery of an aphasic patient.

CONCLUSION

To achieve an efficient and effective stroke outcome audit, information is required on the structure that provides a care programme, the process of that programme and variables which occur during the episode of care being evaluated. TELER provides this within one documentation system and displays that information clearly in a form easily understood by both clinicians and managers. Following this initial pilot study, a catalogue of normal movement (Bobath 1990) indicators has been developed and is presently being validated. A reliable and valid measure of outcome in stroke rehabilitation will then be available to study the effect of that rehabilitation and identify possible patterns of recovery that may occur during its implementation.

REFERENCES

Bobath B 1990 Adult hemiplegia: evaluation and treatment. Heinemann, London
Brott T, Adams H P, Olinger C P et al 1989 Measurements of acute cerebral infarction: a
    clinical examination scale. Stroke 20: 864–870
Department of Health 1989 Working for patients. HMSO, London
Department of Health 1990 The health of the nation. HMSO, London
Department of Health 1993a Clinical audit: meeting and improving standards in health care.
    Health Publications Unit, London
Department of Health 1993b Report of the taskforce on the strategy for research in nursing,
    midwifery and health visiting. HMSO, London
Donabedian A 1966 Evaluating the quality of medical care. Millbank Memorial Federation
    of Quality 44(3): 166–203

Joint Council for Education in Medicine 1992 Making Medical Audit Effective. JCEM, London

Le Roux A A 1993 TELER: the concept. Physiotherapy 79(11): 755–758

Lincoln N B, Leadbitter D 1979 Assessment of motor function in stroke patients. Physiotherapy 65: 48–51

Mahoney F I, Barthel D W 1965 Functional evaluation: the Barthel index. Maryland State Medical Journal 14: 61–65

Mawson S, McCreadie M 1993 TELER: the way forward in clinical audit. Physiotherapy 79(11): 758–761

Murdock C A 1992 Critical evaluation of the Barthel index, part 2. British Journal of Occupational Therapy 55(4): 153–156

Nuffield Institute of Health 1993 Lecture notes measuring health outcomes, July 12th. Leeds

Tallis R 1989 Measurement and the future of rehabilitation. Geriatric Medicine Jan.: 31–40

18. PEP – a positioning education programme for the long-term care team

C. L. Mogensen

INTRODUCTION

Some of the challenges facing the health care team in the management of the severely impaired neurological client are immobility, hypertonicity, poor posture, pressure ulcers and contractures. Obtaining optimal wheelchair and bed positioning, in the presence of these conditions, becomes a very difficult task. In view of the multiplicity of these issues, there is a need to develop therapeutic interventions with a coordinated team approach in order to provide effective care.

The positioning education programme (PEP) has been designed specifically to assist in the management of these problems. The purpose of this chapter is to discuss the major concepts within PEP, to share the results of a PEP quality assurance project, and finally to illustrate PEP with a case study. The major PEP concepts to be addressed are the theory base, the transdisciplinary team approach, and the three primary components of the PEP model of practice.

PEP CONCEPTS

Theory

The theory base is derived from the research findings of Odeen (1981) which demonstrated that long-term elongation of hypertonic muscles for 20–30 minutes was effective in reducing the electromyographic activity of the hypertonic muscles, and in increasing the passive and active range of movement in the opposing muscles. The theory base is also derived from evidence in the literature by Binkley (1989) that supports low load, long-term elongation of muscle and connective tissue to reduce or prevent contracture. The research by Light et al (1984) and Grossman (1982) demonstrated that muscles immobilized in the shortened position lose sarcomeres, whereas immobilizing the same muscles in the lengthened position results in regeneration and the addition of sarcomeres, thus increasing tensile muscle strength. Collectively, this body of knowledge formulates the theoretical basis of the programme, and illustrates the significant role of therapeutic positioning. Positioning muscles in the lengthened position rather than in the shortened position can result in reducing hypertonicity, increasing active and passive movement and increasing muscle strength.

Service delivery model

PEP utilizes an adaptation of the transdisciplinary service delivery model. Within a transdisciplinary team, functions are 'based on the common need for integration of philosophy, personnel and services' (Sparling 1980). The respective disciplines are responsible for initial assessments within their area of expertise. Collectively, the team members then develop a comprehensive individualized therapeutic programme. The interventions are performed by one prime care giver, or possibly two (Ottenbacher 1983, McCormick & Goldman 1979). Key advantages of this model are the increased consistency in the provision of care plans, and a framework which facilitates team problem-solving and team collaboration. Disadvantages of this approach can be the staff's difficulty with the change in their traditional service roles, and staff's concerns with regard to professional security (McCormick & Goldman 1979).

Within PEP's adaptation of the transdisciplinary approach, all disciplines complete their assessments, then collectively team members problem-solve and devise treatment plans. The treatment plans will describe the discipline-specific roles, as well as the bed and wheelchair positioning protocols that have been agreed upon by the team and will be provided by all disciplines in exactly the same manner. This approach enables the various aspects that impact upon optimal positioning to be realized by each discipline (tube feeding, hypertonicity, skin integrity, contractures). All pertinent information can then be incorporated into the design of the positioning protocols to address the client's needs in the bed and the wheelchair, and the client is positioned in a consistent therapeutic manner.

The three primary components of the PEP model of practice

The educational component

The educational component is designed to develop a common knowledge base among team members and to enhance team building and team performance.

It is the author's opinion that basic level training does not prepare health care givers for the complex positioning needs of the severely impaired client; hence the educational sessions are critical to the success of PEP. Some of the principal topics discussed in the educational sessions are:

• the theory
• the transdisciplinary team approach and team building concepts

- terminology review related to position, movement, wheelchairs and wheelchair equipment
- PEP benefits, goals and expected outcomes
- team functions within the transdisciplinary wheelchair seating clinics and bed positioning clinics
- information on how to make cost-effective positioning devices from on-site materials.

At the conclusion of the educational sessions the attendees are recognized as PEP representatives or positioning resource staff. Some of the key roles of the PEP representatives are:

- to educate other staff in the positioning principles
- to assist in the identification of clients who would benefit from PEP
- to participate in the bed positioning clinics and wheelchair seating clinics
- to assist in evaluating the effectiveness of the prescribed programmes
- to ensure charting guidelines are met.

The clinical component

The clinical component provides a framework through wheelchair seating clinics and bed positioning clinics to facilitate the transdisciplinary team approach. Once a seating problem is identified a referral is made to the individual coordinating the seating clinic. In most cases it is the occupational therapist; however this may vary from facility to facility. Team members concerned with the issue are invited to attend the wheelchair seating clinic for their input and assistance in the problem-solving process. If the solution requires new equipment, the process of ordering and obtaining the equipment is begun. Goals and expected outcomes are identified and recorded in the medical chart. Upon receipt of the equipment, reassessments are necessary to ensure that the seating goals are met, wheelchair parts must be labelled, and perhaps most importantly, the client, family and other staff members must receive education in the operation of the wheelchair, and how properly to seat the client in the wheelchair. Ongoing monitoring of the effectiveness of the seating prescription by all team members is important. Should it be found to be ineffective the process must begin again.

The bed positioning clinic membership typically consists of physiotherapy and nursing staff, although all interested parties are welcome to attend at the bedside. Team members share their assessments and concerns with regard to bed posture. Collectively, optimal bed positioning regimes are developed for the left and right 30 degree laterally inclined positions (Seiler et al 1986) and the supine position. Bed positioning goals and expected outcomes are identified and documented. Occasionally commercially made products are purchased, but most often on-site materials are used to assist the client in maintaining the desired positions, e.g. rolled towels, drawsheets, sheets, facecloths, and fire retardant foam cut into the required shapes and appropriately covered. The equipment is labelled and bed positioning pictures are drawn or photographs are taken for display at the bedside, with the permission of the client or family. This information at the bedside greatly enhances the staff's ability to follow the often complex positioning regimes. All of these tasks are shared among the team members.

At each client's first clinic a reevaluation date is set for the purposes of discussing the effectiveness of the bed positioning protocols. The documentation is reviewed as well, and if necessary, revisions are made to the programme.

The evaluative component

Typical PEP client expected outcomes are: the prevention or resolution of pressure ulcers, soft tissue shortening and contractures, a decrease in hypertonicity, enhanced comfort and sitting tolerance, and improved passive and active mobility. As a result, frequent team and facility outcomes experienced are: easier provision of care, fewer treatments required, and ultimately cost savings for the facility.

Table 18.1 and 18.2 provide the positioning programme evaluation results conducted at the Chedoke Continuing Care Centre of Chedoke McMaster Hospital in Hamilton, Ontario, Canada. After the first evaluation (Table 18.1), the audits show the growth of the programme. This was attributed to the impact of the educational courses which enhanced the staff's appreciation of the significant role of optimal positioning. Evaluation 1 shows that, before the first PEP course was instructed, only 8 out of an identified 26 clients (31%) who needed specialized positioning programmes were enrolled in PEP, whereas at Evaluation 3, 12 months after the first PEP course was instructed, 30 out of an identified 33 clients (91%) who required specialized positioning were enrolled in PEP.

The communication of the programme through PEP pictures placed at the bedside greatly improved after Evaluation 1. However, the charting audit revealed that charting is an area which requires attention and improvement.

Each of the evaluative points in the bedside audits were conducted for a 2-week period. Without notification to the staff, an examiner went to the bedside of each client enrolled in PEP at random times in the morning and afternoon, to assess the accuracy of the client's actual bed positioning relative to the prescribed programmes. The accuracy was assessed in terms of 100% accuracy at all four evaluative points, and at Evaluations 2, 3 and 4 the percentage of positioning devices found correctly placed was also recorded. The number of clients found to be in complete agreement changed from 32% to 44% to 71% and finally to 58%. The percentage of equipment found correctly placed improved from 69% to 87% to 82% at the fourth evaluation. These improvements occurred with considerably more clients in the programme at the third and fourth evaluative points.

Table 18.1   Positioning programme evaluation, Chedoke Continuing Care Centre

	Evaluation 1 Pre-PEP course	Evaluation 2 6 months post first PEP course	Evaluation 3 12 months post first PEP course	Evaluation 4 2 years post first PEP course
Number of clients enrolled in PEP	31% 8/26	58% 15/24	91% 30/33	97% 37/38
Number of programmes with:				
Bedside pictures	50%	100%	100%	92% 34/37
Charting re: PEP	100%	100%	77%	84% 31/37
Bedside audit:	42 bedside checks	101 bedside checks	165 bedside checks	145 bedside checks
PEP implemented with 100% accuracy	32%	44%	71%	58%
Percentage of positioning devices found correctly placed	–	69% 270/391	87% 612/703	82% 513/625
Number of PEP representatives on site	3	21	30	36 (42)

One becomes more aware of the complexity of PEP when it is realized that, for example, at Evaluation 4 of the bedside audit during 145 bedside checks, 625 pieces of positioning equipment were required for 37 clients, of which 513 were found to be in the correct position.

The last row in Table 18.1 shows that at the fourth evaluation, 42 staff members had attended the PEP educational courses, of whom 36 still worked at the facility.

Table 18.2 outlines the positioning programme evaluation: client outcomes. The achievement in the identified outcomes is depicted as a fraction. For example, in the third evaluation (E_3), of the 27 clients with the identified goal of preventing a contracture or maintaining range of motion, 26 clients achieved this objective. Cost saving measures are realized through the reduction in the number of physiotherapy treatments required per week for four clients and three clients in the third and fourth evaluations respectively, and through the prevention of pressure ulcers and surgery. Studies (Foster et al 1991, Haley 1986) indicate that the cost to heal pressure ulcers ranges from $3400 to $86 000 in North America. The physiotherapists attributed the reduced levels of hypertonicity and greater range of movement that the clients experienced over time to their ability to reduce the frequency of treatment. It is recognized that PEP is not the only

Table 18.2   Positioning programme evaluation: client outcomes

Client outcome	Achievement	
	E₃	E₄
Prevent contracture or maintain range of motion	26/27	23/26
Increase range of motion	2/2	7/7
Prevent skin breakdown	2/2	5/5
Maintain a balance of muscle tone	12/18	12/15
Reduction in number of physiotherapy treatments required per week	4	3
Prevent surgery	1	–

factor contributing to these outcomes; however, it was felt to play a major role in achieving these outcomes.

The learning experiences of the attendees at the PEP educational courses were also monitored. A multiple choice quiz was administered before the course, immediately after it, and 3 months later. The results showed that there was a 50% improvement in the quiz scores immediately after the course, as well as 3 months later when the scores were compared to pre-course results.

The PEP at Chedoke McMaster Hospital was awarded a certificate of excellence from the Quality Assurance Department in recognition of its contribution to the continuous improvement of staff and client services.

CASE STUDY

The following case study illustrates how the PEP functioned for a particular client.

Client A, with a diagnosis of head injury, was admitted to a long-term care facility 3 years post-injury. He had marked hypertonicity and no voluntary movement in his lower extremities. Flexion contractures were so severe at the hips and knees as to prevent him from being seated in a wheelchair.

After admission, assessments by physiotherapy, nursing and occupational therapy staff were completed and the client goals were stated as follows:

• reduction of lower extremity flexion contractures
• reduction of lower extremity hypertonicity (particularly in the hip adductors and hip and knee flexors)
• prevention of skin breakdown over the greater trochanters
• comfortable seating in a wheelchair
• participation in various programmes in the centre and the community.

Client A was identified as having specialized positioning needs. This initiated his enrolment in the bed positioning clinic where nursing and physiotherapy staff:

• pooled their assessment findings
• developed a therapeutic bed positioning programme

- designed, made and labelled the on-site positioning devices
- completed diagrams of the bed positioning regime for use at the bedside
- completed the charting requirements of the programme in the medical record.

In supine, positioning devices were used to maintain hip abduction with an abductor roll, and as much hip and knee extension as could *comfortably* be attained with a bedsheet drawn taut over the knees and tucked under the mattress. In the 30° laterally inclined position, devices were used to maintain hip abduction with the weight of the body over the glutei muscles rather than over the trochanter.

Because client A had no voluntary movement in his lower extremities, he was positioned as described above by nursing staff at each of the turning sessions, which took place every 2 hours when the client was in bed. Following the exercise programme that was provided by physiotherapy 5 days a week, client A was positioned in the same manner as prescribed in the client's positioning protocol. As the contractures gradually began to reduce, the occupational therapist initiated the wheelchair prescription process by enrolling client A in the wheelchair seating clinic. The assessment findings and expertise of physiotherapy and nursing were sought during the process in order to fully appreciate the skin integrity status, range of motion, muscle tone and comfort level of the client.

Within 1 year the following outcomes were achieved:

- A reduction in contractures. The right and left hip flexion contractures changed from –60° to –35°, and –50° to –23° respectively; and the right and left knee flexion contractures were reduced from –90° to –60° and –95° to –40° respectively.
- A reduction in hypertonicity. Objective measures could not be used because of the client's inability to remain relaxed during testing. Using an ordinal scale the classification of muscle tone changed from severe to moderate.
- Skin integrity was maintained.
- Comfortable seating in a personalized wheelchair was obtained.
- Involvement in centre and community programmes was achieved.

These outcomes were attained without surgery or antispasmodics in an individual who had longstanding contractures and high levels of hypertonicity prior to admission to this facility.

CONCLUSION

The PEP model of practice, within its three primary components: educational, clinical and evaluative, emphasizes the importance of education, a cohesive team approach, and the significant role that therapeutic positioning plays in the management of the severely impaired, neurological client. The framework within this programme is designed to facilitate transdisciplinary team functioning in the bed positioning and wheelchair seating clinics, thereby strengthening team collaboration and team implementation of therapeutic positioning protocols. Team goal setting and measuring outcomes are also important components.

This chapter has illustrated, by means of a quality assurance project, PEP's contribution towards improving programme compliance and enhancing positive client and team outcomes in a long-term care facility.

REFERENCES

Binkley J 1989 Overview of ligament and tendon structure and mechanics: implications for clinical practice. Physiotherapy Canada 41(1): 24–30

Foster C, Frisch S R, Denis N et al 1991 Prevalence of pressure ulcers in Canadian institutions. Canadian Association of Enterostomal Therapy Journal 11(2): 23–31

Grossman M 1982 Review of length-associated changes in muscle experimental evidence and clinical implications. Physical Therapy 62(12): 1799–1807

Haley R W 1986 Managing hospital infection control for cost-effectiveness. American Hospital Publishing, Atlanta, ch 2, pp 3–12

Light K E, Nuzik S, Personius W et al 1984 Low-load prolonged stretch vs high-load brief stretch in treating knee contractures. Physical Therapy 64(3): 330–333

McCormick L, Goldman R 1979 The transdisciplinary model: implications for service delivery and personnel preparation for the severely and profoundly handicapped. American Association for the Education of the Severely Profoundly Handicapped Review 4(2): 152–161

Odeen I 1981 Reduction of muscular hypertonus by long term muscle stretch. Scandinavian Journal of Rehabilitation Medicine 13: 93–99

Ottenbacher K 1983 Transdisciplinary service delivery in school environments: some limitations. Physical and Occupational Therapy in Pediatrics 3(4): 9–16

Seiler W O, Allen S, Stahelin H B 1986 Influence of the 30 degree laterally inclined position of the 'super soft' 3-piece mattress on skin oxygen tension and areas of maximum pressure – implications for pressure sore prevention. Gerontology 32: 158–166

Sparling J W 1980 The transdisciplinary approach with the developmentally delayed child. Physical and Occupational Therapy in Pediatrics 1(2): 3–13

19. A stroke protocol for physiotherapy in primary health care

D. van Ravensberg, J. Halfens, R. Oostendorp

INTRODUCTION

In the Netherlands, health care policy is directed towards a shift from institutionalised care to primary health care (Hendriks & Van Der Wolf 1989). The objective is to provide care 'close to the patient'. The patient and his/her family (spouse, children, non-professional carers) are in a central position. The most important goal is to attain a better 'tuning in' of the care provided by professionals to the needs or wishes of the patient and his/her family.

Care is seen as hierarchically structured. Self-care (a person's ability and initiative to provide his/her own individual need for care or support) gains a primary place in this hierarchy. A secondary place is assumed by the care provided by the partner or children, the family and/or friends. Professional care takes third place.

This way of thinking leads to changes in care models: from professional care to self-care and care by relevant others and, within the professional care, from institutionalised care to home care, and from cure to prevention.

It is expected that this policy will lead to a situation where people are able to stay in their own homes for as long as possible. This policy is directed mainly towards elderly people and those with chronic diseases. People with stroke have a significant place within the latter group.

HOME REHABILITATION OF STROKE PATIENTS

Because of the complexity and severity of the consequences of stroke, among other reasons stroke rehabilitation found its place mainly in institutions such as rehabilitation centres and/or nursing homes. As a result of the shifts in health policy, patients with stroke are now increasingly rehabilitated in primary health care settings, while remaining in their own homes.

Such changes in health care do not take place only in the Netherlands; comparable tendencies are seen in other countries as well (De Pedro-Cuesta et al 1993, Schuling et al 1993, Wade et al 1992).

Notwithstanding some practical problems, rehabilitation care in the home situation is perceived as essential for enhancing the quality of life. This view relates to various aspects of this type of care, such as the practical and moral support of the patient's social environment (family, friends and relatives). Another aspect is the so-called rehabilitation 'together', i.e. the direct participation of the family in the rehabilitation process. A third aspect is the opportunity for a more adequate 'tuning in' of professional care to the needs and/or wishes of patients with stroke and their family, directly related to the specific (home) situation. Further advantages are the maintenance of the normal pre-stroke social contacts and the diminution of problems such as hospital infections and institutionalisation syndromes.

Professionals who generally are involved in home rehabilitation of the stroke patient are a general practitioner (family physician), home nurse, social worker, family carer, physiotherapist, occupational therapist and speech therapist.

Possibilities for home rehabilitation in stroke are related to (Evans et al 1991):

• the current medical status of the patient (cardiovascular and neurological status, the kinds and severity of present impairments and disabilities, the presence of joint contractures and decubitus) and the prognosis on the patient's future (abilities and disabilities)

• the wishes of the patient and his/her family, the estimated physical and psychological load tolerance (namely of the family members), the presence of non-professional support, and the insight of the patients and their family of their situation

• practical considerations: presence of well-trained professionals (with adequate, up-to-date knowledge and skills), and their attitude towards the problems of stroke.

Problems

Several bottlenecks have been identified in home rehabilitation of stroke patients (World Health Organization 1993)

Knowledge and skills

The first bottleneck is the degree of knowledge and skills of professionals in the early recognition and appropriate treatment of the consequences of stroke.

Physiotherapists in primary care settings often lack practice in the rehabilitation of a patient with stroke in the early phases post-stroke. Previously in primary health care, patients were not treated until their condition had stabilised, or were treated a long time after the onset of stroke when they showed any deterioration or had a problem with their shoulder.

In the acute, subacute and rehabilitation stage following stroke, more complex care is needed than in other patient categories within primary health care settings, since stroke comprises a variety of aspects which need various specific and flexible applied forms/methods of physiotherapy.

Coordination and management

The second bottleneck relates to the coordination and management of home care/home rehabilitation.

In home rehabilitation of the patient with stroke, intensive cooperation is needed between the different professionals (general practitioner or family physician, home nurse, social worker, physiotherapist, occupational therapist and speech therapist). A frequent tuning in of activities and tasks between the different disciplines is therefore urgently required. This kind of participation in home rehabilitation settings is new for physiotherapy in primary health care. Physiotherapists have to learn to find their place in this setting, and to define their specific contribution to appropriate home rehabilitation for the patient with stroke.

Insight

The third bottleneck concerns insight into the problems following a stroke, but also into the creativeness and the psychological (and physical) burden placed upon the partner and other family members. There are limits to what can be demanded of non-professional carers.

It is known that the partner and other family members can fulfil many additional demands if they receive appropriate practical help and support. This means that they have to be provided with adequate information on, for example, the problems and changes which occur after stroke, the general prognoses, the individual's expected future abilities and disablement, and the consequences for family life. This also forms a bottleneck in physiotherapy – the physiotherapist in primary health care is not familiar with the tasks of supporting the family of adult patients, training them and giving them tasks in the rehabilitation process, discussing with them the type and content of care and shaping this to the individual needs and wishes of the family.

TOWARDS A PROTOCOL: METHODS

The project was directed towards enhancing the quality of physiotherapy within the home rehabilitation programme of the stroke patient, by developing (and subsequently implementing) a stroke protocol for physiotherapy in home rehabilitation/primary health care.

A stroke protocol is defined as follows:

In the context of quality assurance a stroke protocol is defined as a document, based on relevant literature and using terms from (international) classifications, which provides guidance to physiotherapists for home rehabilitation of the patient with stroke and which leads the decision-making process in common stroke problems.

This protocol serves four goals:

1. To increase the knowledge of the physiotherapist in primary health care on the different phases and aspects of stroke and its treatment in home rehabilitation.
2. To offer a structure for making appropriate decisions on the type and content of physiotherapy intervention, 'tuned in' to the individual patient with stroke.
3. To widen the therapists' eye for the problems and burden (placed upon the partner and/or non-professional carers) in the home situation and to enlarge their knowledge of ways to support them, to give them proper information and to involve them in the rehabilitation process.
4. To enhance the therapists' attention to and participation in the 'tuning in' of care between different disciplines.

A supporting registration form was developed that is to be used together with the stroke protocol. This detailed registration form serves to collect relevant and detailed data about the individual patient with stroke and his/her home situation. These data are considered necessary to follow the subsequent steps of the protocol and to enable the appropriate decisions to be made.

Registered data comprise general information about the person (e.g. age, gender, family network), a description of the medical status, the care given by other disciplines, the health problem as perceived by both the patient and the therapist (past history data and data following the examination of the patient by the physiotherapist), data about the partner and/or non-professional carers and the problems posed for them, and data on the content of the physiotherapy/home rehabilitation programme and an intermittent evaluation of the rehabilitation process and results. This registration form can also be used in interdisciplinary communication.

For the development of these documents (protocol and registration form) an overview of recent literature on stroke and home rehabilitation was used, enriched by physiotherapists' practical knowledge and experience. Furthermore, the terms that are used are expressed in a uniform professional language.

Relevant literature on stroke

Recent literature is screened on topics such as:

• The most recommended therapeutic approaches, known problems in stroke rehabilitation and proposed solutions.

• Opportunities and bottlenecks in home rehabilitation, with special reference to the partner and/or non-professional carers, recommended approaches and prevention of problems.

• Cooperation between different disciplines in primary health care, 'tuning in' of care within primary health care and 'tuning in' and continuation of the care provided in early hospitalization or institutionalization phases as it transfers into the home rehabilitation setting (continuation of care with respect to the process, content and method).

Practical knowledge and experience

For the development of the protocol, practical knowledge of, and experience with, stroke (home) rehabilitation is of the utmost importance. Physiotherapists with considerable experience in the rehabilitation of patients with stroke, and also with home rehabilitation, participated in the development of the protocol. One of the authors is experienced in running practical courses on stroke rehabilitation, based on the Neurodevelopmental treatment (NDT) principle. The Dutch organisation of stroke patients and their partners also participated in the development of the protocol.

A uniform professional language

The different disciplines taking part in the rehabilitation of the patient with stroke often have their own 'professional terms' or 'professional language'. In the exchange of information as well as agreeing on the methods and aspects of treatment, different meanings of words or different terms for the same subject may lead to confusion. This also holds true for intradisciplinary exchange of data.

Uniformity of professional language is a basic prerequisite for adequate communication and, therefore, is essential for providing qualitatively good care. It can be helpful to use International classifications for registration and data exchange.

A thorough description of the health status of the individual patient with stroke is essential. Relevant data for this description are distilled from the medical (referral) data, from the diagnostic process in physiotherapy (patient's complaints, examination findings), and from data provided by other disciplines.

ICIDH

The international classification of impairments, disabilities and handicaps (ICIDH) (World Health Organization 1980) is very useful for the description of a person's health status. The ICIDH can also be used to indicate (indirectly) the goals of rehabilitation and its results (differences in presence and severity of problems between different phases of the rehabilitation).

The ICIDH was edited, in 1980, by the WHO for trial purposes. Since then, it has been used widely (practically applied) in rehabilitation. There is much support for its conceptual framework, but there is criticism of, for example, the unclear classification structure, the level of detail, and the lack of some important categories of disability and impairment (WCC 1993a). In 1993, a formal revision procedure for the ICIDH was started. International criticism as well as proposals for amending the ICIDH are discussed as part of the revision process. One of the proposals for amending the ICIDH was developed in the Netherlands, in close cooperation with the paramedical disciplines of physiotherapy, occupational therapy, kinetic therapy according to Mensendieck, Cesar kinetic therapy, and chiropody (WCC 1993b).

For the development of the stroke protocol and the registration form, and also for use in interdisciplinary communication and exchange of data, a selection of terms was made from the ICIDH that are essential for stroke rehabilitation. This selection was made by, among others, psychiatrists, psychologists, physiotherapists, occupational therapists, speech therapists and social workers, following a proposal, by paramedical staff, for amending the ICIDH.

RESULTS

The protocol and the registration form are now being developed in primary health care settings. Subsequent steps are the attainment of a more general consensus, and further implementation.

The protocol addresses the three topics mentioned earlier in this chapter.

First, the protocol provides the physiotherapist with relevant and up-to-date information about stroke and its (home) rehabilitation; it supports the physiotherapist and helps him/her to make appropriate decisions about the content and nature of his/her treatment.

Secondly, the protocol addresses the general need for information and support for the patient's partner/children/non-professional carer, and the need for training them in their task with respect to the rehabilitation of the patient with stroke.

Thirdly, the protocol addresses the participation of the physiotherapist in the interdisciplinary approach to home rehabilitation of patients with stroke. The added registration form offers items for interdisciplinary communication and data exchange, as well as for the fine tuning of the care provided by the different disciplines.

Within the protocol, specific attention is paid to:

• the different phases in recovery from stroke (the characteristics, prognostic features, outline of treatment in these phases, evaluation of outcomes, indication of phase-specific problems).

• the painful (paretic) shoulder (prevention, differential diagnosis, treatment, advantages and disadvantages of using a supporting sling, instructions to other carers).

• sensibility impairments (characteristics, outline of treatment, specific additional problems).

• impairment of the so-called higher cognitive function (early prevention and recognition, characteristics, diagnosis, additional problems, treatment, transfer of training principles, providing information and instructions to the family and other carers).

• common emotional problems/depression (characteristics, diagnosis, additional problems, treatment, support, providing information to the partner/other carers).

• technical aids and home adaptations (possibilities, indications, different kinds/alternatives, information about proper use of those aids, control on a regular basis).

• a patient's daily activities (priorities, motivation, lifestyle, attitude, social network, recreational activities, work, household tasks).

CONCLUSION

When using the stroke protocol, unwanted and non-intended therapist-related differences in stroke (home) rehabilitation are prevented. Different aspects of the consequences of stroke are outlined in the protocol, and recommendations for treatment are given, based on theoretical views as well as on empirical, practical experience. Treatment approaches to different kinds of problems that are very common in stroke rehabilitation are also discussed.

In addition, guidelines for providing information and support to the patient's partner, family and/or non-professional carers are given. Their proper involvement in the rehabilitation process (giving them specific tasks, monitoring the physical and emotional load placed upon them and their capability, and prevention of overburdening them) is perceived as essential for a favourable outcome of the home rehabilitation process.

The protocol also addresses the participation of the physiotherapist in interdisciplinary home rehabilitation, and by means of the registration form, provides the therapist with data in a uniform language which can be used in interdisciplinary data exchange and communication, and gives support to the 'tuning in' of care given by the different disciplines.

In this way, it is expected that the protocol will contribute to the improvement of the quality of care for patients with stroke, with special reference to the role played by the physiotherapist in home rehabilitation.

REFERENCES

De Pedro-Cuesta J, Sandstrom B, Holm M, Stawiarz L, Widen-Holmqvist L, Bach-Y-Rita
  P 1993 Stroke rehabilitation: identification of target groups and planning data.
  Scandinavian Journal of Rehabilitation and Medicine 25: 107–116
Evans R L, Bishop D S, Haselkorn J K 1991 Factors predicting satisfactory home care after
  stroke. Archives of Physical Medicine and Rehabilitation 72: 144–147
Hendriks J P M, Van Der Wolf J P M 1989 Discussienota substitutie in de
  gezondheidszorg. Nationale Raad voor de Volksgezondheid, Rijswijk, Netherlands
Schuling J, Groenier K H, Meyboom-de Jong B 1993 Thuisbehandeling van patiënten met
  een cerebrovasculair accident. Nederlands Tijdschrift voor Geneeskunde 137: 1918–1922
Wade D T, Collen F M, Robb G F, Warlow C P 1992 Physiotherapy intervention late after
  stroke and mobility. British Medical Journal 304: 609–613
World Health Organization 1980 International classification of impairments, disabilities, and
  handicaps. World Health Organization, Geneva
World Health Organization 1993 Management and rehabilitation of stroke – report on a
  WHO consultation. W Copenhagen
WCC 1993a A survey of criticism about the classification of impairments and the
  classification of disabilities of the international classification of impairments, disabilities,
  and handicaps (ICIDH). Dutch Classification and Terminology Committee for Health,
  Zoetermeer
WCC 1993b Proposals for adaptation of the classification of impairments and the
  classification of disabilities of the ICIDH from the perspective of five Dutch health
  professions. Dutch Classification and Terminology Committee for Health, Zoetermeer

20. A 5-year study of stroke patient recovery

B. Lindmark

INTRODUCTION

Most patients with stroke who need rehabilitation are quite well taken care of during the acute period, up to 3 months post-stroke and during the first year, but after 1 year only a few are offered rehabilitation. For physiotherapists it is also of interest to know how well the functional level is maintained after several years.

There have been few reports on studies in which the progress of patients has been followed up for more than 1 year after a stroke and even fewer have studied the functional recovery.

Brocklehurst et al (1981) studied the effect on the chief carer of stroke patients for 4 years and concluded that carers had a large supervision burden. Wade et al (1984) undertook a 2 year follow-up to identify factors predicting the length of survival and found that the strongest predictors were the severity of the stroke, the pre-existence of cardiovascular disease and the patient's age. Viitanen et al (1988) investigated life satisfaction in a group of patients 4–6 years after the onset of stroke. Persistent motor impairment and ADL disability had a negative effect on several aspects of life satisfaction. Greveson et al (1991) assessed the outcome in 83 stroke patients with stroke more than 3 years post-stroke. Their carers were also assessed and were found to be suffering from emotional stress and social isolation. Collen & Wade (1991) assessed mobility in more than 300 surviving patients with stroke 2–7 years after the stroke and found that more than half of the patients were immobile.

A longitudinal study of 5 years' duration was initiated at the University Hospital in Uppsala, Sweden in 1984 (Lindmark 1988, Lindmark & Hamrin 1989, Hamrin & Lindmark 1990, Lindmark & Hamrin 1994). The main purpose of the study was to follow the changes in functional capacity in terms of motor function and ability and activities of daily living (ADL) during these years. Questions asked were: How many of the patients had survived 1 year and 5 years and did age and sex affect the survival? How many suffered another stroke? How many lived at home? Did the functional level change? Were some motor functions and abilities maintained better than others? Was there any difference in the change in functional performance between men and women? How did the surviving patients rate their health and life situation 1 year and 5 years after their stroke?

METHOD

Subjects

280 acutely ill stroke patients (median age = 76 years, range = 30–96 years, 144 men and 136 women) who were admitted consecutively, during 13 months in 1984 and 1985 to four general medical wards at the Univerity Hospital, Uppsala and survived at least 24 hours, were included in a study of their functional ability.

After 1 year 191(68%) patients (median age at the onset of stroke = 74 years, range = 30–92 years, 102 men and 89 women) were alive and 5 years after the stroke 113 (40%) patients (median age at the onset of stroke = 71 years, range = 30–89 years, 56 men and 57 women) were alive. The median age of the 5-year surviving men was 7 years lower than that of the women. 183 of the 1-year survivors and 101 of the 5-year survivors were visited and assessed.

Assessments

The patients were assessed for functional ability on admission, after 1 week, 3 weeks, at discharge, after 3 months and after 1 year and 5 years. At the 3-month, 1-year and 5-year follow-ups the patients were visited where they resided, which was mostly in their own homes.

The following assessments were carried out on all test occasions:

• Assessment of self-capacity through the activity index (AI) (Hamrin & Wohlin 1982) including mental capacity, motor activity and ADL. The patient was then allocated to one of three score groups.

• Assessment of the ability to perform active movements in supine, sitting and standing, coordination, gross mobility and walking, balance, sensation, joint motion and pain was undertaken with the help of a motor assessment chart developed by Lindmark (Lindmark & Hamrin 1988a). The motor ability of both sides of the body was assessed with a number of variables using a scale from 0 = no function to 3 = normal function. The patient was then allocated to one of four functional groups according to the motor score.

Both instruments have been validated and tested for reliability with satisfactory results (Hamrin & Wohlin 1982, Lindmark & Hamrin 1988a, b).

At follow-up a structured interview was performed according to a schedule constructed by Hamrin (1982). The interview concerned primarily four activity areas: household work, locomotion inside and outside the home, psychosocial function and intellectual activity. Questions concerning overall health and life situation were included at the 1-year and 5-year follow-ups.

Statistical method

Non-parametric statistical methods were used.

Chi-squared method was used to compare distribution between functional groups, and to compare 5-year survivors with those who died between 1 and 5 years after the stroke.

The Mann–Witney U test for independent samples was used to compare men and women and patients with and without further episodes of stroke.

The Wilcoxon matched-pairs signed-rank test was used to investigate change over time.

RESULTS

Survival, age, recurrence of stroke and living conditions

68% of the patients' were alive after 1 year and 40% 4 years later. The median age of the 5-years survivors at the onset of stroke, 71 years, was 5 years lower than the median age of all patients included in the study. The difference was significant ($p < 0.001$). The median age of the women was significantly higher than that of the men at each stage ($p < 0.001$). At the onset of stroke the difference was 4 years, 1 year after the stroke the differece was 6 years and 4 years later the difference was 7 years (Lindmark & Hamrin 1994).

Of the 101 5-year survivors who were visited, seven reported that they had suffered at least one transient ischaemic attack (TIA), 10 had had just one more minor stroke, with almost no new residual symptoms, and five had a further severe stroke during the 5-year period (Lindmark & Hamrin 1994).

One year after the stroke 24% of the 183 assessed 1-year survivors lived alone in their own home, 52% with a spouse, 7% in homes for elderly people and 16% in hospitals for long-term care (Lindmark & Hamrin 1989). Of the 101 assessed 5-year survivors 26% lived alone, 62% with a spouse, 4% in homes for elderly people and 9% in hospitals for long-term care 1 year after the stroke. Four years later 26% of the 101 5-year survivors still lived alone, 56% with a spouse, 12% in homes for elderly people and 7% in hospitals for long-term care (Lindmark & Hamrin 1994).

Changes in motor performance

All measured function and ability, i.e total motor ability, balance, mobility, walking and function in different parts of the paretic side, improved significantly during the first year for the group as whole (Lindmark 1988).

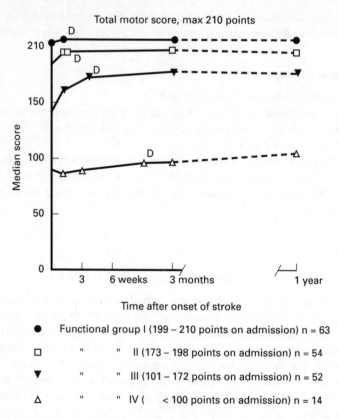

Fig. 20.1 Improvement of median total motor score evaluated with the motor assessment, in 1-year survivors of different functional groups. D = median discharge time for each group. (Adapted from the Scandinavian Journal of Rehabilitation Medicine, with the permission of Scandinavian University Press.)

There were significant improvements between admission and discharge (the median length of stay in hospital was 10 days) and between discharge and 3 months, but not between 3 months and 1 year after the stroke. Balance, walking and coordination did not improve as well as the other functions measured.

The patients of functional group I (minor to no impairment) improved most during the first week after the stroke. The improvement in the total motor scores between admission and discharge (median length of stay in hospital = 6 days) was significant, but the improvement between discharge and 3 months or between 3 months and 1 year was not significant (Fig. 20.1) (Lindmark 1988). In functional group II (moderate impairment) the greatest improvement again occurred during the hospital stay, but the patients continued to improve slowly for up to 3 months. This group showed significant improvement in the total motor scores between admission and discharge (median length of stay in hospital = 10 days) and between discharge and 3 months, but not between 3 months and 1 year (Fig. 20.1) (Lindmark 1988).

In functional group III (moderately severe impairment) the improvement pattern was similar to that of functional group II. The improvement in the total motor scores between admission and discharge (median length of stay in hospital = 24 days) and between discharge and 3 months was significant in both cases, but the improvement between 3 months and 1 year was not significant (Fig. 20.1) (Lindmark 1988).

Patients belonging to functional group IV (severe impairment) improved slowly throughout the year. The improvement in the total motor scores between admission and 3 weeks was not significant, but when admission scores were compared with the scores on discharge (median length of stay in hospital = 58 days) significant improvement was found. Even though there was a slow improvement after discharge up to 3 months and 1 year after the stroke, the improvement was not significant. One reason for this may have been the small number of patients in this functional group, 14 patients, who survived 1 year (Fig. 20.1) (Lindmark 1988).

When the functional groups were divided into a younger half and an older half, the younger halves improved more rapidly and better than the older halves, especially in functional groups III and IV. This was most evident for mobility and balance (Lindmark 1988).

At the onset of stroke the 280 patients were evenly distributed over all functional groups with about 25% of the patients in each group.

Both at 3 months and 1 year after the stroke about 50–55% of the surviving patients belonged to functional group I, 25–30% to functional group II, 10–15% to functional group III and less than 10% to functional group IV (Lindmark & Hamrin 1988).

The median total motor score obtained for all 101 assessed 5-year survivors was 188 on admission, 204 after 1 year and 196 after 5 years. The changes in total motor score between admission and 1 year and between 1 year and 5 years were significant ($p < 0.0001$) (Lindmark & Hamrin 1994).

Figure 20.2 shows the distribution of all assessed 5-year survivors into different functional groups on admission, after 1 year and after 5 years. During the first year after the stroke there was a significant improvement, with most patients in the two best functional groups at 1 year, but between 1 and 5 years there was instead a significant decline in motor performance ($p < 0.0001$). The majority of the patients were still in the best two functional groups 5 years after the stroke but a larger proportion was in group III (Lindmark & Hamrin 1994).

There were no significant differences in motor performance at the 5-year follow-up between patients who had suffered a further stroke or TIA and those without such episodes (Lindmark & Hamrin 1994).

The median score for gross mobility for the 101 assessed 5-year survivors was 25 on admission, 27 at 1 year and 26 after 5 years. The median score

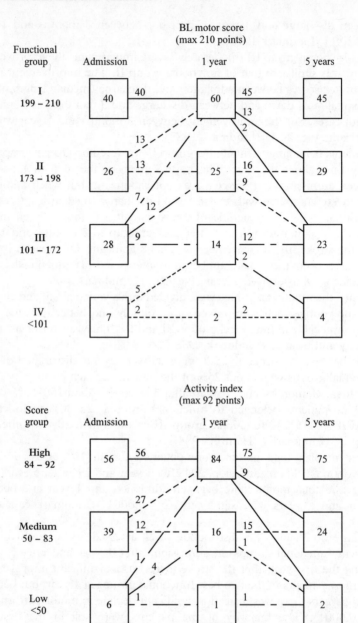

Fig. 20.2 The distribution of all 5-year survivors into functional groups according to motor assessment and activity index score groups on admission and 1 year and 5 years after the stroke (N = 101). (Adapted from Clinical Rehabilitation, with the permission of Edward Arnold.)

for balance was 14 on admission, 19 after 1 year and 17 after 5 years. The median score for walking ability was 4 on admission, 6 after 1 year and 5 after 5 years. All the differences were significant (p < 0.001) (Lindmark & Hamrin 1994).

No differences were found between men and women. Both men and women improved during the first year and deteriorated slightly but significantly in the last 4 years.

Changes in self-capacity assessed with activity index

On admission 37% of all 280 patients included in the study belonged to the high score group according to the activity index, 41% to the median score group and 22% to the low score group (Hamrin & Lindmark 1990). Both at three months and one year after the stroke about 70–80% of the survivors belonged to the high score group, about 20% to the median score group and just a few to the low score group (Lindmark & Hamrin 1989). There was a significant change between admission and 3 months (p < 0.0001) but not between 3 months and 1 year after the stroke.

The distribution of the 101 5-year survivors into different activity index score groups is given in Figure 20.2. During the first year there was improvement with 84% of the patients in the highest score group at 1 year. Between 1 and 5 years there was a slight but significant decrease (p < 0.001) and at this time 75% of the 5-year survivors were still in the highest score group (Lindmark & Hamrin 1994).

No differences were found between men and women (Lindmark & Hamrin 1994).

Changes in ADL based on structured interviews

There was a decrease in all investigated instrumental ADL activities between the time just before the stroke and 3 months after the stroke which was significant in both men and women (p < 0.001) with very few exceptions. No significant changes were then seen between 3 months and 1 year after the stroke. The activity level was maintained during this time (Lindmark & Hamrin 1989). Between 1 and 5 years some significant decreases occurred among the 5-year survivors. The results of the structured interviews concerning some activities at 1 and 5 years in men and women who survived 5 years are given in Table 20.1.

In household activity, a pronounced decrease of the activity in all variables (making coffee, cooking simple meals, washing the dishes, making the bed, cleaning, doing the laundry) is seen for both men and women 5 years after the stroke compared with 1 year after the stroke. The women were traditionally more active but they also had a significant decrease (p < 0.01) in their household activity. The decrease in the women's activity was larger than the decrease of the men's activity between before the stroke

Table 20.1 Instrumental activities of daily living in assessed 5-year survivors before the stroke and 1 year and 5 years later (52 men, 49 women)

Activity	Managed and did without help Men Before %	1 year %	5 years %	Women Before %	1 year %	5 years %
Household work						
Make coffee	77	65	61	96	78	61
Cook simple meals	44	50	33	94	73	65
Wash the dishes	54	56	39	90	73	65
Make the bed	56	44	44	90	65	51
Clean	42	37	31	57	37	33
Do the laundry	35	31	21	80	55	43
Locomotion						
Move from bed to chair	100	94	85	100	90	80
Move about at home	100	100	90	100	98	88
Manage stairs	100	83	73	92	59	57
Walk outdoors	96	81	79	90	53	55
Unlock and close entrance door	100	94	88	98	90	82
Psychosocial activities						
Write letters	37	27	25	37	24	22
Use the telephone	90	79	69	96	86	71
Visit friends	83	75	63	84	49	37
Use public transport	77	60	50	49	31	29
Visit public premises	56	52	48	47	27	20
Go shopping	87	65	63	73	49	31
Intellectual activities						
Read newspaper	94	83	85	94	88	78
Listen to news on radio/TV	100	94	90	100	94	86
Read books	40	35	40	55	45	31
Manage finances	81	65	71	78	59	45

and 1 year after the stroke ($p < 0.05$) in some household activities such as making coffee, cooking and washing the dishes (Lindmark & Hamrin 1994).

The locomotion ability (moving from bed to chair, moving about at home, managing stairs, walking outdoors, unlocking and closing the entrance door) was better maintained, but both men and women had a significant decrease in managing the stairs between 1 and 5 years post-stroke ($p < 0.05$). The women showed a significantly greater decrease in outside activities than the men from the time before the stroke to 1 year after the stroke. The women who were older had more problems with the activities of locomotion even before the stroke (Lindmark & Hamrin 1994).

Even before the stroke the women, especially, needed help from someone else with most of the psychosocial activities (writing letters, using the telephone, visiting friends, using public transport, visiting public premises). After the stroke these activities deteriorated in both sexes. Between 1 and 5 years after the stroke there was a significant decrease in the ability to use the telephone for both men and women ($p < 0.05$) and the men became less active in visiting friends ($p < 0.05$) and women in shopping without company ($p < 0.01$) (Lindmark & Hamrin 1994).

Most of the men continued with the intellectual activities (reading the newspaper, listening to the news on radio/TV, reading books, managing finances) on about the same level, but the women showed a significant decrease in activities such as reading newspapers and books and managing finances ($p < 0.05$) between 1 and 5 years post-stroke. Very few of the patients read books even before the stroke and many also had help with their finances before the stroke (Lindmark & Hamrin 1994).

Satisfaction with health and life situation

One year after the stroke 75% of the 1-year survivors regarded their health to be good or very good and 79% regarded their life situation to be good or very good (Lindmark & Hamrin 1989).

Of the 101 assessed 5-year survivors 81% were satisfied with their health and 84% with their life situation 1 year after the stroke. The corresponding figures for 5 years after the stroke were 82% and 88% (Lindmark & Hamrin 1994).

DISCUSSION

The median age of the 5-year survivors was lower at the onset of stroke than the median age of all patients included in the study, and the patients who died between 1 and 5 years post-stroke were older than the 5-year survivors. This is in agreement with Wade et al's conclusions about age being one of the predictors for long-term survival (Wade et al 1984). The men were on average younger than the women. Men seem to suffer from stroke earlier and tend not to live as long as women after a stroke.

The living conditions of the 5-year survivors did not change significantly between 1 and 5 years. A few more lived in homes for elderly people.

Changes in motor performance

The pattern of improvement of motor function and ability during the first year was in accordance with the findings of other authors (Skilbeck et al

1983, Torngren et al 1990). Most of the improvement occurred during the initial period of hospitalization and recovery and then continued at a slower rate for up to 3 months. Improvement after that time was noted mostly among the severely affected patients (Lindmark 1988).

Among the 5-year survivors there was a slight but significant decline in all function between 1 and 5 years post-stroke, especially in the ability to perform active movements, to maintain balance and to walk (Lindmark & Hamrin 1994). The decrease in median motor score from 204 to 196 does not seem large. However, this is a median score which means that quite a large group had an even greater decline. A decline of more than 10 points has clinical importance for patients. They may not be able to use the paretic arm or may have lost the control of a leg, which could lead to walking and mobility problems. Whether this decrease is a normal consequence of age or whether the decrease in activity is more pronounced in victims of stroke still has to be investigated. With increasing age some of the abilities such as maintaining balance and walking may normally be affected in the course of 4 years. Some of the patients had suffered a further stroke or TIA, but only 5 of the patients had suffered further severe strokes and when these patients were excluded there was still a similar and significant decline. One explanation could be, for example, that the patient stopped using an arm if the activity was not functionally useful and then forgot about the little activity that remained. The activities that seemed to be maintained best were those that were carried out every day such as gross mobility.

Few patients had received rehabilitation later than 1 year after the stroke. Whether late rehabilitation helps the patients to maintain their ability still has to be proven. Some promising but unpublished results of late rehabilitation have been obtained in Sweden. However, Wade et al (1992) found that late physiotherapy intervention improved mobility but that the improvement was not maintained.

Changes in ADL behaviour

Most of the improvement in self-capacity score with the activity index occurred in the first 3 months and the ability was then maintained for up to 1 year after the stroke (Lindmark & Hamrin 1989). Between 1 and 5 years post-stroke there was a slight decrease, but this was not as pronounced as in motor performance (Lindmark & Hamrin 1994). Many of the activities assessed with the activity index have to be carried out daily, and are very important for the patient's independence and are therefore maintained.

The decrease in instrumental ADL between the time before the stroke and 3 months after the stroke is of course explained by the stroke-induced impairment. The activities were then maintained up to 1 year after the stroke (Lindmark & Hamrin 1989).

The findings that the women had a larger decrease than the men in household activities is explained by the fact that women were more active before the stroke in household activities. This was also true after the stroke, but more women needed help then before. Men were more capable in activities that demanded balance and ability to move around outside both before and after the stroke. The men were on average younger and women usually had more problems with knees and hips with increasing age.

Between 1 and 5 years post-stroke ability to perform many of the activities declined (Lindmark & Hamrin 1994). This could to some extent be explained by increasing age, but was also due partly to relatives and home care services taking over many of the household duties which the patients could have performed themselves, if they had been given time, leading to overprotection. A more rehabilitation directed help might have been better, where the patients and the helpers did the household work, for instance, together.

One question that arose was whether patients with stroke needed more help than a similar group of healthy elderly people. Compared with such a group from the same province the stroke group in our study needed more help. Surviving patients with stroke seemed to be more fragile, and in need of more help than 'ordinary' healthy elderly people.

Satisfaction with health and life situation

The high proportion of patients both at 1 and 5 years post-stroke who felt satisfied with their health and life situation, in spite of motor impairment and a high level of dependence, was surprising but gratifying. The patients seemed to have adapted to their functional level over the years. In some cases neglect and poor insight may be contributory. However, many older people regard good health as equivalent to absence of symptoms of sickness and pain, and good life situation as living in one's own home, with relatives around and access to the help required.

Conclusion

The main part of the improvement of motor ability and ADL occurred during the acute stage up to 3 months after the stroke. Between 3 months and 1 year the functional level was maintained. During the following 4 years a significant decrease in almost all measured variables occurred and the patients with stroke were to a large extent dependent upon someone else. In spite of that, the majority of the patients were satisfied with their health and life situation.

Acknowledgements

This investigation was supported by grants from the Swedish Medical Research Council, the Delegation of Social Research, the King Gustav V and Queen Victoria Foundation, The Medical Faculty of Uppsala

University, Swedish Society of Medicine and 1987 Foundation for Stroke Research.

REFERENCES

Brocklehurst J C, Morris P, Andrews K, Richards B, Laycock P 1981 Social effects of stroke. Social Science Medicine 15A: 35–39
Collen F M, Wade D T 1991 Residual mobility problems after stroke. International Disability Studies 13: 12–15
Greveson G C, Gray C S, French J M, James O F W 1991 Long-term outcome for patients and carers following hospital admission for stroke. Age and Ageing 20: 337–344
Hamrin E 1982 III. One year after stroke: a follow-up of an experimental study. Scandinavian Journal of Rehabilitation Medicine 14: 111–116
Hamrin E, Wohlin A 1982 I. Evaluation of the functional capacity of stroke patients through an activity index. Scandinavian Journal of Rehabilitation Medicine 14: 93–100
Hamrin E, Lindmark B 1990 The effect of systematic care planning after acute stroke in general hospital medical wards. Journal of Advanced Nursing 15: 1146–1153
Lindmark B 1988 The improvement of different motor functions after acute stroke. Clinical Rehabilitation 2: 275–280
Lindmark B, Hamrin E 1988a Evaluation of functional capacity after stroke as basis for active intervention. Presentation of a modified chart for motor capacity assessment and its reliability. Scandinavian Journal of Rehabilitation Medicine 20: 103–109
Lindmark B, Hamrin E 1988b Evaluation of functional capacity after stroke as a basis for active intervention. Validation of a modified chart for motor capacity assessment. Scandinavian Journal of Rehabilitation Medicine 20: 111–115
Lindmark B, Hamrin E 1989 Instrumental activities of daily living in two patient populations three months and one year after acute stroke. Scandinavian Journal of Caring Sciences 3: 161–168
Lindmark B, Hamrin E 1994 A five-year follow-up of stroke survivors: motor function and activities of daily living. Accepted for publication in Clinical Rehabilitation
Skilbeck C E, Wade D T, Langton-Hewer R, Wood V A 1983 Recovery after stroke. Journal of Neurology, Neurosurgery and Psychiatry 46: 5–8
Torngren M, Westling B, Norrving B 1990 Outcome after stroke in patients discharged to independent living. Stroke 21: 236–240
Viitanen M, Fugl-Meyer K S, Bernspång B, Fugl-Meyer A R 1988 Life satisfaction in long-term survivors after stroke. Scandinavian Journal of Rehabilitation Medicine 20: 17–24
Wade D T, Skilbeck C E, Wood V A, Langton-Hewer R 1984 Long-term survival after stroke. Age and Ageing 13: 76–82
Wade D T, Collen F M, Robb G F, Warlow C P 1992 Physiotherapy intervention late after stroke and mobility. British Medical Journal 304: 609–613

21. A study of reaching movements in stroke patients

P. van Vliet,   D. G. Kerwin,   M. R. Sheridan,
P. Fentem

INTRODUCTION

The experiment reported here is one of a series, which aim to clarify the main differences between the way stroke patients perform goal-directed movements in comparison with normal people. A common therapeutic aim is to help the stroke patient to regain movement that is as normal as possible. In order to do this, it is necessary to know what the details of these differences are. Detailed analyses of stroke patients' and normal people's movement can be used to formulate hypotheses about underlying control processes and treatment strategies can be formulated on this basis. One way to obtain these detailed analyses is to measure the kinematics of movements, including displacement, velocity and acceleration.

This study aims to begin to determine whether stroke patients' reaching kinematics reflect the preservation of normal movement organisation for reaching or whether they employ very different organisational strategies. One characteristic of normal reaching that emerges clearly from the literature is that the kinematics of reaching alter according to task constraints. The task being performed appears to be a major factor in the formulation of a motor programme for movement. In this chapter, an experiment is reported which investigated the ability of stroke patients and normal subjects to adapt the kinematics of their reaching movements to different task constraints.

Two distinct phases have been identified in normal reaching movements. First, a high-velocity ballistic movement of the hand towards the target, and secondly, a low-velocity phase as the hand nears the target (Jeannerod 1981, 1984). Experiments examining the two phase structure of aimed movements have involved manipulation of the speed or distance moved, or the accuracy requirements of tasks. These experiments have shown that there is a trade-off between speed and accuracy, where the more accurate a movement is, the slower it will be. Fitts (1954) showed that in tasks where subjects moved a stylus between two targets as quickly as possible, movement time increased with both the distance separating the targets and the narrowness of the actual targets.

During reaching movements, the peak velocity of the hand is usually achieved within the first 50% of the movement time where the movement consists of one bell-shaped velocity profile (Jeannerod 1984, Marteniuk et al 1987), but this can vary according to task constraints. Marteniuk and his colleagues (1987, 1990) studied the kinematic characteristics of normal reaching when grasping discs of different sizes and when grasping a fragile object (a lightbulb) versus a soft resilient object (a tennis ball). They found that the peak velocity, expressed as a percentage of movement time, occurred earlier in the trajectory when more precision was required, allowing for a longer deceleration phase. Different tasks performed with the same object were also compared. Subjects grasped a disc to either throw it into a large box or place it in a tight fitting well. The peak velocity occurred earlier in the more precise fitting task. Thus the proportion of time spent in each phase can vary according to the task. These findings support the view that the task is an important factor in the formulation of a motor programme. The main question addressed by this study is, can patients with stroke adapt their movement kinematics for different task constraints?

METHOD

Subjects

Eight stroke and eight normal subjects participated in the experiment. The stroke group was homogenous in the following respects:

1. Subjects had a total anterior circulation infarct (TACI) or partial anterior circulation infarct (PACI) according to the Bamford classification for cerebral infarction (Bamford et al 1991). This classification is based on clinical signs and symptoms and TACI and PACI indicate ischaemia in the territory of the middle and anterior cerebral arteries. For five out of the eight stroke subjects, the involvement of the middle cerebral artery was confirmed by computed tomography scan.

2. None of the subjects had had a previous cerebrovascular accident.

3. Subjects' arm function scored between 3 and 5 on the arm section of the Rivermead motor assessment (Lincoln & Leadbitter 1979). A score of 3 is described as 'Lying; holding extended arm in elevation with some external rotation, the subject is able to flex and extend the elbow. The elbow must extend to at least 30 degrees of full flexion.' A score of 4 is described as 'Sitting; elbow is held unsupported and at right angles into side – pronate and supinate at least three-quarters of normal range.' A score of 5 is described as 'Reach forward, pick up large ball with both hands and place down. Ball is on table in front of the patient.'

General characteristics of the stroke subjects are shown in Table 21.1. Spasticity was measured using the modified Ashworth scale (Bohannon & Smith 1987). The scale ranges from 0 to 4, where 0 is 'no increase in muscle

Table 21.1 Patient characteristics

Subject	Age	No. of weeks since stroke	Side of lesion (CVA)	Hemianopia	Arm function	Spasticity			Sensation					Neglect	Spatial ability	Pain
						Elbow	Wrist	Fingers	Touch	Pressure	Kinematic	2-pt palm	2-pt finger			
1	64	1.5	R	No	4	2	0	1	2	2	2	1	1	49	16.5	0
2	67	19	L	No	4	2	2	0	1	1	1	1	0	54	31	0
3	72	6	R	Yes	4	0	0	1	2	2	3	1	2	54	21	0
4	63	3.5	R	Yes	4	2	0	0	2	2	3	1	1	52	21.5	0
5	63	30	R	No	4	1+	3	2	2	2	3	0	0	53	32	2
6	75	4	R	No	3	1	0	1	1	1	1	0	1	50	15	0
7	77	9	R	No	4	1+	0	0	2	2	2	0	1	37	20.5	2
8	70	8	L	No	4	2	0	0	2	2	3	1	1	53	13	0

tone' and 4 is 'affected part rigid in flexion or extension'. In most cases, the body part could be moved easily, with often a slight, or a more marked increase in the muscle tone felt by the examiner. Sensation was measured using the Nottingham sensory assessment (Lincoln et al 1991). The subject scores 0 if the sensation is absent on testing, and 2 or 3 if the sensation is normal. The presence of visuospatial neglect was tested using the Star cancellation test (Wilson et al 1987). Normal scores lie between 51 and 54. Spatial abilities were tested by the Rey figure copy (Rey 1959). Normal scores for this test are between 31 and 36 points. The present pain intensity, from the McGill pain questionnaire (Melzack 1987) was used to determine the presence of shoulder pain, both before the experiment and after an initial practice session. On this scale of 0 to 5, a score of 0 equals no pain.

Normal subjects were matched to the stroke subjects for age and whether their dominant or non-dominant hand was used in the experiment, and for sex, where possible. The mean age of the normal subject group was 64.6 years. There were 5 females and 3 males in this group. The mean age of the stroke subject group was 68.9 years and there were 4 females and 4 males in this group.

Equipment

A two-dimensional video technique was used to measure the reaching movements. A single video camera, positioned above the seated subject, recorded the reaching movements with the aid of photographic lighting. A calibration object of known dimensions was placed in the field of view and recorded prior to testing each subject. Data were collected at 50 Hz. Once recorded, video data were manually digitised and filtered using computer software designed for this purpose (Kerwin 1993). A Butterworth filter with a cut-off frequency of 5 Hz was used.

Experimental set-up

Subjects were seated at a table, with their waist resting against the table edge and their wrist resting on the starting position, a predetermined distance from a cup in front of them. The distance for the stroke subjects was the maximum distance they could reach and still make an attempt to grasp the cup. The stroke subjects reached different distances according to their ability. The distance for normal subjects was determined by placing the cup in a position where the subjects would have their elbow 10 degrees short of full extension when grasping the cup, so the distance was calibrated to the individual subject for normal subjects also. The distance was measured and a marker placed on the table in the end position. At the start of each movement, the subjects' forearm was in a mid-pronated position and the tips of the index finger and thumb were lightly touching. An adhesive paper marker was placed on the radial styloid to indicate wrist position and all measures were derived from the position of this marker. The subjects were instructed to perform the movements in their own time.

Procedure

The experimental design for both normal and stroke subject groups was a one way block design. Each subject performed five trials under each of four conditions. The conditions were as follows:

1. Reach forward to pick up an empty cup and place it on the table closer to them (behind a marked line).
2. Reach forward to pick up a cup half-filled with water and place it on the table closer to them (behind the marked line).
3. Reach forward to pick up a cup three-quarters filled with water and place it on the table closer to them (behind the marked line).
4. Reach forward to pick up a cup three-quarters filled with water and take a drink from it, then place it back on the table (behind the marked line).

To minimise learning from previous trials and to minimise fatigue, the conditions occurred in a random sequence. To familiarise the subjects with the movements required and thereby to further reduce any learning effect, the subjects practised each movement at least twice before recording began. Subjects were given a 5-minute rest after this practice and then 2 minutes' rest between each condition in the experiment.

Data analysis

A standard software application (Excel 4) was used to analyse the data. The dependent variables were movement time (duration of the movement), average velocity, peak velocity, and the time at which peak velocity occurred as a percentage of movement time. The movement time was defined as the time at which the maximum distance of the wrist was first reached, minus the time at which the wrist first moved forward. Although the tasks involved grasping, the analysis was performed only on the approach to the cup (the reaching phase). Statistical analyses were performed on these measures using analyses of variance with supplementary Newman Keul's tests to determine between which conditions any significant differences lay. Analysés were performed on the mean scores of each condition for each subject. To test whether the subsequent task (drinking or moving) had any effect on the kinematics, a separate analysis of variance was performed on conditions 3 and 4.

Direct comparison of the measures between the stroke and normal groups was not appropriate as, of necessity, individuals in the two groups moved different distances, and distance could affect the measures chosen rather than any inherent differences between the two groups. It was thought that there may be a difference in the variability of performance between normal and stroke subjects, so an analysis of variance on the coefficients of variation of each measure was performed. The coefficient of variation was calculated by dividing the standard deviation by the mean for each condition for each subject.

RESULTS

Stroke subjects moved shorter distances than normal subjects (approximately 5–10 cm shorter); they were much slower than normal subjects and were not always successful at grasping the cup.

Table 21.2 shows the means of the eight stroke subjects compared to the means of the eight normal subjects, for each of the measured variables.

For the normal subjects, there was a significant difference between conditions for movement time, $F(3,21) = 3.165$; $p < 0.05$ and average velocity, $F(3,21) = 4.762$; $p < 0.05$. This result arose from condition 1 being different from each of the other conditions. There were no differences between conditions 2, 3 or 4. In condition 1, where subjects picked up the empty cup, the movement time was shorter and the average velocity was higher.

For the stroke subjects, there were no significant differences between conditions for any of the variables tested in the main analysis of variance. The separate analysis for conditions 3 and 4 however, showed a significant difference for movement time, $F(7,7) = 11.25$; $p < 0.01$, where movement time was shorter for grasping the three-quarter full cup to drink as opposed to moving it. Average velocity was higher for drinking than for moving but

Table 21.2 Means and standard deviations (in parentheses) of movement time (MT), peak velocity (PV), % peak velocity/movement time (% PV/MT) and average velocity (AV), in each condition, for normal and stroke subjects

		Condition 1	Condition 2	Condition 3	Condition 4
MT (s)	Normal	0.87 (0.16)	0.93 (0.23)	0.95 (0.21)	0.94 (0.18)
	Stroke	5.98 (3.61)	5.42 (2.57)	5.85 (2.19)	4.64 (1.75)
PV (m/s)	Normal	0.65 (0.14)	0.62 (0.13)	0.55 (0.23)	0.6 (0.11)
	Stroke	0.144 (0.74)	0.145 (0.064)	0.126 (0.036)	0.14 (0.026)
%PV/MT	Normal	35.5 (3.46)	34.2 (4.3)	34.7 (4.9)	32.7 (5)
	Stroke	33.1 (17.9)	31.9 (15)	27.3 (12)	26.1 (14.1)
AV (m/s)	Normal	0.314 (0.054)	0.298 (0.055)	0.283 (0.044)	0.277 (0.04)
	Stroke	0.045 (0.025)	0.044 (0.026)	0.035 (0.020)	0.045 (0.023)

the difference was not significant. Six out of eight subjects increased their average velocity, and two subjects decreased their velocity (subjects 7 and 8). Subject 7 had the greatest decrease in average velocity. Table 21.1 shows that this subject was the only one with an obvious visuospatial neglect, and also was one of the two subjects with shoulder pain.

The variability of the stroke subjects was significantly greater than that of normal subjects for all the variables tested including percentage time of peak velocity, $F(1,14) = 36.91$; $p < 0.01$, movement time, $F(1,14) = 17.343$; $p < 0.01$, peak velocity $F(1,14) = 21.05$; $p < 0.01$ and average velocity, $F(1,14) = 11.06$; $p < 0.01$. Stroke subjects also differed significantly from each other for percentage time of peak velocity, $F(7,21) = 3.63$; $p < 0.05$, movement time, $F(7,21) = 40.22$; $p < 0.01$, peak velocity, $F(7,21) = 4.04$; $p < 0.05$ and average velocity, $F(7,21) = 17.11$; $p < 0.01$.

DISCUSSION

There is some evidence of a trade-off between speed and accuracy in the normal subjects as picking up the empty cup, the easiest task in terms of precision and complexity, was performed with more speed. The other three tasks were different from the first in terms of the amount of water in the cup and the task to be performed with the cup. The increased level of difficulty of each of these tasks was insufficient to cause normal subjects to alter their strategy.

It was anticipated that stroke subjects would find these tasks more difficult and so differences between tasks would be sufficient to affect the reaching kinematics. This was not the case however as there were no differences between the stroke subjects' scores when all conditions were compared. The two tasks concerned with the difficulty of the subsequent task, moving or drinking from the three-quarter full cup, were different however. The more difficult task of drinking, which involved first drinking then placing the cup back on the table close to the subject, was performed with a higher average velocity (though not significantly higher) and shorter movement time. Normal subjects, had the tasks been sufficiently different, would have been expected to respond in the opposite way.

Variability was greatly increased in stroke subjects compared to normal subjects. Normal subjects tend to become more variable when moving either longer distances or with greater force. Schmidt et al (1979) found a greater variability in end-point accuracy when moving longer distances. Stroke subjects moved shorter distances than normal subjects. Normal subjects moving shorter distances would be expected to have decreased variability, but the stroke subjects' variability increased in all of the measured variables. Variability of performance appears to be a major problem with stroke subjects. Given the amount of variability, it is not surprising that there were few differences between their performance in different tasks.

Individual stroke subjects were able to perform the movement quite well on some occasions, but on others would do something very different, implying that the basic mechanism for reaching was present, although they could not perform the task consistently. This emphasises the need, in measuring reaching performance for clinical or research purposes, to assess not only that stroke patients can perform the task, but also that they can repeat it.

One of the differences between reaching of stroke subjects and normal subjects is their lower peak velocity. Trombly (1993) has shown that the amplitude of peak velocity can increase in stroke subjects over the course of time. Average velocities were not reported in Trombly's study. It is interesting that the stroke subjects responded to the drinking task by increasing their average velocity. Increasing the average velocity is a reasonable therapeutic goal, if the aim is to train patients to move as normally as possible. It may therefore be useful sometimes to increase the functional demands of a task to improve performance in terms of increasing the overall speed. It is possible that increasing the speed of performance could make the movement smoother also, as an improvement in smoothness accompanied an increase in the amplitude of peak velocity in Trombly's study. Alternatively, increasing the average velocity might also have detrimental effects, such as increasing the variability of the movement. To check this, the coefficients of variation for average velocity for the drinking and moving tasks were compared and the drinking task had no greater variability than the simple moving task.

In conclusion, the group of stroke patients in this study, who were developing the ability to reach forward and attempt to grasp a cup, were not able to adapt their reaching kinematics to different tasks in the way that normal subjects can. These stroke subjects demonstrated considerable variability in their reaching movements, making it difficult for them to alter their reaching strategy for different tasks. They showed some differences in their performance for drinking from a cup compared to moving it, but their response to the more difficult task was different from normal.

Acknowledgement

This work was funded by the Stroke Association, UK.

REFERENCES

Bamford J, Sandercock P, Dennis M, Burn J, Warlow C 1991 Classification and natural history of clinically identifiable subtypes of cerebral infarction. Lancet 337: 1521–1526
Bohannon R W, Smith M B 1987 Interrater reliability of a modified Ashworth scale of muscle spasticity. Physical Therapy 67: 206–207
Fitts P M 1954 The information capacity of the human motor system in controlling the amplitude of movement. Journal of Experimental Psychology 47: 381–391

Jeannerod M 1981 Intersegmental coordination during reaching at natural objects. In: Long J, Baddeley A (eds) Attention and performance IX. Erlbaum, Hillsdale NJ, pp 153–169

Jeannerod M 1984 The timing of natural prehension movements. Journal of Motor Behaviour 26(3): 235–254

Kerwin D G 1993 High resolution video digitisation. In: Yeadon M R (ed) Proceedings of the British Association of Sports Sciences, Biomechanics section. Loughborough University of Technology, Loughborough, 18: 25–28

Lincoln N B, Leadbitter D 1979 Assessment of motor function in stroke patients. Physiotherapy 65: 48–51

Lincoln N B, Crow J L, Jackson J M, Waters G R, Adams S A, Hodgson P 1991 The unreliability of sensory assessments. Clinical Rehabilitation 5: 273–282

Marteniuk R G, MacKenzie C L, Jeannerod M, Athenes S, Dugas C 1987 Constraints of human arm trajectories. Canadian Journal of Psychology 41(3): 365–378

Marteniuk R G, Leavitt J L, MacKenzie C L, Athenes S 1990 Functional relationships between grasp and transport components in a prehension task. Human Movement Science 9: 149–176

Melzack R 1987 The short-form McGill pain questionnaire. Pain 30: 191–197

Rey A 1959 Le test, de copie de figure complexe. Editions Centre de Psychologie Applique, Paris

Schmidt R A, Zelanznik H N, Hawkings B, Frank J S, Quinn J T Jr 1979 Motor output variability: a theory for the accuracy of rapid motor acts. Psychological Review 86: 415–451

Trombly C A 1993 Observations of improvement of reaching in five subjects with left hemiparesis. Journal of Neurology, Neurosurgery and Psychiatry 56: 40–45

Wilson B, Cockburn J, Halligan P W 1987 Behavioural inattention test. Thames Valley Test Company, Titchfield, Hants

22. Comparison of two motor function scales (FIM/RMA)

M. L. Seisenbacher

INTRODUCTION

Rehabilitation of people with stroke is an important medical and social need. The ultimate goal is to enable the patient to perform, as fully as possible, activities of daily living despite continued impairment (WHO 1989). In Austria this is accomplished by early rehabilitation measures while the patient is in the acute hospital (in a special stroke unit, or in the general neurological or medical ward); in addition, the patient may be transferred to an inpatient rehabilitation centre and finally after discharge from being an inpatient may be treated on an outpatient basis in special rehabilitation and physiotherapy centres.

Since rehabilitation can be costly and admission to special rehabilitation facilities is limited, various criteria and prognostic measurements of impairment and disability have been developed (Alexander 1994, Granger & Hamilton 1990, Ottenbacher 1993). Furthermore, in the light of increasing costs and limited resources and findings, evaluation of rehabilitation outcome is becoming increasingly important (Kesselring & Gamper 1992, Gloag 1985, Wade 1992b). In the future it will be necessary to provide information about the patient's functional change during rehabilitation, the speed with which gains are obtained and the degree to which the individual patient's potential to function was obtained. This quality assessment and quality assurance will have an effect on patient care, on comparing rehabilitation services in different settings, on the selection of patients for specialized rehabilitation units and on the availability of sufficient funding (Wade 1992a).

COMPARISON STUDY

There are a variety of scales to evaluate possible effective outcome during the rehabilitation phase. The Barthel index and the more recent functional independence measure (FIM) are prototypes of disability measures which assess functional skill and try to document rehabilitation measures uniformly (Keith et al 1987).

The Rivermead motor assessment (RMA) is another test to measure motor function after stroke (Lincoln & Leadbitter 1979). The scale mixes impairments (arm, leg, trunk) and disabilities (gross function).

These two standard scales of functional recovery were compared in an inpatient rehabilitation centre which admits the patient approximately 2–3 months after the onset of acute stroke.

122 (55 female, 67 male) consecutive patients admitted to the Grossgmain-Salzburg neurological rehabilitation centre were evaluated on admission and again at discharge. Each patient was evaluated by the rehabilitation team using the FIM and the RMA.

Functional independence measure

The FIM is an 18 item rating scale of functional capacities in dressing, walking, toileting and communication. For purposes of comparison of motor function, a 13 item score (A–M), eliminating items referring to communication and cognitive function (N–R), was used. A seven-point scale was used to reflect the burden of care required. The underlying rationale for classifying an activity as 'independent' or 'dependent' is whether another person (a helper) is required, and if help is required, how much.

Rivermead motor assessment

The RMA is divided into three sections: gross function, leg and trunk function and arm function. The first category deals with functional movement and assesses a range of movements from sitting, and sitting to standing to transfers and ambulation. The second category deals with the degree of control of movement. The third category concerns both motor control and functional movement of the arm.

Results

54 patients had a left cerebral lesion, 64 had a right cerebral lesion and four had other (frontal pons) lesions. Patients ranged in age from 13 years old (77x ± SD, 52 ± 13 years). The average length of inpatient rehabilitation was 36 days.

All patients were treated by a team of physiotherapists and occupational therapists experienced in neurological rehabilitation using the concepts of Bobath, PNF and Perfetti.

Professor Perfetti's approach is based on the awareness of sensorimotor input (Perfetti 1986). For instance, the patient's limb is led over various surfaces or objects, such as geometrical figures. The patient is then asked to interpret the tactile and kinaesthetic information (i.e. a cognitive therapeutic exercise). This attention drawn to the hemiplegic side causes a potent facilitatory stimulus for arm, trunk or leg and adaption of the muscle tone.

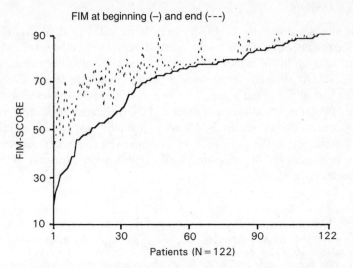

Fig. 22.1 Change of score from the initial to final examination in the individual patients assessed by the FIM.

If the patient is already able to carry out selective movements without spasticity, a carefully monitored extension of the exercise programme is possible.

The average period of individual therapy was 2 hours per day. Results are given in Figures 22.1 and 22.2 for each method of evaluation in the 122 patients treated in an inpatient neuro-rehabilitation centre.

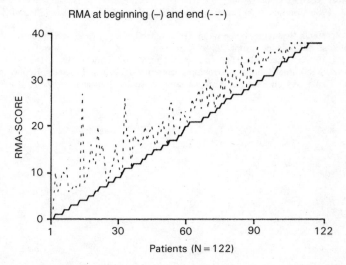

Fig. 22.2 Change of score from the initial to final examination in the individual patients assessed by the RMA.

CONCLUSION

In this study changes in the FIM scores from initial to final examination were seen mainly in patients with a marked depressed initial score, whereas patients with an initial higher score (> 70) showed only minor changes.

The RMA showed improvement from initial to final evaluation independent of the initial score. The format of the RMA assesses both the degree of impairment in motor control and the qualitative functional aspects of movement. Therefore, the RMA adds qualitative aspects of movement, is of importance in the evaluation of patients with less severe impairment and is preferable in the assessment of rehabilitation measures weeks or months after the stroke.

REFERENCES

Alexander M P 1994 Stroke rehabilitation outcome. A potential use of predictive variables to establish levels of care. Stroke 25: 128–134

Gloag D 1985 Rehabilitation after stroke: What is the potential? British Medical Journal 290: 699–701

Granger C V, Hamilton B B 1990 Measurement of stroke rehabilitation outcome in the 1980s. Stroke 21 (suppl. II): 46–47

Keith R A, Granger C V, Hamilton B B, Sherwin F S 1987 The functional independence measure: a new tool for rehabilitation. In: Eisenberg M G, Grzesiak R C (eds) Advances in clinical rehabilitation, Springer Verlag, New York, vol 1, pp 6–18

Kesselring J, Gamper U N 1992 Vom Nutzen der Neurorehabilitation. Schweizer Medizinische Wochenschrift 122: 1206–1211

Lincoln N B, Leadbitter D 1979 Assessment of motor function in stroke patients. Physiotherapy 65: 48–55

Ottenbacher K J, Jannell S 1993 The results of clinical trials in stroke rehabilitation research. Archives Neurology 50: 37–44

Perfetti C 1986 Condotte terapeutiche per la rieducazione dell'emiplegico. Ghedini Editore, Milano

Wade D T 1992a Evaluating outcome in stroke rehabilitation. Scandinavian Journal Rehabilitation Medicine, suppl. 26: 97–104

Wade D T 1992b Stroke: rehabilitation and long term care. Lancet 339: 791–793

WHO 1989 Recommendations on stroke prevention, diagnosis and therapy. Report of the WHO Task Force on Stroke and other cerebro-vascular disorders. Stroke 20: 1407–1431

23. Measurement in neurological rehabilitation (abstract)

D. T. Wade

USES OF MEASURES

Neurological rehabilitation is a reiterative problem-solving process, and measurement is a vital part of this. First, measures may be useful to identify and quantify problems. Secondly, they may help in understanding the situation. Thirdly, they may help prioritise problems (or patients). Lastly, and most importantly, measures should be used to evaluate the effectiveness of interventions both in research and in day-to-day clinical practice.

CHOOSING A MEASURE

The most important single question to consider when choosing a measure is: 'What do I really want to know and why?'

Measures should never be used unthinkingly; it wastes your time and the patient's time.

Once the reason for measuring has been considered, then a measure can be chosen. For each measure considered one should ask:

• Will it measure what I want it to measure?	Validity
• Will anyone else believe the results?	Validity and reliability
• How much will the result vary from time to time?	Reliability
• Will it detect the change/difference I am interested in?	Sensitivity
• Will I or anyone else be able to use it regularly?	Simplicity
• Will anyone else understand the results?	Communicability

When choosing a measure, start by discovering what suitable measures exist. In most circumstances there will be several available. If at all possible choose and use an existing measure – it saves time and effort.

Finally, be sure to distinguish between measures of process and measures of outcome. In general, measures of outcome will be at the level of disability or handicap, whereas measures of impairment will be measures of process. While it is easier to measure impairment, and it can be reasonable, in most contexts it is important to measure outcome in functional terms.

24. Quality management in physiotherapy: challenges to clinicians

T. B. Buene

INTRODUCTION

Health personnel strive to meet increasing expectations from patients and other users of health services. It is a constant challenge to meet requirements set by authorities, politicians and society at a time when budget control and budget cuts seems to be more important than patient satisfaction.

Health personnel are also challenged to meet professional and ethical standards set by themselves and their own associations. Research and new technology reveal a never-ending list of new opportunities as to what could be done for each individual 'if only ... '. The gap between everyday practice and technological possibilities seems to be wider than ever.

Quality in health services can be described as satisfying patient's needs, fulfilling professional standards or meeting requirements set by authorities. The task sometimes seems overwhelming. Up until now too little has been done to clarify what is good and acceptable physiotherapy practice according to accepted professional standards. In this chapter an overview is given of the principles in quality management.

Quality management can act as a tool to better practice in accordance with professional standards for physiotherapy services. The main purpose of the Copenhagen conference was to give updated knowledge of what was known about stroke and the effect of physiotherapy upon patients with stroke. This, in turn, can give a common platform for further development if one dares to accept something as good and to reject other treatments as not acceptable.

FROM HEALTH PROMOTION TO LONG-TERM CARE

Physiotherapists seem to care too little about being involved in health promotion as a means of prevention of stroke. Quality policy on a national level or for an individual community should include aims and quality goals as well as a total concept of services for patients with stroke, and should contain a chain of care from activities related to health promotion, and prevention, through acute treatment and rehabilitation to long-term care.

Society needs the know-how and the expertise which physiotherapists have, in order to create a better environment for people who have to live with the consequences of a stroke. Physiotherapists must bring their knowledge to the attention of administrators and politicians in order to promote adequate, updated and ethical, acceptable health services and care for patients with stroke.

Health services for patients with stroke are a multidisciplinary task. All team members have a common challenge to develop updated, scientifically-based and well documented services for patients with stroke.

The main task for health personnel is to meet the patients expectations for a better life following the incidence of a stroke. The patients' main concerns will be:

• Who can help me to be the person I used to be?
• What can I do to recover as soon as possible?

A wide variety of different modalities and techniques have been offered to patients with stroke. For people to gain confidence in physiotherapy services, it is necessary to reduce the variation in the wide range of services that are currently accepted by the profession. Physiotherapists themselves must clarify what is accepted as *good* physiotherapy practice, what is outdated, and what cannot be accepted. Physiotherapists must clarify benefits, risks and the cost of acceptable services and systematically explore, test and revise what is done in order to improve quality.

Today many patients with stroke will not be offered adequate medical help. Some patients are offered adequate acute medical services, but no follow-up rehabilitation or help in adjusting to social life. A policy statement relating to stroke management can be:

All patients with stroke shall be offered adequate medical services as soon as possible and a rehabilitation programme that enables them to reach the highest level of health and function possible, in accordance with their medical condition.

This is an individual approach to the challenge.

Most politicians, economists and bureaucrats are likely to add: 'fully meeting requirements at the lowest cost'; or, as Øvretveit states (1992):

Fully meeting the needs of those who need the service most, at the lowest cost to the organization, within limits and directives set by higher authorities and purchasers.

This is a political approach – and both approaches are necessary.

There will always be discussion about priorities in health services. Priorities cannot be left to the individual care giver and the patient alone. Physiotherapists must present what they can accomplish according to updated knowledge. Politicians and administrations will present their priorities, and very often the conclusion is:

'All that could be done cannot be done because of lack of resources.'

Physiotherapists must accept cost–benefit analyses as obligatory on the priority list. Quality management in health services, and in physiotherapy, will not only be to plan for an optimal service. Each hospital, clinic or individual physiotherapist will have to consider what can be done with the knowledge and the resources available today, and may clarify what could be done with more resources. Nevertheless, future patients with stroke will not demand less, expect less, or ask for less help than today's patients!

To achieve excellence, physiotherapists have to contribute to their department's system for planning and organization, as well as delivery and evaluation of services. The department has to decide which quality goals will be acceptable. Quality must be described, characterized or defined in order to become an explicit goal for which to aim.

Quality is the totality of characteristics of an entity that bear on its ability to satisfy stated and implied needs. Quality is the ability of the organization – or of a professional – to satsify patients' stated or implied needs. The challenge is to plan, produce and deliver adequate services according to acceptable professional guidelines in accordance with the needs of the individual stroke patient.

QUALITY MANAGEMENT

Quality management is the overal approach of an organization to meet quality requirements. The attainment of the desired quality requires the commitment and participation of all members of the organization, whereas the responsibility for quality management belongs to top management:

All activities of the overall management function which determine the quality policy, objectives and responsibilities and their implementation by means such as quality assurance and quality improvement within the quality system. (ISO/DIS 8402)

Top management will always be responsible for the decision to implement a quality policy and develop a quality improvement process, but no

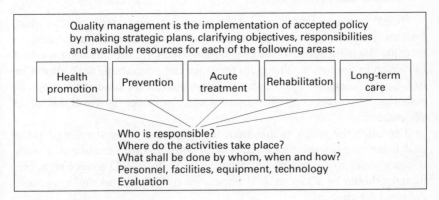

Fig. 24.1 Quality management.

management can implement a process without the commitment of all employees. Excellence is a state of mind, a dedication to do better and a common striving towards accepted goals.

Quality management is all the activities undertaken by the management to determine a quality policy, setting objectives and giving responsibilities to employees. The implementation requires means, such as planning, control and quality assurance systems, and commitment of a continuous process of improvement. No important changes will take place without the participation and dedication of all members of the organization.

Activities and efforts towards improvement will benefit the organization itself, its staff, its user (patients), and society as a whole.

QUALITY POLICY

Quality policy is the intention and stated expression of an organization with regard to quality. To achieve this policy, the organization needs a system for implementation, which states structure, responsibilities, procedures, processes and resources. There will be no progress made by the organization if quality policy and implementation is left to the imagination of each employee.

THE SYSTEM

The system has to strive to achieve excellence in the following:

- organization and administration of services
- staffing
- policies and procedures
- staff development and education
- facilities and equipment
- quality assurance programme
- evaluation and monitoring.

Quality management is a tool for employers and employees to make 'visions become reality'. Systematic work and outlined plans need to vizualize the main lines and the direction in which the organization may wish to turn to in the future. The main focus for the programme shall always be to keep the client's, or the patient's, best interest in mind throughout all activities. The main question for any activity must be: 'how will this affect the patient?'

Too often the reality is that *what we believe we do* – and *what we really wish to do* – are not *what we actually do*. Too often the evaluation of a piece of work seems to document that activities and effects did produce what one thought should be achieved. It is imperative to face realities and appreciate the need for change.

There is a need for a more integrated decision-making process based on research, documentation, evaluation and integrated decision-making rather than on individual choice, beliefs and preferences.

In order to 'do the right thing right the first time', it is necessary to know what the 'right thing' is. How do we know what is right for a person suffering from a stroke? What examinations must be done? Which signs lead to the right differential diagnoses? It is hoped that the Copenhagen conference gave some guiding principles as to what is good, current, acceptable and advisable treatment for patients with stroke at different stages; thereby creating a more common platform for what can be specified as good and acceptable physiotherapy practice throughout Europe.

GUIDELINES

Guidelines, or standards for good practice, can be set at a national level or for a certain hospital or a clinic. Guidelines can be set for a multidisciplinary team or for a group of professionals, e.g. physiotherapists. The recommendation will be to have guidelines for a multidisciplinary team handling patients with stroke and supplementary guidelines and procedures for each profession.

Guidelines and procedures should be at hand in a book available to everybody in the department. Guidelines are:

• the guiding principles for preventive, diagnostic, therapeutic or management procedures
• a written abstract of actual current professional knowledge representing a professional position generally agreed upon
• comments to present to practitioners regarding acceptable practice according to a given diagnosis
• a way to present professional knowledge to patients, other staff members or the public
• a tool for everyday practice and a prerequisite for quality assurance.

Guidelines state in a more overall manner than a procedure:

• what to do
• how to do it
• who can do what
• equipment
• documentation.

Guidelines can be developed by a multidisciplinary expert team or by a team of professional experts with various backgrounds and experiences.

The team must work out a proposal for guidelines based upon knowledge from scientific research (literature search), professional knowledge, clinical and empiric traditions, practice patterns, documentation from clinical research, equipment available and accepted technology.

The team must take into consideration known benefits from different regimes, known harmful effects or side-effects of different regimes, and the cost of different alternatives.

A proposal presenting goals, methods, expected effects and benefits of the guidelines must be presented to a large number of clinicians and evaluated by them before being accepted as, for example, national guidelines regarding stroke management. Someone must be responsible for continuous updating, re-evaluation and revision of the guidelines if they are to have any impact as a tool in a quality improvement process. Guidelines and procedures can be a tool for more standardized examination, handling and treatment, and can help in a quality improvement process.

PROCEDURES

Procedures are written documents held within a department which, for a certain activity, state in detail:

- what will be done by whom
- when it will be done
- where it will take place
- how it will be done
- how to document non-conformity.

A procedure also contains a list of necessary equipment and how this equipment will be controlled and maintained.

A procedure is established to ensure that intended activities will be achieved. The procedure must have the acceptance of everybody working within the organization, and its intention is that all activities shall:

- meet well defined or implied needs
- satisfy patient expectations
- comply with applicable and acceptable standards/guidelines
- comply with requirements of society, including cost considerations (alternative costs).

A procedure is made explicit and written down to make it more likely that the process undertaken will give the expected outcome, and that every person involved will act the same way.

QUALITY ASSURANCE

Quality assurance is all those planned and systematic actions necessary to provide adequate confidence that a product or a service will satisfy given requirements for quality. In health services the aims of quality assurance systems are to reflect the needs of patients. An organization, i.e. a hospital or a clinic, should seek to accomplish the following objectives with regard to quality:

- achieve and sustain the quality of the service so as to continually meet the patient's stated or implied needs
- give confidence to its own management that the intended quality is being achieved and sustained
- give confidence to the patient that the intended quality is being or will be achieved.

Quality management for stroke patients has to include systematic plans to ensure that all patients receive appropriate service from the first stage of acute-intensive care until they have settled back in their own home, where many will have to cope with the lasting effects of the stroke for the rest of their lives.

Rehabilitation should give appropriate service at the right time. The patient should be subjected to the same guiding principles of care when moved from hospital to nursing home. There should be no change in the overall guiding principles for patients when moved from one clinic to another, or to home care.

The same guiding principles, the same procedures and the same concept of progress towards self-sufficient care, should be a part of the individual care plan to instil in each patient confidence in the services offered.

It is known that most patients with stroke will be taken care of by a multitude of health personnel and are likely to meet several physiotherapists during a rehabilitation process. The challenge to physiotherapists is to present the same common ideas throughout the process concerning what is offered as current physiotherapy and as acceptable health services.

FURTHER READING

Buene T B 1992 Kvalitet i Fysioterapi. Fysioterapeuten 9: 3–7
Donabedian A 1993 Envisioning quality assurance in physical therapy. Quality Assurance in Physiotherapy. Conference papers, Valkenberg, Netherlands
Field M J, Lohr K N 1992 Guidelines for medical practice. National Academy Press
ISO/DIS 8402 In: ISO 9000 1993 International standard for quality management, 3rd ed. ISO Central Secretarial, Geneva
Kaasenbrood A 1993 Guidelines for good physiotherapy practice. Quality Assurance in Physiotherapy. Conference papers, Valkenberg, Netherlands
McIntosh J 1993 Sketching the contour for quality assurance in physiotherapy. Quality Assurance in Physiotherapy. Conference papers, Valkenberg, Netherlands
Øvretveit J 1993 Health service quality. Blackwell Scientific, Oxford

Psychological aspects and management of change

25. Organization of rehabilitation

I. Lie

INTRODUCTION

Before discussing organization of rehabilitation one should try to define rehabilition. The concept of rehabilitation may have a variety of meanings, and to date there seems to be a lack of common agreement on a standard definition to guide the development of organizational models.

DEFINITION OF REHABILITATION

Rehabilitation may be described as a three-step process, starting with medical treatment of actual impairment, followed by training and/or compensation of remaining functional disability functions, and ending with an attempt to obtain an optimal level of integration into the local community (Fig. 25.1).

Until now, professional education and practice have focused mainly on step 2, i.e. post-medical improvement of disability.

However, during the last decade there has been an increasing ideological and political concern about equal rights for all people to participate in common activities of daily life according to their capabilities, needs and interests. The old paradigm of more than 50 years' standing of institutional care and education has been replaced by the new paradigm of integration. With reference to the three-step rehabilitation model illustrated in Figure 25.1, a change of primary focus has taken place from improvement of disability to self-management of daily life. Accordingly, solving existential life quality problems has become the ultimate concern of the rehabilitation process.

This paradigm shift challenges conventional rehabilitation practice and calls for great changes in professional routine as well as in attitudes towards rehabilitation work.

Diagnosis and treatment in rehabilitation

Quite different diagnostic and treatment regimes exist in the two professional paradigms.

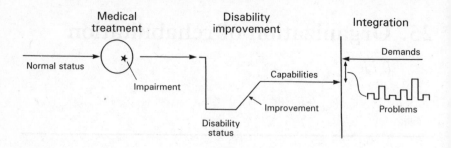

Fig. 25.1   A three-step model of the rehabilitation process.

Diagnosis

In working with disability improvement, the diagnostic reference is the deviation from normal function. The main concern is to measure and characterize the type and amount of deviation from some normal standard.

In working with integration, diagnosis is not, perhaps, an appropriate term to use. Instead, the professional concern is to *identify* and *describe* the concrete problems the person encounters in coping with his/her physical and social environment when attempting to maintain his/her own wishes as regards their quality of life.

This kind of problem analysis should be performed according to the principles of standard ergonomic analysis of man–environment interactions: the everyday life of any person may be sorted into a number of problems to be solved. Each problem may be described in terms of the relationship between the functional demand generated by the design of the environment and the person's individual ability. A problem exists when there is a mismatch between ability and demand.

Usually, individuals adjust to this relationship in two principle ways: by learning/training and by selection of activities. Human ability is known to be trainable to a large extent, and in modern society a tremendous amount of both organized and unorganized learning takes place. For most people, there also exists freedom to choose life conditions that match the level of individual ability so that problems tend to be avoided.

However, heredity, illness and accidents, for example, may change the functional ability to such an extent that ordinary strategies for matching ability and demand are insufficient to avoid severe problems in functionally important areas of life such as education, transport and work. In these cases the person has to be considered a handicapped person.

A handicap may be defined accordingly as the aggregate sum of concrete problems resulting from the daily mismatches between environmental demand and individual ability.

Treatment

The disability improvement approach is aimed at normalizing the functional status by training and/or compensation for impaired function, while the integration approach is aiming at normalizing life management through problem-solving.

A problem is solved when the ability matches the demand. The match may sometimes be most effectively attained by functional improvement of ability, and in other instances by adaptation of environmental demand to the existing ability or by using technical aids. Most often a combination of remedial action is required. It should be noticed that within the integration approach, improvement of inferior functions is of interest only when contributing effectively to solving specific integration problems.

Professional attitudes in rehabilitation

As far as professional attitudes are concerned one may, in fact, speak about two different cultures controlling the relationship between the professional worker and the handicapped person. When focusing on disability, the handicapped person is treated as a patient who is told what is found about their situation, and what to do in order to obtain the best result. When focusing on integration, the handicapped person is no longer a patient in the traditional manner of speaking, but is rather a person who has problems with planning their future.

A handicapped person may be legally competent or legally incompetent. In the case of a legally competent handicapped person it is the individual who is responsible for planning his or her future life. In the case of a legally incompetent person the responsibility for rehabilitation planning is formally transferred to their guardian.

The role of professionals in rehabilitation planning

It may seem simple to leave the responsibility of rehabilitation planning to the individual handicapped person or to a guardian. However, few handicapped people possess the necessary competence to perform qualified rehabilitation planning by themselves.

Such planning is primarily a psychological process, which starts in the medical hospital as a cognitive and emotional reaction to expectations of an unavoidable inferior position of status for the rest of one's life. Anxiety, frustration and grief may develop into early self-devaluation and pessimistic life prospects from the very start of rehabilitation planning. This pessimism may easily escalate further into a stripping process by which activities of the previous life are omitted when they cannot be maintained in the future, leaving the person with an adaptation to a restricted 'rest-of-life'. This kind of stripping process may be considered to be one of dehabilitation rather than rehabilitation.

A case illustration

Erik, a 35-year-old teacher, was involved in a traffic accident. He suffered a brain injury resulting in a moderate expressive aphasia and hemiparesis. After medical treatment he was transferred to a rehabilitation hospital for further functional diagnosis, training and assessment for possible provision of technical aids.

Erik was known as a very active person. He loved his job and pursued many leisure activities; he was an eager hunter and salmon fisherman, and he was the manager of a local amateur theatre group. He was unmarried, and lived on a small arable farm (without domestic animals).

In the beginning, he denied the situation and believed that he would soon recover. However, during his stay at the rehabilitation hospital he gradually realized the permanency of his disability. He began to acknowledge, for example, that he would not be able to continue his job as a teacher, that he could no longer go hunting or fishing and that he could not carry on as an instructor in the theatre.

This 'stripping' of job and leisure activities made him feel that the basis for a meaningful life, for self-confidence and dignity, was crumbling away. Thus, a self-devaluation process had started, and during the next few weeks he began to adapt to the thought that possibly he would be satisfied if he could manage to stay in his own home with a minimum of help from others. He also recognized that the situation could have been much worse, and that compared to other patients he had seen in the hospitals, he should in fact be happy and should not complain at all. He had always been fond of reading; he could still read, and now he would have plenty of time for reading.

When he was discharged from the hospital he stayed in a nursing home for some time while his home was rebuilt for 'wheelchair locomotion'.

In this case the handicapped person is an intelligent legally competent and previously active person who has taken on the responsibility for planning his life following trauma. The professional services have focused on disability improvement and ergonomic adaptation of home conditions in order to obtain independent management of his activities of daily living. This case may perhaps be a representative example of the best solution that a majority of handicapped people can possibly be offered in most western countries today. However, is this case a good model for how to organize rehabilitation?

Erik has the same personality as before the accident. The only difference is that he has severe communication and mobility problems. The majority of his psychological and physical capacities are intact, and his basic needs and interests are unchanged. Taking into account that he is still a person with plenty of resources, there is an obvious gap between untapped resources and the restricted life he is left with as a result of stripping previous activities. In discussing rehabilitation models this gap should be recognized as the great challenge, calling for reorientation of life goals to be the key concept in rehabilitation.

As already discussed, the professionals do not have any legal right to take over the goal-setting for individual rehabilitation. However, the professionals should take responsibility for assisting the handicapped person to develop the competence necessary for a real freedom of choice in planning the future. Erik did not receive such assistance.

ORGANIZATION OF REHABILITATION

In view of the above considerations, the nature of rehabilitation may be acknowledged as the existential process of planning and shaping future life. If this ideological perspective is agreed upon, rehabilitation should be organized to optimize the possibilities for developing and implementing individual rehabilitation plans, directed, under professional guidance, by the handicapped person concerned. The logical steps of such a procedure are as follows (Fig. 25.2):

1. formulating and specifying the goals of rehabilitation
2. identification of and an ergonomic description of the problems that hamper the goals to be reached
3. suggesting remedial action for solving the problems
4. evaluation of the results of the total rehabilitation procedure
5. follow-up evaluation of rehabilitation status over time.

In practice it may be seen to be necessary to go back and forth between these steps in order to get the rehabilitation process started. Nevertheless, the statement of the goal of rehabilitation should be given ultimate priority, before any remedial action is taken, except in the case of post-traumatic functional training that is expected to facilitate physiological recovery of function.

In step 1, the handicapped person has to be 'the boss'. The professional is the assistant who is responsible for ensuring that the handicapped person

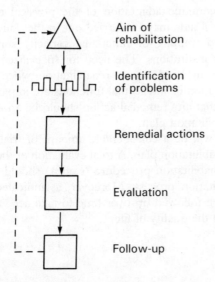

Fig. 25.2 A five-step individual rehabilitation plan.

becomes competent to become a qualified director of planning for his/her future.

How this assistance should be offered depends upon the individual case. It is not possible, of course, to describe general procedures for this kind of guidance work. Nevertheless, some basic elements of rehabilitation competence may be pointed out:

- knowledge of one's own resources, basic needs and interests
- knowledge about one's own impairment, disability and prognosis
- knowledge of the rehabilitation potential of technical aids, ergonomic measures, training and re-education
- knowledge of public services and support facilities.

The considerations so far have been with regard to legally competent handicapped people. Step 1 becomes considerably more difficult where the legally incompetent handicapped person is concerned. In principle, the guardian takes over the 'boss' function. In practice, however, this will not be a satisfactory solution because the guardian can never be a substitute for the handicapped person's own personality. As yet, the author cannot see how to formulate basic principles for rehabilitation guidance of legally incompetent people. This is a question that challenges moral, ideological and psychological thinking. In the meantime, it may be necessary to maintain a more pragmatic position, trying to formulate rehabilitation goals in accordance with the common ideas about sharing equal rights to live and participate in a welfare state, i.e. aiming at obtaining maximum integration in normal life situations.

As to steps 2 and 3, thematic and methodological complexity may often require interdisciplinary and interdepartmental cooperation. Some remedial action, such as ergonomic adaptation of the physical environment and provision of technical aids may be carried out in the daily living situation, while diagnosis and training of functional capacity sometimes may be offered in specialist institutions. The need for specialized services may be especially pertinent in head injury rehabilitation when specific motor, sensory, communication or intellectual functions are impaired. It should be stressed, however, that any remedial action should be an integrated part of the individual rehabilitation plan.

Normally, there will be a considerable amount of trial and error when implementing a rehabilitation plan. A total evaluation of the practical results of the complete rehabilitation procedure (step 4) should be an obligatory part of the rehabilitation process. Moreover, as indicated by step 5, the evaluation should be followed up over time to take account of changes in disability status and the quality of life.

26. The acute treatment of stroke

F. Bakke

INTRODUCTION

Several studies have shown that patients treated in stroke units have a better outcome than patients treated in general medical wards (Garraway et al 1980, Hamrin 1982, Wood-Dauphinee et al 1984, Stevens et al 1984, Strand et al 1985, Sivenius et al 1985, Aitken et al 1993). One of these studies has been performed in Trondheim, and the results from this trial and the treatment model used are presented here (Indredavik et al 1991).

A group at the University Hospital of Trondheim (1986–1988) conducted a randomized controlled trial to evaluate the clinical outcome of treatment of patients with acute stroke in a stroke unit compared with treatment in a general medical ward. Outcome was measured at 6 weeks and 52 weeks after the stroke by the proportion of patients at home, the proportion of patients in an institution, the mortality, and the functional state.

Conscious patients with acute focal neurological deficits of vascular origin were included in the study. Patients living in nursing homes, patients from other health districts, and patients with subdural hematoma, subarachnoid haemorrhage or brain tumour were excluded. Patients' fulfilling the inclusion criteria were then randomly assigned to treatment in the stroke unit or general medical wards using sequentially numbered sealed envelopes. 102 patients were allocated to treatment in the stroke unit, and 104 to the general medical ward.

No significant difference existed between these groups with regard to sex, age, marital status, medical history or functional impairment on admission.

For management of acute stroke in the stroke unit a programme was constructed that was standardized with regard to diagnostic evaluation and medical care, systematic observation and very early and intensive stimulation/mobilization. The Barthel index was used to assess the patient's ability to perform activities of daily living. The other score that was used was a neurological score called the Scandinavian stroke scale. The main aims were to minimize the brain injury, avoid complications, retrain function, and individual adjustment to lasting neurological deficit.

RESULTS

Some of the main results from this trial are shown in Table 26.1. After 6 weeks, 59.8% of the patients treated in the stroke unit (SU), and 34.6% of the patients treated in general wards (GW) were at home, and after 52 weeks, 64.7% and 46.2% respectively were at home. After 6 weeks, 33.3% from the SU and 49% from the GW were still in an institution and after 52 weeks, 22.1% were still in an institution in the GW group compared with 10.8% in the SU treated group. All these differences were significant. The acute mortality was also significantly reduced – 6.9% in the SU group and 16.4% in the GW group died within 6 weeks – but after 52 weeks the difference in mortality was no longer significant. The differences in acute mortality were examined more carefully and it was found that there were no changes in mortality between the SU and the GW for the first 5 days. The difference in mortality was present in the subacute period between day 5 and day 42 and was due mainly to three clinical diagnoses (pneumonia, new strokes, and pulmonary embolism).

Patients who died within 42 days had the following characteristics compared with patients still alive: higher mean age and higher incidence of reduced consciousness and dysphagia.

Significant treatment variables were shorter time to systematic mobilization, medication to reduce fever, and more intravenous infusion which probably caused more stable diastolic blood pressure in the SU group.

As physiotherapists were involved in the research, particular attention was paid to the score on the Barthel ADL index in the two groups: after 6 weeks, the mean score was 79.7 in the SU group and 65.8 in the GW group, and after 52 weeks it was 84.7 and 72.4 respectively. All differences were significant.

In conclusion, this study showed that a combination of acute medical treatment and early intensive rehabilitation in a stroke unit is probably the most effective treatment that can be offered to stroke patients today.

Table 26.1 Number and proportion of patients allocated to stroke unit and general medical wards at home, in institution, and deceased after 6 weeks and 52 weeks

Time	SU No.	(n = 102) %	GW No.	(n = 104) %	p
6 weeks					
Dead	7	6.9	17	16.4	0.037
In institution	34	33.3	51	49.0	0.012
At home	61	59.8	36	34.6	0.0003
52 weeks					
Dead	25	24.5	33	31.7	0.220
In institution	11	10.8	23	22.1	0.0076
At home	66	64.7	48	46.2	0.001

Value of p by log-rank test

THE STROKE UNIT TODAY

This study is now complete, and this chapter describes in more detail this 'package' as used in the existing stroke unit in Trondheim, which is based upon the results from the study, and contains the same elements with some adjustments.

MEDICAL CARE AND ELEMENTS TO MINIMIZE BRAIN INJURY

The stroke unit is organized with a team approach. When a patient is admitted, a diagnostic and functional evaluation is performed immediately and a treatment plan is made. The professionals in the team are a physician, nurses and a physiotherapist. During the first few days in the stroke unit all patients receive a standardized systematic examination and observation of neurological deficits, blood pressure, cardiac and pulmonary disorders, fever, glucose level, and fluid and electrolyte balance. Most patients receive at least 1000 ml saline solution intravenously in order to avoid dehydration and to stabilize their blood pressure, which is not allowed to fall during the acute stage. Decreasing temperature, avoiding glucose infusion and using oxygen therapy in somnolent patients are shown to be very important for the final outcome. The nurses in charge examine closely the patients' neurological deficits on an observation scale during the first 3 days. Treatment with anticoagulants is indicated in patients with a progression of neurological deficits and with a CT scan which does not show signs of haemorrhage.

The physiotherapist monitors the neurological deficit, the level of consciousness, the patient's ability to orientate him or herself and undertakes a brief survey of any language problems using the Scandinavian stroke scale.

COMPLICATIONS RELATED TO THE STROKE

Pneumonia

One of the most common and serious complications is pneumonia. In the Trondheim trial it was found that early mortality was reduced to 58%, and one of the main causes of death was pneumonia.

To prevent this, it was necessary right from the start to watch closely the patient's position in bed. It is necessary to vary the position often and to observe the working condition of the diaphragm, to ensure that deep respiration is possible and that the patient is able to cough and get rid of secretions. It is known that pneumonia is often caused by aspiration, and it is crucial to make great efforts to prevent aspiration. Food and drink should not be offered until the staff are quite sure that the patient is awake and aware enough to swallow normally. The patient has to be brought to an upright position and supported in such a way that the neck and head are held at an optimal angle, and then the patient should practise swallowing his own saliva. If the patient has reduced production of saliva, the therapist may try to stimulate this by placing a little taste of honey or jam on the tongue and encouraging smacking of the lips. Gradually, thickened liquid and food of a variety of textures are tried. In addition, the physician prescribes early use of antibiotic medicine if aspiration is suspected.

Contractures

Another complication is contractures of the joints on the affected side. The resting position should be chosen and observed very carefully and should not allow the muscles to shorten. Muscles to be observed in particular are the calf muscles, the hip flexors, and the finger, wrist and elbow flexors. If considerable work is put into this at the beginning, a better functional recovery may be gained and the gait disorder due to the stroke may be reduced to a minimum at a later stage.

In the very early mobilization programme within the Trondheim stroke unit, emphasis is placed upon bringing the patient to a standing position as soon as possible, stressing weight bearing through the affected leg. The other joints have to be examined, because the patients are mostly elderly, and the hip or knee, for example, on the unaffected side, may be stiff and painful and could develop a contracture.

Resting positions must be observed and varied often to prevent pressure sores. Early standing with weight through the affected leg and stimulation of voluntary muscle activity will stimulate blood flow and prevent deep venous thrombosis in the leg.

Passivity and immobility may be the origin of all mentioned complications in acute stroke patients. In addition, passivity also may be regarded as a complication, causing the patient to be understimulated, depressed and more dependent than necessary.

THE ROLE OF THE PHYSIOTHERAPIST

The physiotherapist, in the stroke unit in Trondheim, works in conjunction with the nurses, assistant nurses and patients during all care and nursing throughout the day and this team work is, in fact, one of the important aspects of the acute stroke treatment package.

A physiotherapist in this special stroke unit has the opportunity to be close to the patients in many situations during the day, e.g. personal toilet, dressing and feeding. This enables the therapist to assess the patient's function, psychological condition, perceptual praxis and cognitive deficits in daily activities. Their language problems and disorders of speech and comprehension during an everyday conversation are noted and the physiotherapist tries to find out what their needs and thoughts are concerning the future.

As a result of this approach, the physiotherapist is capable, in a short time, of planning the main objectives which should be contained in individual therapy sessions. There has been found to be a great advantage in using the four steps of the motor relearning programme for stroke (Carr & Shepherd 1987).

A great deal of time is spent discussing with and instructing the staff how to give a patient both challenge and support, and finding tasks he/she can practise without struggling too much, but which encourage the patient to be an active participant.

It is useful to have all staff members informing and helping each other, aiming at understanding the reasons for various types of behaviour and attitude demonstrated by stroke patients, as well as the emotional effects of stroke. Thinking as a team helps to keep everyone inspired and optimistic.

It is important to educate the relatives about the pathophysiology of stroke, the meaning of symptoms, the adaptability of the brain, the physical and emotional effects of stroke, and thus to make them capable of participating in the rehabilitation process.

The patients will be affected by shock, and will be depressed about their lost function, and although the staff are not psychologists, it is important to know the patient's individual ways of reacting. In particular, when the patient undergoes the stage when he/she is beginning to understand what has happened, he/she will often try to protect him or herself by pretending that nothing has happened. The patient may then be misunderstood and considered to be confused and even senile.

The physiotherapist has to be professional, and must show a great deal of understanding and empathy, provide comfort, and give the patient tasks to solve. It is crucial that the patient is successful in solving the early tasks, as this will encourage, motivate and lead to acceptance at a later stage.

Therefore, early assessment procedures are used to consider all aspects of recovery from the stroke, and behavioural methods are used to encourage motor learning and to facilitate the learning of new motor skills. The methods must also consider cognitive and language deficits. Recent research has shown that a separation between motor processes and cognitive processes is not possible. Motor behaviour is the result of a complex integrated and adaptive information-processing system closely linked to its environment. Emphasis is placed on setting the patient tasks of graded difficulty, practised in a variety of contexts, using plenty of feedback on performance to ensure that learning takes place (Mulder 1993).

The patient and the patient's family are active participants in rehabilitation, and the staff in the stroke unit are more involved in practising activities of daily living than in other general medical wards. It is crucial that every normal situation throughout the day is utilized to practise motor skills, dependent upon the patient's medical condition. The nurses are responsible for the assessment of the patient's ability to dress and feed, for example, and the Barthel ADL index is used for this evaluation.

The Barthel index is assessed at day 1 and every week until discharge, and gives important information as to the patient's level of function.

Although the nurses and the physiotherapist overlap in terms of the daily functional training, the physiotherapist has to develop the physiotherapeutic problem-solving process: recognition, analysis, decision-making, action-taking and re-evaluation, and must keep in mind human interrelations with sensitivity, awareness, intuition and interaction.

As soon as the patient is well enough and functional potential is achieved in the stroke unit, the patient is transferred to a rehabilitation clinic where it is possible to practise in a more motivating environment than in a hospital.

Patients with minor strokes and with lesser deficits are discharged directly home and and if necessary, domiciliary services are organized.

Case history

To illustrate the physiotherapist's approach, the case history of a typical patient will be used as an example

A 79-year-old man is found lying on the floor in his home. When he is admitted to the stroke unit, the diagnostic evaluation and acute medical treatment are commenced according to general procedures.

The patient is somnolent; he is difficult to rouse and to keep awake. He moves his right arm and leg spontaneously; his left arm and leg seem to be paralysed. He is holding his head turned to the right, and it seems that his awareness of the left side of his body, is diminished.

This patient is seriously brain injured, and he is at the stage where he is unaware of his own needs. A systematic observation plan and medical care must be organized, and simultaneously great emphasis is placed on preventing complications as described earlier, with particular regard to chest and lung function.

Traditionally such patients are kept in bed, immobile, until they regain consciousness, because it is thought that their level of consciousness is too low to get a response. However, experience shows that he has to be mobilized in order to raise his level of consciousness.

The patient is brought to an upright position at the side of the bed to stimulate awareness and mental alertness, by speaking to him clearly and by making him open his eyes. There are two aims: first, to make contact with him, inform him about what has happened and some of the problems the stroke has caused and, in simple words, inform him about plans for his care and the reasons for it; secondly, to keep him awake and in this position, using methods to activate his flaccid muscles, e.g. his knee extensors.

This man has suffered a brain injury; he feels generally ill and uncomfortable, often dizzy and nauseated. Nevertheless, he has to be mobilized and at the same time has to regain function and relearn how to use his injured motor system. Therefore, he must understand from the very beginning that he has abilities to relearn and the importance of his own participation. He must then be taught how to perform, or start to perform, the tasks.

It is very important that communication is established early, making sure that the physiotherapist and the patient understand each other, and that the patient understands that the physiotherapist wants the best for him.

These stimulation procedures must be carried out while ensuring that the patient's medical condition is closely observed. If he becomes pale, clammy and feels pain, he must of course be laid down again, and his blood pressure and pulse must be monitored.

The results of this trial show that there is no evidence that this approach, in the critical phase, may increase the brain damage. On the contrary, the conclusions are that this element, in the acute care package, reduced complications and was important for the final outcome.

When the patient's level of consciousness becomes a little higher, and he is able to respond, one of the first concerns is to teach him to change his position in bed, and how to manage to sit up over the side of the bed. At this early stage, the aim is to enable him to perform this by using as little effort as possible. It is important that he is successful, because this will encourage him and keep him motivated to go on with the training programme.

The stroke patient in our example is stimulated continuously to turn his head to the left, to make eye contact with people addressing him, and to be aware of what is happening at his left side. Within a few days the patient attempts to stand. He is usually 'off balance', but he has to start postural adjustment, be aware of the centre of gravity, and feel that small movements of the head or limb change the centre of gravity. A rapid regaining of balance in standing increases awareness of bilaterality and position in space and of body parts, which is particularly important for people with unilateral spatial neglect or diminished kinaesthetic sensibility. Standing may prevent contractures, provides motivation and self-confidence and enables the patient to start training in walking skills.

The patient in this example is now able to stay awake for longer periods. He spends more time out of bed, and starts to regain the ability to perform motor tasks such as transferring from bed to wheelchair and other activities of daily living which are of great importance and meaning to the patient.

CONCLUSION

In the Trondheim stroke unit, acute stroke patients are offered a combination of acute medical treatment and early intensive stimulation, mobilization and rehabilitation. This treatment package increases the proportion of patients able to live at home, improves functional outcome, reduces the need for institutional care, and reduces early mortality. The very early start of mobilization seems to be one of the most important aspects in this treatment package and the physiotherapist plays a significant role in this very acute stage. However, in this integrated approach, acute medical treatment and early stimulation/mobilization are closely linked, and it is difficult to determine which specific aspect is most important. A contribution to a successful outcome may also be made by the psychological aspect, because the stroke unit can be envisaged as a therapeutic community in which the close relationship between the patients and the staff plays an important part in achieving a high level of functional independence. It is difficult to evaluate the importance of these aspects.

However, the approach to acute stroke care which has been developed in the Trondheim stroke unit seems to be an effective way of treating patients with acute stroke.

Acknowledgements

I wish to thank Dr Bent Indredavik, Pt. Hild Fjærtoft and Pt. Turid Aasheim for their assistance in the preparation of this paper.

REFERENCES

Aitken P D, Rodgers H, French J M, Bates D, James O F W 1993 General medical or geriatric unit care for acute care? A controlled trial. Age and Ageing 22 (suppl 2): 4–5
Carr J H, Shepherd R B 1987 A motor relearning programme for stroke, 2nd edn. Butterworth-Heinemann, Oxford
Garraway W M, Akhtar A J, Hockey L, Prescott R J 1980 Management of acute stroke in the elderly: preliminary results of a controlled trial. BMJ 280: 1040–1044
Hamrin E 1982 Early activation after stroke: does it make a difference? Scand J Rehabil Med 14: 101–109
Indredavik B, Bakke F, Solberg R, Rokseth R, Haaheim L L, Holme I 1991 Benefit of stroke unit: a randomised controlled trial. Stroke 22: 1026
Mulder T 1993 Current topics in motor control: implications for rehabilitation. In: Greenwood R, Barnes M P, McMillan T M, Ward C D (eds) Neurological rehabilitation. Churchill Livingstone, Edinburgh, ch 11, pp125–132
Sivenius J, Pyorala K, Heinonen O P, Salonen J T, Riekkinen P 1985 The significance of intensity of rehabilitation after stroke – a controlled trial. Stroke 16: 928–931
Stevens R S, Ambler N R, Warren M D 1984 A randomised controlled trial of a stroke rehabilitation ward. Age and Ageing 13: 65–75
Strand T, Asplund K, Eriksson S, Hagg E, Lithner F, Wester P O 1985 A non-intensive stroke unit reduces functional disability and the need for long-term hospitalisation. Stroke 16: 29–34
Wood-Dauphinee S, Shapiro S, Bass E et al 1984 A randomised trial of team care following stroke. Stroke 5: 864–872

27. Rehabilitation of chronic stroke patients – experiences from Sätra Brunn

S. Lind,   M. Loid

INTRODUCTION

Sätra Brunn is a centre for rehabilitation, owned by the University of Uppsala in Sweden and situated in the countryside west of Uppsala. It is one of the oldest health resorts in Sweden and was donated to the university in 1747 for clinical teaching and training purposes. It has been in constant use since the beginning of the 18th century and has been developed into a modern centre for rehabilitation. Today it offers specially designed rehabilitation programmes for diagnoses such as stroke, rheumatoid arthritis, fibromyalgia, ankylosing spondylitis and other musculoskeletal problems. Approximately 200–250 patients are referred simultaneously for three periods of 4 weeks each every summer.

Sätra Brunn is special for its way of combining old traditions, such as using the healing power of the spring water, medical baths, stroll in the park and concerts, with modern methods of treatment and rehabilitation. It is like a small village where the patients and the staff stay in red cottages dating back to the 18th and 19th centuries. The houses are surrounded by lawns, beautiful flowers, old trees, pathways and woodland scenery.

THE STROKE PROGRAMME

The stroke programme at Sätra Brunn started in 1987. In each 4-week period, no more than 48 patients with stroke or other brain injuries are accepted. Of these, 15 will have aphasia. They come from all parts of Sweden. The staff consists of four occupational therapists and four physiotherapists, one speech pathologist, three assistants, one nurse, one physician (part-time) and a consultant in neurology. To participate in the programme the patients have to fulfil the following criteria:

- The time after onset should be at least 6 months (1 year for patients with aphasia).
- They should be living at home and in need of intensive treatment, not only recreation.

• They should be mainly independent in personal activities of daily living (ADL) skills due to the limitation of nursing staff.

The programme is designed primarily for patients with sensorimotor deficits and slight perceptual and behavioural problems. A few patients with severe brain damage who bring their own nurse can also attend. The aim of the programme is that the patients will improve their functional ability to further enhance their level of independence and social activity and, hopefully, decrease their need for continuous physical training.

The philosophy of the treatment is based on the Bobath concept (Bobath 1990, Davies 1985, 1990), which in the short term means stimulating sensorimotor and perceptual learning; this is incorporated in functional everyday skills to make it possible for the patients to improve their quality of life. Important aspects are to increase motor function and balance, to teach the patients to use their whole body in different activities, and to guide them into strategies for problem-solving (Affolter 1991, Carr & Shepherd 1987).

Rehabilitation after brain damage is a lifelong elarning process (Bach-y-Rita 1981) and what has to be found out is how these 4 weeks of training at Sätra Brunn should be used in the most effective way for each patient. These patients, who have had their problems for a long period of time, have different complications, e.g. established compensatory movement patterns, shortening of muscles, soft tissue and joint structures, hypertonia and pain. Many of the patients are also in the process of trying to cope with their new functional ability in all of life's different situations. This means that the majority of them are seeking help in learning how to move and to function more normally. In order to fulfil these needs treatment focuses on trying to regain a more normal biomechanical alignment as one of the basic prerequisites for developing postural adjustment and more selective movement (Carr & Shepherd 1987, Davies 1990, Mohr 1990). Another link is to regain the awareness of the body as a whole and to relearn how to use the different parts. Daily activities offer many opportunities for the therapist to guide the patients in using their whole body and to promote cognitive processes (Horak 1991). By working on these three levels the patients are given the opportunity to learn to apply the functions they already have as well as to develop new ones. It also incorporates the gaining of new strategies for problem-solving.

Sätra Brunn provides a good learning atmosphere by means of its stimulating setting, the competence of the therapists who have at least a basic Bobath course (IBITAH 1992), the fact that there is a group of patients working together, and the structure of the programme (Carlsson 1988).

The structure and content of the programme

The stroke programme is built upon individual occupational therapy and physiotherapy in combination with group treatment with different aims and directions. Before the real training period starts a thorough assessment of the patients is carried out by the team. The physician examines the patients and the speech pathologist assesses the patients with aphasia and maps out their ability to communicate from a linguistic and neuropsychological approach. The nurse inquires about the psychosocial conditions. The occupational therapist and physiotherapist make a common assessment of each patient. They register the functional level related to the following questions:

- What can the patient do? How is it achieved?
- What can the patient not do? Why not?

This level should be related to daily living skills that are important for the patient. The therapists make an analysis on the basis of the following data:

- assessment of motor performance of transfers, walking and ADL skills
- voluntary movement
- oro-facial function
- balance reactions
- muscular tone – associated reactions
- other problems of relevance
- perceptual and cognitive function.

The patient's main problems and assets can now be formulated. Based on this the patient and the therapists set up the functional goals that will be relevant for the 4 weeks of training. The goals should be measurable so that any progress can be registered at the end of the period. Then the schedule for the training period can be designed. The frequency and the length of the treatment sessions in the different departments are almost standardized but the content is individualized and the programme offers:

- individual treatment twice a week for 30–40 minutes in the occupational therapy and physiotherapy departments respectively
- ADL treatment one to four times a week for between 45 and 75 minutes
- speech therapy five times a week, in a group for 1 hour
- group treatment two to three times a week for 1 hour in the occupational therapy and physiotherapy departments respectively
- group treatment one to two times a week for 1–2 hours led by an occupational therapist and a physiotherapist together
- positioning in bed two to three times a week for 30 minutes
- guidance in daily routines, various
- leisure activities, various
- medical baths twice a week for 45 minutes
- patient education twice, for a period of 1 hour
- information from patient organisations once, for a period of 2 hours
- information to relatives; this varies.

An example of a schedule for a patient without aphasia is shown in Figure 27.1. For the patients with aphasia, speech therapy in a group is added daily, which means that some of the other activities might be excluded.

The occupational therapist and physiotherapist decide how to tackle the patient's main problems within their treatment programme, in relation to the function that the patient has to be prepared for in order to be able to reach the planned goals.

Individual physiotherapy

Physiotherapy is focused mainly on helping the patient to gain a range of motion through different techniques (Ada & Canning 1990), in order to obtain a better biomechanical alignment as a preparation for facilitating posture and voluntary movement. Another important part of physiotherapy is the reinforcement of body awareness as a whole or for specific parts of the body by using, e.g., tactile kinaesthetic stimulation (Carey et al 1993). The physiotherapist also guides the patient to use his/her improved balance for safer transfers and for walking with less support in different situations. One way of introducing functional activities can be to let the patient participate in arranging the treatment equipment by fetching the different objects required.

Individual occupational therapy

The occupational therapist concentrates on guiding the patient step by step into practical more or less familiar activities. The aim of this is that the patient learns to control and use the whole body as well as the different parts in activities of varying complexity, which means learning to integrate more

Monday	Tuesday	Wednesday	Thursday	Friday
ADL	ADL	ADL	ADL	ADL
Breakfast	Breakfast	Breakfast	Breakfast	Breakfast
OT ind	PT ind	PT group stretching	OT ind	Creative activities
Positioning	OT group stretching	Positioning	Walk	OT group arm/hand
Lunch	Lunch	Lunch	Lunch	Lunch
Mini golf	Free activities	Creative activities	PT group balance	PT ind
Med. bath		Med. bath	Positioning	
Dinner	Dinner	Dinner	Dinner	Dinner

Fig. 27.1   Training schedule.

normal movement in performing a task. To make it possible for the patient to succeed, the occupational therapist often has to guide the movement manually. This is also a way of stimulating the tactile kinaesthetic information as a part of perceptual and cognitive training (Affolter 1981). Occupational therapy also deals with building up more selective movement especially in the upper extremity in preparation for functional activities.

It is very important that the occupational therapy and physiotherapy programmes overlap with each other in this learning process. The occupational therapist must ensure that the patient has a well prepared motor function for performing a task; meanwhile the physiotherapist has to introduce activities in the patient's treatment to make movement goal-directed (Gleiner 1985). This implies that there are some very fundamental problems which have to be worked upon by both the occupational therapist and physiotherapist:

• The abnormal muscular tone has to be normalized to enable new functions to develop or to be controlled by the patient to increase the functional use of the body.

• The asymmetrical use of the body has to be diminished in all daily activities in order to help the patient to maintain muscular length, increase balance and promote weight bearing on the affected side as well as incorporate the awareness of the hemiplegic side of the body.

ADL treatment

ADL treatment is given by both the occupational therapists and physiotherapists. The aim is for the patient not only to gain independence but to increase the quality of the performance by, for example, working in a more symmetrical way, using both hands and working on a higher level of performance. It can also be a part of perceptual and cognitive training.

Speech therapy

The patients with aphasia are divided into three groups on different communication levels. The general aim is to improve the patients' communication skills all the way from increasing a non-verbal communication to learning to use their verbal ability in more complex situations.

Group treatment

The groups have different aims and to make them more effective there are only four patients, with approximately the same functional level, in each group which means that each type of group exists on different levels. The general aim is to reinforce some of the functions which the patients are learning in the individual sessions on a higher level of independence. The intention when working in groups is for patients to learn from each other and also to have fun.

Physiotherapy. Stretching groups have the aim of increasing range of motion, mastering abnormal muscular tone and gaining muscular control. By transferring from a standing to a lying position and vice versa the patient is practising the above mentioned functions. By moving the body against the floor and in space the patient has the opportunity to increase body awareness in relation to different sensory inputs.

Balance groups have the aim of facilitating balance and the perception of the body in different positions and situations. This incorporates learning a more dynamic way of weight bearing in, for example, transfers, moving the body in relation to different objects in the room and moving on different surfaces.

Occupational therapy. Stretching groups have the same aim as physiotherapy stretching groups, but with the focus on the upper trunk and extremities. This is done both in sitting at a table and in standing.

Balance groups have the aim of increasing postural adjustment mainly in sitting and directed towards dressing activities and transfers.

Arm and hand function groups have the aim of learning to control the arm against the body as the first step of being able to use the arm and hand for holding on to things, to fixate them or to use the arm and hand in a more dynamic way. This is done in both sitting and standing positions.

Hand groups have the aim of practising manipulation of different familiar objects including working on two-hand function. This implies a rather high level of selective voluntary movement in the hand.

Occupational therapy and physiotherapy. ADL problem-solving groups have the aim of increasing strategies for problem-solving. This is done by making use of the patient's own experiences of different problems in their daily life. Therapists and patients try to solve the problems together and in a way where the whole body is active. Examples might be carrying things in a bag with the affected hand, peeling a hot potato, handling a vacuum cleaner and making a bed.

Free activity groups have the aim of encouraging the patients to do things they normally would not dare to do or think that they are able to perform. This is done in a group of 10 patients and it takes place outside the occupational therapy and physiotherapy departments. Walking in a forest carrying a rucksack, sitting down on a rock or on the grass handling a cup of coffee and a cake can be a great challenge as well as a practical problem-solving exercise.

Positioning in bed

Positioning in bed is used to teach the patient one way of maintaining their muscular length and normalizing tone. For some of the patients this can be part of their home programme.

Guidance in daily routines

This is the next step for the patient in carrying over functions that have been practised in the individual and group sessions in the occupational therapy and physiotherapy departments into different daily activities. The assistant guides them in activities such as dressing, transfers, walks, carrying a plate at mealtime, shopping, picking flowers or riding a bicycle.

Leisure activities

Sport and creative activities indoors as well as outdoors are encouraged with the aim of having fun, moving around a little bit more or faster than normally, cooperating and being social with other people. The purpose can also be finding a new hobby. Examples might be mini golf, badminton, darts, oil painting, woodcraft or card games. Sätra Brunn also offers a variety of social and cultural activities such as dancing, parties and concerts.

Medical baths

The aim is purely relaxation and to attain a balance between activity and rest.

Patient education

This is held in small groups and is led by the doctor. The aim is to inform and to answer questions concerning brain damage and its consequences.

Information from the patient organizations

The patients as well as their relatives have the possibility of obtaining information from the patient organisations with regard to their different activities and their network in the patient's home district.

Information to relatives

The relatives are invited both to a common information session about the programme and to follow their relative during treatment.

CONCLUSION

Working with patients with chronic stroke in accordance with a programme such as this, which combines individual treatment sessions with different group treatments and makes it possible for the patients to apply their newly gained function in daily activities, has many advantages especially for the learning process (Carr & Shepherd 1987, Horak 1991). Built into the programme is the requirement that the patients have to participate very actively in reaching their goals as the individual treatments are relatively few during the period. They are also encouraged to become aware of their resources and problems in order to be able to carry over and develop their function at home. It has been found that working in groups also has a very beneficial effect on the learning process since the patients relate to and learn so much from each other in a way which can never be created by the therapists. All this, together with the very stimulating and not very adjusted environment at Sätra Brunn and the fact that the patients live very close together and away from home, makes it possible for them to learn new abilities in many situations in the short time of 4 weeks. The results of an evaluation of the programme showed that patients had maintained their functional level even 6 months later (Carlsson 1988). A longitudinal study of the programme began in 1990 and the results are ongoing (Carlsson et al 1994).

REFERENCES

Ada L, Canning C 1990 Anticipating and avoiding muscle shortening. In: Ada L, Canning C (eds) Key issues in neurological physiotherapy. Butterworth-Heinemann, London

Affolter F D 1981 Perceptual processes as prerequisites for complex human behavior. International Rehabilitation Medicine 3(1): 3–9

Affolter F D 1991 Part III Learning in a Wirklichkeit. In: Perception, interaction and language. Interaction of daily living. The root of development. Springer Verlag, Berlin

Bach-y-Rita P 1981 Brain plasticity as a basis of the development of rehabilitation procedures for hemiplegia. Scandinavian Journal of Rehabilitation Medicine 13: 73–83

Bobath B 1990 Adult hemiplegia. Evaluation and treatment, 3rd edn. Heinemann, London

Carey L M, Matyas T A, Oke L E 1993 Sensory loss in stroke patients: effective training of tactile and proprioceptive discrimination. Archives of Physical Medicine and Rehabilitation 74: 602–611

Carlsson M 1988 Effekter av behandling enlight Bobath konceptet. Untvärdering av strokebehandlingen på Sätra Hälsobrunn sommaren 1987. FoU-rapport Vårdhögskolan, Uppsala

Carlsson M, Lind S, Loid M et al 1994 En utvärdering av Sätra Brunns stroke program, en longitudinell studie. To be published

Carr J H, Shepherd R B 1987 A motor relearning programme for stroke. Heinemann, London

Davies P 1985 Steps to follow. A guide to the treatment of adult hemiplegia. Based on the concept of K. and B. Bobath. Springer Verlag, Berlin

Davies P 1990 Right in the middle. Selective trunk activity in the treatment of adult hemiplegia. Springer Verlag, Berlin

Gleiner J A 1985 Purposeful activity in motor learning theory. An event approach to motor skill acquisition. American Journal of Occupational Therapy 39: 12

Horak F 1991 Assumptions underlying motor control for neurological rehabilitation. In: Contemporary management of motor control problems. Proceedings of the II Step conference. Foundation for Physical Therapy, American Physical Therapy Association, Alexandria

IBITAH 1992 Byelaws, rules and regulations. International Bobath Instructors/Tutor Association Adult Hemiplegia.

Mohr J D 1990 Management of the trunk in adult hemiplegia: the Bobath concept. In: In touch, topics in neurology, lesson 1. APTA Educational Department, Alexandria

28. Rehabilitation at home after stroke: a pilot study

L. Widén Holmqvist, J. de Pedro-Cuesta

INTRODUCTION

Before major changes in the health care system can be designed and implemented, exploratory case studies, where individual patients are studied in depth, are often needed to assess which type of changes are feasible and show greatest promise. This pilot study is part of the research project: 'Development and evaluation of rehabilitation at home after stroke in south-west Stockholm', and originates from the Division of Neurology, Department of Clinical Neuroscience and Family Medicine, Karolinska Institute, Huddinge University Hospital, Huddinge, Sweden. Five papers have already been published (Bach-y-Rita & de Pedro-Cuesta 1991, de Pedro-Cuesta et al 1992, de Pedro-Cuesta & Widén Holmqvist 1993, de Pedro-Cuesta et al 1993, Widén Holmqvist et al 1993). The purpose of this pilot study was to find out if it was feasible to substitute institutional rehabilitation with early discharge combined with rehabilitation at home and to lay a foundation for a large formal experiment. At the present time, a randomized controlled trial is being conducted where rehabilitation at home after stroke is compared with accepted, customary rehabilitation in different departments.

Based on a set of pilot cases, the objectives of the present study were:

1. to identify, on a population-based background, characteristics of the target incident patients
2. to describe the structure, process and outcome of the implemented rehabilitation programme
3. to perform a health-economic evaluation.

During the 9-month study period, 658 patients were admitted to the Department of Neurology at Huddinge Hospital (HH) with the diagnosis of acute stroke on 910 different occasions. On 403 occasions, the patients were discharged within 5 days of hospitalization. Based on the remaining 507 occasions, 173 patients were evaluated with regard to the Katz index of activities of daily living (ADL) (Katz et al 1963) between 5–12 days of hospitalization. A subsample of the 173 patients, the size of sample being limited by the availability of therapists, was offered rehabilitation at home as an alternative to sustained rehabilitation at the HH Neurology Department, or transfer to different rehabilitation or geriatric units for continued rehabilitation.

MATERIAL AND METHODS

Criteria for inclusion in the intervention sample were:

- age < 80 years on day of admission
- independence in toileting at time of discharge according to the Katz index of ADL
- mini-mental state examination (Folstein et al 1975) score > 23, indicating cognitive function within normal limits.

A home rehabilitation programme, individually planned by the staff physiotherapist, and occupational and speech therapists associated with the HH Neurology Department, was drawn up for each patient who passed the entry criteria and was willing to participate. After discharge, one of the therapists was selected to be *case manager*, using the other therapists on a consultant basis. The case-manager was responsible for:

- most of the therapy at home
- coordination between HH therapists
- contact with the relatives and home service assistants.

Education and individual counselling (Evans et al 1988) were systematically offered to spouses and home service assistants. The model of neurological rehabilitation used in this study was based on the *task-oriented approach* (Carr & Shepherd 1987), which assumes that control of movement is organized around goal-directed and functional behaviour rather than on muscles and movement patterns. The patient and the family were encouraged to be active participants in the rehabilitation programme and *adherence to structured training between therapy sessions was promoted* (Ada et al 1990). The patients were asked to keep diaries recording the time spent on training and the type of this training undertaken between therapy sessions.

Follow-up visits were scheduled 3, 6 and 12 months after stroke. Interviews and assessments were conducted using the following procedures:

1. Since it has been suggested that certain personality traits will affect desirable health behaviour, such as adherence to therapeutic regimes, and that self-motivation is highly correlated with attraction to physical activity and perception of exercise as having value for health, the sense of coherence questionnaire was used (Antonovsky 1987). The scores were compared with normative data from a population sample in Stockholm and the patients' adherence to structured training between therapy sessions was examined taking the individual scores into account.

2. Lifestyle activities, i.e. other than personal care, undertaken by the patients before and after stroke were measured using the Frenchay activities index (Wade et al 1985).

3. Information about dependency on another person in performing personal and instrumental ADL was recorded using the Katz index of ADL extended with cooking, shopping, cleaning and transport (Hulter Åsberg & Sonn 1989).

4. Motor ability on the paretic side was assessed using the chart developed by Linkmark & Hamrin (1988).

5. Walking speed was tested by asking the patients to walk 10 metres inside their home or, if possible, on the level outside their home (Wade et al 1987).

6. Self-reported verbal behaviour in the speech situation was measured for patients with dysphasia and dysarthria (Währborg & Borenstein 1988).

Using this sample of 15 patients in the pilot study, various health-economic aspects were assessed, i.e. patients' satisfaction with care, patients' subjective assessment of their own health status, family involvement, consequences and cost and cost and resource use and cost of health care.

In order to identify which aspects of the present organization of the rehabilitation programme were acceptable and which aspects needed improvement, patient satisfaction was measured using a questionnaire (Bendtsen et al 1993). The questionnaire contained the following dimensions: art of care, technical quality of care, accessibility/convenience, finances, availability, continuity, efficacy/outcome of care, and active participation in discharge and rehabilitation planning. Changes in the patients' subjective assessment of their health status during the first year after stroke were measured using the sickness impact profile (SIP) (Bergner et al 1981) in interview form, 3 and 12 months after stroke.

This intervention may have implied transfer of burden to family caregivers. The subjective health status for spouses living with the patient, was assessed by means of the SIP in interview form, 3 and 12 months after stroke. The time and cost for family caregivers giving assistance with personal and instrumental ADL was also estimated

Resource utilization and direct cost calculations were done for the following health-related cost items: hospital care and outpatient care, medication, technical aids, home adaptation, home service, health-related transport service and rehabilitation at home.

RESULTS

Admitted patients

15 stroke patients, with a mean age of 68.2 (range 45–79 years) – six females and nine males, seven with right hemiparesis, including one with dysphasia,

eight with left hemiparesis – were offered early discharge and rehabilitation at home. 10 patients were living with their spouse and five were living alone. 10 patients were retired and five were in gainful employment. Before inclusion in the pilot study, the planned rehabilitation for five patients was continued rehabilitation at HH Neurology Department, for another five patients transfer to different rehabilitation units, and for the other five patients transfer to geriatric units.

Intervention

The time for discharge from the Department of Neurology and the frequency of contact with different paramedical professions during both hospital stay and home-based rehabilitation for each of the patients are shown in Figure 28.1. The mean number of therapy sessions at home was 11 (range 4–27). The intensity varied from four home visits per week after discharge, to one per 2–3 weeks at the end of the rehabilitation period, evincing a general pattern of the gradual process of discharge from therapy. The length of the rehabilitation programme varied from 4 to 19 weeks after discharge, depending on the needs of the patient and spouse.

The most frequently used task-specific activities in the rehabilitation programme at home were activities using manual dexterity, e.g. writing, handicraft, carpentry, followed by different pastime and leisure activities, e.g. cooking/washing up, and walking indoors and outdoors.

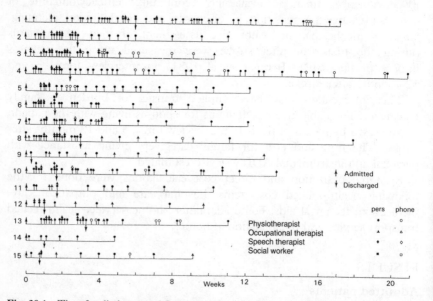

Fig. 28.1   Time for discharge and frequency of personal (pers) and telephone (phone) contacts with paramedical professionals during hospital stay and rehabilitation at home for consecutive patients in the pilot study.

14 patients with sense of coherence scores within normal range in comparison with the population sample, reported adherence to training between therapy sessions. One patient with a low score was not motivated to do so. According to diaries kept by the patients, the mean time spent in training per day was 1.2 hours (range 0.5–2.8).

Outcome

All patients took part in the 3 months follow-up. Only 14 of them were alive and able to participate in the interview and assessment 6 and 12 months after stroke.

The median percentage of scores for lifestyle activities, ADL and motor capacity at different time points, before and after stroke, are shown in Figure 28.2. All patients were already restricted in lifestyle activities before their stroke. Such activities were affected 3 months after stroke, but not at later evaluations. There was an improvement in personal and instrumental ADL capacity from 60% at discharge to 100%, 3 months after stroke. 12 months after stroke, the median ADL capacity had decreased slightly. Improvement in motor capacity occurred from discharge to 3 months after stroke. Minor improvement occurred between 3 and 12 months.

The majority of patients were satisfied with all measured dimensions of care.

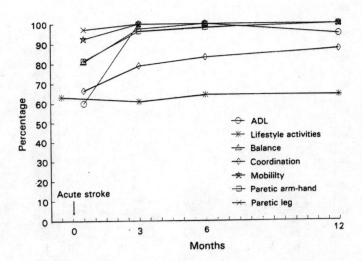

Fig. 28.2   Median percentage of scores for 14 surviving patients in pre-stroke lifestyle activities and personal and instrumental ADL, motor capacity and lifestyle activities at discharge and 3, 6 and 12 months after stroke. Time-point for discharge after stroke plotted at the mean interval-value (14 days).

According to the median scores for subjective dysfunction for patients 3 months after stroke, recreation and pastimes were most affected, followed by home management, ambulation, emotional behaviour, sleep and rest.

11 of the 15 patients received assistance from an informal caregiver in personal and/or instrumental ADL during the rehabilitation programme at home.

Median scores for different categories of subjective dysfunction for spouses were low. Five spouses reported dysfunction in social interaction, emotional behaviour and recreation and pastimes due to giving care to the patient with stroke.

In the sample of 173 patients evaluated by the Katz index of ADL, 49% of the patients had ADL-grade A–E and 51% had ADL-grade F–G, 1 week after stroke. Grade A indicates complete independence in personal ADL and grade G indicates complete dependence.

The median duration of hospital stay by ADL-grade for patients discharged to their own home within 6 months, for patients in the pilot study and for patients not affected by the intervention are shown in Figure 28.3. Patients in the pilot study were only recruited among patients with ADL-grades A–E. The mean duration of hospital stay for patients in the pilot study was 14 days and for patients with ADL-grade A–E, but not affected by the intervention, it was 29 days.

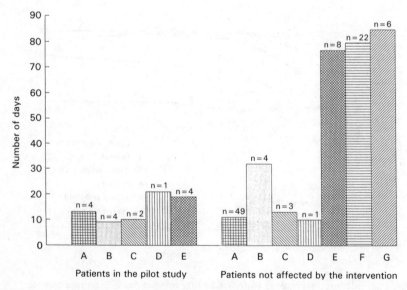

Fig. 28.3 Median duration of hospital stay by ADL-grade for patients in the pilot study and for patients not affected by the intervention discharged to their own home within 6 months after an acute stroke episode.

The cost of rehabilitation at home for each patient, based on the mean number of home visits, corresponds to the cost of 4–5 days of hospital care at HH Department of Neurology.

CONCLUSION

This pilot study indicates that, in Sweden, the target group for rehabilitation at home 3–4 months after acute stroke, determining a considerable reduction of hospital stay, are patients with persisting residual deficits at least 1–3 weeks after stroke, patients with ADL-grade A–E according to the Katz index 1 week after stroke, and patients with a mini-mental state examination score > 23.

Gender, age, family situation, professional status, mild defective visual scanning and medical history do not seem noticeably to limit the patients' participation in such a programme.

The study shows that a considerable proportion of patients with stroke can:

- safely undergo early discharge and rehabilitation at home
- actively participate in task-specific training with frequently structured training between therapy sessions
- regain function following similar patterns as reported from other stroke patients.

REFERENCES

Ada L, Canning C, Westwood P 1990 The patient as an active learner. In: Ada A, Canning C (eds) Key issues in neurological physiotherapy. Butterworth-Heinemann, Boston

Antonovsky A 1987 Unraveling the mystery of health. Jossey-Bass, San Francisco

Bach-y-Rita P, de Pedro-Cuesta J 1991 Neuroplasticity in the ageing brain: development of conceptually-based neurological rehabilitation. In: Proceedings of the VI Congress of the International Rehabilitation Medicine Association, Madrid. Elsevier, Amsterdam

Bendtsen P, Bjurulf P, 1993 Perceived need and patient statisfaction in relation to care provided in individuals with rheumatoid arthritis. Quality Assurance in Health Care 5: 243–253

Bergner M, Bobbit R, Carter W, Gilson B 1981 The sickness impact profile: development and final revision of a health status measurement. Med Care 8: 787–805

Carr J H, Shepherd R B 1987 A motor relearning model for rehabilitation. In: Carr J H, Shepherd R B, Gordon J, Gentile A M, Held J M (eds) Movement science: foundation for physical therapy in rehabilitation. Aspen, Maryland

de Pedro-Cuesta J, Widén Holmqvist L, Bach-y-Rita P 1992 Evaluation of stroke rehabilitation by randomized controlled studies: a review. Acta Neurol Scand 86: 433–439

de Pedro-Cuesta J, Sandström B, Holm M, Stawiarz L, Widén Holmqvist L, Bach-y-Rita P 1993 Stroke rehabilitation: identification of target group and planning data. Scand J Rehab Med 25: 107–116

Evans R L, Matlock A-L, Bishop D S, Stranahan S, Pederson C 1988 Family intervention after stroke: does counselling or education help? Stroke 19: 1243–1249

Folstein M F, Folstein S F, McHugh P R 1975 Mini-mental state: a practical method for grading cognitive state of patients for clinicians. J Psychiatric Res 12: 189–198

Hulter Åsberg K, Sonn U 1989 The cumulative structure of personal and instrumental ADL. Scand J Rehab Med 21: 171–177

Katz S, Ford A B, Moskowitz R W, Jackson B A, Jaffe M W 1963 The index of ADL: a standardised measure of biological and psychosocial function. J Am Med Assoc 185: 914–1919

Lindmark B, Hamrin E 1988 Evaluation of functional capacity after stroke as a basis for active intervention. Presentation of a modified chart for motor capacity assessment and its reliability. Scand J Rehab Med 20: 103–109

Wade D, Leigh-Smith J, Langton-Hewer R 1985 Social activities after stroke: measurement and natural history using the Frenchay activities index. Int Rehabil Med 7: 176–181

Wade T, Wood V A, Heller A, Maggs J, Langton-Hewer R 1987 Walking after stroke: measurement and recovery over the first 3 months. Scand J Rehab Med 19: 25–30

Währborg P, Borenstein P 1988 Verbal performance rating scale. In: After stroke. Behavioral changes and therapeutic intervention in aphasics and their relatives following stroke. Thesis. University of Gothenburg, Gothenburg

Widén Holmqvist L, de Pedro-Cuesta J, Holm M, Sandström B, Hellblom A, Stawiarz L, Bach-y-Rita P 1993 Stroke rehabilitation in Stockholm. Basis for late intervention in patients living at home. Scand J Rehab Med 25: 173–181

29. The stroke patient as a person: body-image and sexuality

E. Greve

INTRODUCTION

This subject is very important and yet very underestimated in stroke rehabilitation today. It has been said, that sexuality – broadly defined – is the most important part of rehabilitation, because of its close relationship to self-confidence, self-esteem, body-image, interpersonal attachment and motivation. Motivation, in turn, is the most important of these relative to rehabilitation. Sigmund Freud, for example, defined mental health as the ability to love and to work.

Today, sexual health should be an integrated component of all rehabilitation programmes, as the importance of sexual information to patient and family has been clinically documented.

WHAT IS SEXUALITY?

Everybody longs for emotional union with other human beings. One may achieve this union with or without sexual activity, but sometimes it is very difficult because of the barriers which are set up between individuals. Sexual activity may facilitate such an emotional union, if the partners are able to give up the resistance against the feeling of being lost. In healthy people sexuality is an integrated part of life. Sexuality is the ability to give and receive emotions, tenderness and intimacy, and to express femaleness or maleness in every aspect of life.

This broad definition of sexuality leads one to the conclusion that no-one is too disabled to be sexual and that everyone has the right to develop the fullest potential in all aspects of life. Disabled people are not asexual and do not lose their sexuality after stroke. These negative opinions are functions of an individual's own prejudgements. People with disabilities have a feeling of isolation and helplessness, and if others deny their sexual problems after stroke, these feelings are increased.

In reality sexual problems among people with disabilities are not so different from problems in the healthy population. Maybe one too often looks for differences instead of recognizing the similarities between able and disabled people. The sexual rights and responsibilities of people with disability are identical to those of all people.

THE PATIENT WITH STROKE IN CRISIS

In the rehabilitation of patients with stroke the staff encounter many very difficult problems. Although compliance with hospital structures and organization may be appreciated by the staff, it may not be related to maximum rehabilitation results, because a successful return to independent life requires active and autonomous behaviour, and not passivity and dependence. Therefore, the difficult patients are sometimes the best in terms of potential for successful rehabilitation.

The changes in the stroke patient create a crisis that affects his/her entire life, and also that of family and friends. This is the reason why the patient with stroke often goes through a period of reduced sexual drive and denial of essential feelings.

Normal feelings of grief as a reaction to serious illness are feelings of fear, anxiety, shock, denial, anger and blame. These feelings are best dealt with by acknowledging them and expressing them. In this way they can be worked out instead of stored. Unhealthy denial and storing of feelings often leads to a protracted grief reaction and interferes negatively with rehabilitation. These feelings need to be replaced with acceptance of the disability if progress is to occur. The patient with stroke has to learn to value his or her new sexual abilities as opposed to trying to regain the same sexual life as before. Therefore, success in sexual rehabilitation results from working on the remaining strengths, thus patients may learn to value their bodies again.

PHYSICAL PROBLEMS AFTER STROKE

What is going wrong for the patient with stroke? Why do so many patients with stroke reduce or cease their sexual activities? Probably some of the reasons are physical problems with catheter, incontinence, hygiene, speech, salivation, vision, hearing, sensibility, dressing or pain. A few have more specific sexual disturbances such as partial or absent erection, retarded or retrograde ejaculation, decreased vaginal lubrication, vaginal pain or reduced sensation in the genital areas.

The reduced or ceased sexual life might also be associated with specific stroke disabilities such as neglect, weakness, spasticity, soiling, decreased ability to touch or fatigue.

PSYCHOLOGICAL PROBLEMS AFTER STROKE

The psychological effects after stroke are perhaps the most significant when patients give up their sexual life. Some of these problems are the result of organic pathology as mentioned earlier, and others have their origin in deep psychological issues such as identity, dependency, self-esteem and values.

Identity

Identity refers to questions of who one is, and was and can become in the face of altered physical capacities. Identity is about who one is as a sexual person.

Dependency

Dependency involves not only dependence on help from others, but also emotional issues about personal power and degree, and about locus of control. If the patient with stroke feels dependent both physically and mentally, this may create serious relationship conflicts and inability to take responsibility for their own sexual needs and behaviour.

Self-esteem

Self-esteem is seriously challenged by disability. Self-esteem and self-confidence depend on body-image and accurate evaluation of one's own behaviour. Self-esteem is necessary for sexual functioning, for being able to feel attractive. If a person does not feel attractive, they may not care so much about their appearance or self, which in turn, really makes them appear unattractive.

Values

Values means ethical principles of behaviour including, e.g. respect, confidence and honesty. Values are also concerned with the meaning of life and deeper spiritual considerations. Sexual values decide a person's sexual behaviour and awareness of these values leads to more honest choices in sexual life.

If these four issues are bothering the patient with stroke, he or she may feel them as disturbances in desire, pleasure, comfort or competence, even when genital function is normal. The patient with stroke may also feel decreased libido, enjoyment, excitement or decreased ability for communication.

Other important aspects of rebuilding emotional and sexual life after stroke could be personal changes, which may be very serious as a background for conflict in a relationship leading to emotional and sexual disturbances, normal grief reaction which may be protracted if feelings are stored, depression, anxiety, or concerns about appearance and disability of the negative kind, which set up limits for the patients, causing them to feel rejected or upset by role changes. Sometimes psychotherapy is needed to solve these problems.

The patient with stroke may fall into a vicious circular reaction such as: how one perceives oneself influences how one acts and therefore what is drawn from other people. How others perceive one, in turn influences how one perceives oneself. If stroke patients have negative images of themselves, this reaction mode may run in the family and among friends, and may be the reason for their withdrawal from the patient.

FAMILY INVOLVEMENT IN REHABILITATION

Previous problems in the family may be worsened by the illness, thus causing rifts, but the crisis can also be managed successfully. Much too often the relatives forget their own grief and only take care of the patient and his reaction to the illness. Staff can have an important role in telling the relatives that it is quite natural that they themselves feel grief. The illness also creates a loss for the close relatives.

Good family adjustment can improve rehabilitation success by providing warm, loving, consistent support to the patient. Therefore, rehabilitation ought to include the family and friends early; this means active inclusion of relatives and not only as visitors. The rehabilitation team can involve the relatives in many ways, e.g. through meetings with the staff in different situations and through family support groups.

HOW TO COPE WITH STROKE

The process of coping following stroke varies from patient to patient and depends on a great number of factors including: previous psychological adjustment, quality of the support system, age at onset; physical health and the patient's own beliefs and expectations.

'Red able' theory is a theory used in quality studies. 'Red ables' in contrast to 'green ables' are the good ones. In the 'red able' theory, one concentrates on the patients that manage well; they could be called the 'super-patients'. It is these patients who succeed in rebuilding their lives with families, friends and perhaps even work.

Consider the super-patients with regard to their ability to succeed in emotional and sexual life after stroke. These are the patients who regain sexual identity, integrity and functioning.

They have some specific abilities; first, they have realized that everyone has a repertoire of behaviour that can communicate sexual feelings. They know that love has no limits and does not care about disability, age or anything else, and that sexuality is being together, emotionally close and is not a question of performance. They know that trust, confidence and tenderness are of great importance and that no sex is better than sex without emotion.

These patients have good premorbid sexual and social adjustment, and they are sensitive to emotional changes in themselves and in others. They know their needs for physical touch and are willing to work for it, because they have an active attitude towards problems and want to fulfil their own wishes.

They know and like their bodies and how they feel and act. They are sensitive to the new signals from their bodies. This gives them self-confidence and self-understanding. They continue with physical training after discharge and are aware of personal hygiene, dressing and appearance.

They respond supportively to necessary role changes and are able to keep separate the roles of caretaker and partner to preserve intimacy. They develop skills in wordless communication and intimacy, because they know that specific and immediate communication between sexually involved partners is essential for a satisfactory relationship.

Most importantly, they develop a willingness to experiment with love, romance, intimacy and techniques. They use their fantasy constructively and value non-genital erogenous zones such as ear, neck, tongue, knee, hand and foot. They are secure enough to realize that not every experiment will work out.

CONCLUSION

The attitude of the rehabilitation team towards these issues is of great importance. Staff should be informative about emotional and sexual problems connected with stroke, they must be aware of the patients' needs for tenderness and body contact, and the spirit of the department should be open-minded and sensitive, so that the patients and their relatives, in turn, feel secure enough to discuss any problem with the rehabilitation team.

FURTHER READING

Boller F, Frank E 1982 Sexual dysfunction in neurologic disorders. Raven Press, New York
Ducharme S, Gill K, Biener-Bergman S, Fertitta L 1993 Sexual functioning: medical and psychological aspects. In: DeLisa J A, Gans B M (eds) Rehabilitation medicine, 2nd edn. Lippincott, Philadelphia
Gill K, Ducharme S 1992 Sexuality and the elderly. In: Calkins E, Davis P J, Ford A B, Katz P (eds) The practice of geriatrics, 2nd edn. Saunders, Philadelphia
Glass D D, Padrone F J 1978 Sexual adjustment in the handicapped. Journal of Rehabilitation 44: 43–47
Humphrey M, Kinsella G 1980 Sexual life after stroke. Sexuality and Disability 3: 150–153
Imes C 1984 Interventions with stroke patients. Cognitive Rehabilitation 2(5): 4–17
Keller S, Buchanan D C 1984 Sexuality and disability: an overview. Rehabilitation Digest 15: 3–7

McIntyre K, Elesna-Adams M 1984 Sexual limitations caused by stroke. Journal of Sex Education and Therapy 10: 57–59

Masters W, Johnson V, Kolodny R 1986 Masters and Johnson on sex and human loving. Little Brown, Boston

Monga T, Lawson J S, Inglis J 1986 Sexual dysfunction in stroke patients. Archives of Physical and Medical Rehabilitation 67: 19–22

Muckleroy R N 1977 Sex counseling after stroke. Medical Aspects of Human Sexuality 1: 115–116

Renshaw D S 1975 Sexual problems in stroke patients. Medical Aspects of Human Sexuality 9: 68–74

30. Early and late rehabilitation of stroke: current approaches including assessment of the quality of outcome

M. Kaste

INTRODUCTION

The annual incidence of stroke in Europe including first and recurrent stroke varies from 150 to 280 per 100 000, the variation being for the most part due to differences in the age structures of the populations involved. The incidence rates rise sharply with advancing age. One-third fall under the age of 65, and two-thirds under the age of 75. The degree of disability in this large group of patients varies from catastrophic, with total dependence upon others, to minimal and manageable disability. At least half of this group has significant neurological residua that limits independence and one-quarter is totally dependent. Application of rehabilitation techniques can reduce the number of patients who are left dependent after stroke.

The physician is almost always asked about the outcome of a specific patient. Figure 30.1 shows items which may help in construction of the statement about outcome.

EARLY REHABILITATION

40% of patients with stroke need active rehabilitation services. Immediate rehabilitation of a victim with stroke is started as soon as it is logistically possible. This means that the patient should be brought to a hospital with

---

1. If the level of consciousness is reduced together with hemiplegia, the mortality is about 40%, and immediate prognosis is poor until actual improvement begins.
2. Rapid onset (less than 5 minutes) of maximal neurological deficit – paralysis in contrast to weakness, then persists for 72–96 hours – generally means that normal function will not return.
3. If there is any movement in the leg during the first week the probability that the patient is able to walk independently is 80%.
4. If there is no meaningful distal motor function in the hand during the first week the likelihood that the hand will recover in performing higher-skilled activities is 20%.

Fig. 30.1 A few guidelines on how to estimate the outcome of a stroke patient.

such facilities as soon as possible not only because of acute diagnosis and therapy but also because of early rehabilitation. If a patient remains at home, which almost never happens in acute stroke in Scandinavia, treatment is initiated as soon as suitable personnel can be recruited to start providing rehabilitation at home.

The intensity of the actual rehabilitation programme depends on the status of the patient and the degree of the disability. If the patient is unconscious the rehabilitation is passive to prevent contractures and joint pain and to prevent distress for the patient when movement is restarted after immobilization. With passive rehabilitation one can also minimize the risk of bed sores and pneumonia. All joints on the paralyzed side are moved through the full range of motion several times a day (3–4 times at least). When the patient recovers consciousness and is able to cooperate or if she/he has a normal level of consciousness from the onset of symptoms, then they are encouraged to take an active part in the rehabilitation programme.

Patients rarely need to be immobilized in bed for more than 1 or 2 days after the stroke unless they have a major decrease in the level of consciousness. Prolonged immobilization and hemiplegia carry a risk of deep venous thrombosis and the complication of pulmonary embolism. In hemiplegic patients and those stroke patients who must be immobile for any reason for more than a day or two, a low dose heparin of low molecular weight heparinoid therapy should be given subcutaneously. After 2 or 3 days most patients who are alert can be moved out of bed with safety and placed in either a wheelchair or fixed chair for a substantial part of each day.

Rehabilitation programme

Once the initial phase of stroke has passed, usually a matter of 2–3 days, but sometimes as long as 2 weeks, the patient should be carefully assessed for the degree of disability and a detailed rehabilitation programme should be devised. The assessment of the patient's situation includes intellectual impairment including specific cognitive deficits such as aphasia, agnosia, apraxia, mood, motivation, the degree of motor weakness, sensory loss and visual loss, as well as the magnitude of problems facing the patient such as finances, return to social activities and work, living at home, sexual function, and the need for care, which all influence the outcome of the rehabilitation programme.

The stroke team

The personnel usually required to provide adequate rehabilitation for victims of stroke, i.e. a stroke team, includes: the patient's physician, who is interested in and trained for stroke, the patient's nurse, who is experienced in stroke management, a physiotherapist trained in stroke rehabilitation, an occupational therapist skilled in stroke, a speech therapist familiar with speech problems in stroke, a neuropsychologist accustomed to stroke rehabilitation, and a social worker familiar with the problems of patients with stroke.

Of course most hospitals treating patients with stroke do not have all these specially trained stroke experts, but the core of the stroke team, i.e. a physician, a nurse and a physiotherapist, can be found in most hospitals and they can provide a decent rehabilitation programme if they rise to the challenge.

Prediction of outcome

All patients with stroke do not have identical potential for recovery. The factors listed in Table 30.1 suggest less optimal outcome after rehabilitation.

The more of the predictors for poor outcome which the patient has (Table 30.1), the less optimal a candidate he/she is for rehabilitation. If there is a local shortage of money and/or rehabilitation services the resources should be allocated to those patients who are most likely to be able to take advantage of the resources invested in them. The aspects of neurological dysfunction that are used to predict outcome are valid for large groups of patients. For individual patients, the variation in outcome may be great. In view of this, it is generally recommended that a 2-week trial of the rehabilitation programme should be carried out to assess a patient's potential for becoming independent. This is particularly rewarding when a patient who is believed to have no rehabilitation potential responds to treatment and becomes independent or less dependent.

Monitoring progress

When the assessment of a patient with stroke has been performed by the members of the stroke team and the rehabilitation programme for him/her

Table 30.1 Factors the presence of which increase the likelihood of poor outcome

Poor outcome	Probably poor outcome
Reduced level of consciousness for longer periods	Hemisensory defect
Incontinence for more than 2 weeks	Right hemispheric injury
Dementia	Marked pre-existent loss of cognitive ability
Marked receptive dysphasia	Marked depression
Severe hemiparesis/hemiplegia with no recovery of motor function within a month	High age
Serious pre-existent systemic disease, especially heart disease	Previous stroke
Neglect with no recovery	Poor socioeconomic background Absence of a family or inability of existing family to help

has been tailored in the rehabilitation meeting, the progress of the patient needs to be followed on a daily basis by the different members involved in the rehabilitation. Once a week the members of the stroke team should meet and analyze the progress of individual stroke patients. Should there be a block in any of the subplans of the rehabilitation programme, the reason for it needs to be established and corrected. The individual patient and the members of their family should be accepted as members of the stroke team and they should be taught stroke rehabilitation; the members of the family also need to be taught when not to help the patient in order to optimize the progress of the rehabilitation plan. As soon as the patient's condition allows they should visit their own home, or their family home, in order to smooth the transit to home and to increase their motivation to do their best in rehabilitation. The occupational therapist, if there is one (if not, a physiotherapist) should undertake the home visit together with the patient to evaluate the changes needed at home in order to support the patient's homecoming.

If the patient needs a longer rehabilitation period within the acute hospital they should be transferred to a special rehabilitation hospital if such a place is available locally, and if the question of who pays for it has been settled. When the patient is transferred to a rehabilitation hospital, it is of the utmost importance that all members of the stroke team who were involved in his/her rehabilitation transfer to the members of the stroke team of the rehabilitation hospital all appropriate documentation of the patient's progress in his/her rehabilitation programme. After institutional rehabilitation, or if the patient does not need such care, the rehabilitation programme can be taken over by the outpatient rehabilitation clinic, if one exists locally. This ensures the smooth transfer of the patient to the next rehabilitation step on the road back to normal life.

The total length of the rehabilitation period in the acute stage of stroke depends upon the severity of the stroke, the financial possibilities and locally available stroke rehabilitation services. The acute stage of the rehabilitation programme should not last longer than is actually needed for a successful outcome, which usually is 12 weeks and seldom more than 24 weeks if the cost–benefit ratio is considered, although it is by no means exceptional for the members of the stroke team to wish to continue with the patient for longer periods than those needed for a good and cost-effective outcome of rehabilitation.

LATE REHABILITATION

The fastest recovery of neurological deficit occurs during the first 3 months after the onset of symptoms. This is also the optimal time for rehabilitation. Active rehabilitation should be administrated as long as objective improvement in the neurological dysfunction is observed. This usually takes from 2 to 6 months.

Patients who have mild to moderate disability generally show more improvement during the first year after discharge from hospital than do patients with severe neurological disability. Even after a 5-year follow-up period there is a consistent but small group of patients who show improvement. This holds true especially for cognitive function.

After most of the improvement in neurological dysfunction has occurred and the active rehabilitation programme has come to an end, the patient with stroke needs a long-term rehabilitation programme which should include a twice-yearly series of 15–20 physiotherapy sessions. This is to guarantee that the functional status which has been achieved during the acute rehabilitation programme is sustained. Should the functional outcome of a patient be in jeopardy, an active, more comprehensive rehabilitation programme is needed, and sometimes it is reasonable to readmit the patient for a more intensive inpatient rehabilitation period.

Assessment of the quality of rehabilitation

The results of rehabilitation programmes for patients with stroke are usually measured by whether the patient can return home and by the degree of independence achieved in activities of daily living (ADL). The quality of life is less seldom assessed and there is no generally accepted scale to evaluate the quality of life of stroke patients.

Activities of daily living (ADL)

The instrument used most often to measure ADL of a patient with stroke is the Barthel index. Although it is far from optimal it is one with which everyone is familiar, which is a distinct advantage and makes it suitable for comparisons not only between individual patients but also between institutions and countries.

The clinical impression

The clinical impression of a patient can be evaluated by using the Rankin scale. This is a 5-grade scale which gives an overall impression of the life situation of a patient. It is quite often used in evaluating the recovery of patients with stroke and allows the comparison of different strategies in stroke management.

Mood

Depression after stroke is common. The mood of a patient can be assessed by using the Hamilton rating scale for depression or the Beck depression inventory, although these include some items which are not useful for patients with stroke. Furthermore they are not suitable for reliable assessment of patients with stroke with major speech problems. It may be useful to perform a dexamethasone suppression test in such patients if they offer evidence of depression through facial expression, attitude, interest in food, prevalence of constipation, tears and sleeplessness. If depression is present, it should be treated. Not only does the treatment of depression affect the quality of life of the patients, but also treated patients show more improvement in rehabilitation programmes than do those who are not treated for depression.

Is there evidence that rehabilitation programmes are indicated?

Rehabilitation programmes do not change the neurological deficit, but patients can become ambulatory and largely independent. Of more importance is the fact that the majority of patients are able to be at home and so do not require nursing-home care. The age of the patient is not a limiting factor, nor is the severity of the dysfunction; on the contrary, elderly patients with stroke and those severely affected can be effectively rehabilitated. Younger patients and those with milder strokes who most often get the major share of rehabilitation resources also have a better outcome without strenuous rehabilitation, whereas elderly patients and those more severely affected have a potential for recovering with rehabilitation but may not do so without rehabilitation.

In Helsinki University Central Hospital, the effects of systematic stroke management in the elderly were assessed in a controlled randomized trial. The study revealed that elderly patients with stroke (no patient was excluded because of severity of stroke, pre-stroke diseases or social factors) were able to leave hospital an average of 16 days earlier (24 vs 40 days), went directly home more often (75% vs 62%) and were more often fully independent in ADL (76% vs 59%) 1 year after the onset of stroke if they had been diagnosed, treated and rehabilitated systematically by a stroke team, as compared with ordinary, less systematic stroke management.

A better outcome of stroke is of benefit in both human and economic terms. That such results can be achieved with systematic stroke management and not by chance is verified by identical results from the University Hospitals of Umeå, Sweden and Trondheim, Norway.

FURTHER READING

Dombovy M L, Sandok B A, Basford J R 1986 Rehabilitation of stroke: a review. Stroke 17: 363
Gresham G E 1992 Rehabilitation of the stroke survivor. In: Barnett H J M, Mohr J P, Stein B M, Yatsu F M (eds) Stroke: pathophysiology, diagnosis and management, 2nd edn. Churchill Livingstone, New York, pp 1189–1201
Indredavik B, Bakke F, Solberg R, Rokseth R, Lund-Haaheim L, Holme I 1991 Benefit of a stroke unit: a randomized controlled trial. Stroke 22: 1026–1031
Kaste M, Palomäki H 1992 By whom should elderly stroke patients be treated? Stroke 23: 163

Langhorne P, Williams B O, Gilchrist W, Howie K 1993 Do stroke units save lives? Lancet 342: 395–398
McDowell F 1987 Rehabilitation from stroke. In: Millikan C H, McDowell F, Easton J D (eds) Stroke. Lea & Febger, Philadelphia, pp 205–220
Norris J W, Hachinski V C 1986 Stroke units or stroke centres? Stroke 17: 360–362
Rissanen A 1992 Cerebrovascular disease in the Jyväskylä region, central Finland. Series of Reports, Department of Neurology, No. 23. University of Kuopio, Kuopio
Sivenius J 1982 Studies on the rehabilitation, epidemiology and clinical features of stroke in east central Finland. Series of Reports, Department of Neurology, No 6. University of Kuopio, Kuopio
Strand T, Asplund K, Eriksson S, Hägg E, Lithner F, Wester P O 1985 A non-intensive stroke unit reduces functional disability and the need for long-term hospitalization. Stroke 16: 29–34
Strand T, Asplund K, Eriksson S, Hägg E, Lithner F, Wester P O 1986 Stroke unit care – who benefits? Stroke 17: 377–381
Viitanen M, Fugl-Meyer K S, Bernspång B, Fugl-Meyer A R 1988 Life satisfaction in long-term survivors after stroke. Scan J Rehab Med 20: 17–24

31. Wheelchairs and seating in stroke

B. Engström

INTRODUCTION

The goal in the rehabilitation process after stroke is to harmonize the return of muscle tone for functional postural reactions and purposeful movement. Designing the treatment and training sessions for the restoration of functional gait is one important priority. Although gait may be a main goal there are many stages preceding the skill of independent walking.

A stage many stroke patients cannot avoid is sitting in a wheelchair. Prescription of a wheelchair, individually fitted, may not be done in the acute or subacute stage. One reason for this is that the aim of the rehabilitation plan is for walking, not for using a wheelchair.

There are, however, some valid reasons why wheelchairs should be individually fitted for more patients early in their rehabilitation programme. These reasons are postural stimulation, physical activity and for psychological reasons.

Many of the patients change dramatically after a stroke. They become not only physically inactive but are also affected mentally and socially. One critical value in life is to maintain mobility. Mobility is a part of social interaction. A patient who experiences great difficulty in maintaining mobility will probably become psychologically less positive than a patient who can move around 'effortlessly' from the beginning of the rehabilitation process. A positive state of mind facilitates the acceptance of a long-term training period. It is easier to convince a patient who is positive that even if the wheelchair is easy to move and feels comfortable, the goal is, after some time, to leave the wheelchair behind and begin walking again.

The patients referred to mainly are the ones who may become debilitatingly inactive, physically, mentally and socially if they spend too much time in bed or sit in poorly fitted, heavy wheelchairs which restrict mobility.

Mobility is one of two reasons for fitting a wheelchair early in the rehabilitation plan. The other reason is so that the patient may experience the upper body in space for the stimulation of postural correction in sitting. Both reasons are part of the therapeutic goals to balance muscle tone and to stimulate dynamic postures for activities of daily living (ADL) and mobility.

This chapter will explore some of the difficulties encountered when sitting in and propelling a wheelchair, with one hand and one or both feet. It will also point out how some of these difficulties can be corrected to improve and stimulate a more functional response.

Foot propulsion when seated is an odd and difficult activity. Patients with stroke are often given a wheelchair without sufficient attention being paid to how the wheelchair is set up. A wheelchair can make the difference between active and efficient training and a postural disaster leading to fatigue and increased spasticity. The wheelchair is, if it is set up correctly, a training tool for 'seated walking' for the stimulation of ADL and mobility, not for only half an hour but for the entire day.

ELDERLY HEMIPLEGIC PATIENTS

Many persons suffering from dysfunction due to stroke are elderly.

Before a decision is made to prescribe a personal wheelchair, many therapists like to 'wait and see' if the ability to walk returns. It is a sensitive decision. There are many factors to consider in the rehabilitation of elderly hemiplegic patients. Age is one important factor; the other is sitting-time.

The rehabilitation programme and the expected outcome for a 50-year-old person, who is still working, is different from the expectations and the approaches used when treating an 80-year-old person. Elderly people may have not only impaired function due to the stroke, but also impaired senses such as vision and hearing, impaired joint mobility, decreased postural reactions and low muscular endurance. This is often a challenge when treating older patients. The difficulty lies in keeping them active.

In order to encourage elderly hemiplegic patients to become more active and ADL-functional they need to participate as much as they can, and they need individually adjusted wheelchairs for that purpose. Even if the intentions are good in the non-prescription of a personal wheelchair, some questions need to be asked:

- How is this elderly person sitting and performing during the day?
- How will this influence the person in the long term?

Many elderly patients with stroke slide down in their wheelchair with little chance of sitting up and they may not be able to propel their wheelchair because it is too heavy to propel.

A couple of months is not a long time for most people, but for a fragile 80-year-old suffering from stroke it may be a very long time. That amount of time can be sufficient to make an elderly person physically and mentally inactive and totally dependent. In the future there will be more and more elderly people to care for and many of them will have had a stroke.

Elderly people improve and maintain their physical and mental functions more readily if they are stimulated to be active from the beginning, after a stroke, and not after some 'observation time'.

For the elderly patients with stroke there are *only* two choices for the future, and they both have a price-tag.

Do it right from the beginning

This option is the stimulation of ADL function and mobility with correctly adjusted wheelchairs early in the rehabilitation process. This may be more costly today, but will probably save money in the future as there will be fewer problems to correct.

'Wait and see'

This option is inefficient physical, mental and social activity caused by poor seating and restricted mobility as a result of low-cost, short-term thinking. This may save money today, but will probably result in considerably more money being spent in the future to correct poor seating and the problems created by inactivity.

FOOT PROPULSION PRINCIPLES

In order to be able to set up a wheelchair for foot propulsion it is necessary to understand some of the forces involved and how they influence the patient when he/she is working with various muscles to move the wheelchair.

One of three basic principles applies when the foot increases the pressure against the floor. The only force direction creating friction is downwards, perpendicular to the floor. An oblique force direction, under the horizontal plane, makes the wheelchair move in the opposite direction to the force applied. The oblique force is a combination of the perpendicular force and the force parallel to the surface; down and sideways.

If the direction of movement of the foot is downwards and backwards the wheelchair moves forward. The downward and forward direction of the foot moves the wheelchair backwards. When the foot direction is downwards and sideways the wheelchair turns.

The relationship of the seat unit, the body position, the rolling resistance and the friction between the foot and the floor decide how much a patient's muscles need to work to move the wheelchair. Muscle force and efficiency change when the position of joints change. The most important leg muscles used in foot propulsion run over the hip joint (gluteus maximus) or the hip and knee joint (hamstring muscles). These muscles' lengths and strengths are dictated by the position of the involved joints and the position of the pelvis. Changes made to the angle of the seat and the backrest change the interrelationships between the pelvis, trunk and hips and the feet. The goal when adjusting a wheelchair's seat unit for foot propulsion is to increase the *cooperation* between the lower body and the upper body.

The leg muscles responsible for performing foot propulsion forwards are hip extensors and knee flexors. They are attached to the pelvis. When they work they tend to tilt the pelvis backwards. If the trunk is not correctly positioned in relation to the pelvis, and to gravity, it is difficult to avoid this pelvic tilt which results in sliding on the seat and slouched sitting. This is a key problem for patients with hemiplegia.

When one foot increases its pressure against the floor, in an attempt to move the wheelchair forwards, the pelvis is easily tilted backwards and/or dragged down on the seat. When one or both arms push forwards on the handrim the tendency is the same – trunk flexion and backward pelvic tilt. This means that there are always forces trying to tilt the pelvis backwards when one propels a wheelchair forwards.

The forces tilting the pelvis backwards need to be 'neutralized' by opposite forces. Stabilizing the pelvis is normally done by leaning the trunk forwards, so adjusting the seat unit for the hemiplegic patient focuses on creating that possibility. The setting up of the wheelchair's seat unit determines how easy or difficult it will be to lean forward.

COMMON COMPENSATIONS IN HEMIPLEGIA

The tilted seat unit and the reclined backrest

A backward tilted seat unit creates two problems, even with a correct seat height. The tilt-in space makes it difficult for the trunk to lean forwards and the front of the seat often restricts the foot in reaching the floor in front of the seat. When the heel or the toes reach the floor the pelvis is forced out of position; it slides down on the seat. A reclined backrest also increases sliding; the pelvis is easily 'dragged' down by the hamstring muscles.

The seat is too low

A seat height for hemiplegic users may be too low, resulting in insufficient thigh support. Active hip flexion is then necessary to lift and move the foot forwards on the floor. Both heel and toe propellers have a tendency to slide down in the chair. Sliding down and moving the foot/feet forwards when foot-propelling makes it less tiring for muscle groups such as iliopsoas (less work), hamstrings (elongation) and dorsiflexors (less dorsiflexion).

The seat is too high

The goal in reaching the floor is to find the functional foot–ground contact. A *motivated* user who cannot reach the floor often compensates by sliding down. Excessive use of toes on one side may stimulate the user to rotate the trunk towards the opposite side and also to press it against the backrest.

THE BACKREST – AN ORTHOSIS FOR THE TRUNK

Many reports are written about seating and the risk of developing pressure sores. Techniques to prevent excessive pressure have resulted in a number of different seat cushions.

Some manufacturers have developed adjustable *seating systems*. Other manufacturers have designed wheelchairs with *built-in* adjustments of the seat and the backrest. There are many useful products on the market and many users are in a far better situation today in terms of sitting in appropriate seating. However, many wheelchairs still have ergonomically ineffective backrests.

In using the term 'backrest', advanced moulded backrests for severely involved users are not included. The backrests referred to are for the majority of wheelchair users – those who do not need special equipment, but need to sit without developing injuries in the long term.

A splint for a paralysed hand is different from the splint for a spastic hand, or a splint for a rheumatic hand. A similar situation exists with a wheelchair backrest for long-term use. The function of the backrest is to support and balance the user's upper body. Users, paralysed from a spinal cord injury, have different upper body needs from hemiplegic users, or rheumatic users. Their major differences and problems, from the seat and upwards, are solved by the seat unit's backrest.

The balance of a person's upper body is individual, from the ischial bones to the head. The effective backrest has contours which follow the contours of the user's spine and trunk to create pressure distribution, balance and stability. The goal with a backrest is to support and facilitate the function of the upper body. The reason why this is so extremely important is time. If a user leans against a backrest 10 hours a day, it must be perfectly fitted or it will begin to cause problems.

BACKREST CONTOURS

Step 1: the pelvis

Make sure that there is sufficient room for the pelvis to efficiently position the sacral bone. It is better to leave the lowest part of the backrest a little loose rather than too tight. If there is insufficient room for the pelvis the user will slide down. Make sure that the sacral part of the pelvis is supported, but be aware of the pressure against this area. Too much pressure also creates sliding.

Step 2: the thoracic spine

Let the contours of the *balanced* extended thoracic spine act as guide. Ensure that the contact area with the thorax is smooth and that the upper part of the backrest allows for thoracic extension.

Supporting the lower and lateral parts of the thorax often stimulates natural extension and makes upright sitting easier. The supporting surfaces in contact with the trunk are efficient if they are shaped according to the contours of the thorax.

Step 3: the lumbar spine

Good contact is ensured by contouring from side to side and following the lordosis. Do not create pressure. Too much pressure causes overextension of the spine or stimulates sliding.

The backrest's *primary support* against the spine should, for most people, be on the sacrum and the pelvis.

Step 4: the cervical spine and the head

A functional, balanced cervical spine and an optimal head position are created by an efficient alignment and balance of the spine, based on a correct position of the pelvis.

SLOPING OF THE SEAT

The trunk response when a foot increases the pressure against the floor depends on *which part* of the foot is used, the foot's *pressure direction* and the *position in space* of the trunk in relation to the active foot.

Backward sloped seat/tilt-in space

A seat sloped backwards makes the pelvis tilt backwards if the seat-to-backrest angle is 90°. An angle of less than 90° positions the pelvis in a more upright position.

Foot pressure against the floor, in an attempt to move the wheelchair *forwards*, activates the gluteal muscle and the hamstring muscles. These muscles simultaneously tilt the pelvis backwards.

Heel pressure stimulates the abdominal muscles to flex the trunk *and* also tilt the pelvis backwards which, in a reclined position, makes it very difficult for the trunk to lean forwards. Toe pressure in this position stimulates the trunk to extend against the backrest which interferes with the leaning of the trunk forwards.

The backward sloped seat makes it difficult to move a wheelchair forwards *without* sliding down, even when the seat-to-backrest angle is less than 90°.

The horizontal, contoured seat

A horizontal, contoured seat and an upright, contoured backrest ensure a more erect position of the pelvis and trunk, making it easier for the user to lean forwards. If the pelvis tilts backwards it can be stabilized by moving the trunk forwards.

The forward sloped, contoured seat

The forward sloped contoured seat tilts the pelvis forwards which facilitates the foot to increase the pressure against the floor and stimulates the trunk to extend and the lean forwards. The response is the same whether it is the heel *or* the toes creating the pressure against the floor, but the heel stimulates a more natural 'gait' response.

Ischial support on the seat

A contoured seat supporting the ischial tuberosities prevents the pelvis from being dragged down by the hamstring muscles, thus preventing the pelvis from tilting backwards, which facilitates forward flexion of the trunk.

Sacral support against the backrest

Such a support prevents the strong gluteal muscles from tilting the pelvis backwards. The support assists the pelvis to maintain an upright position which facilitates the forward flexion of the trunk performed by the abdominal muscles.

ROLLING RESISTANCE

The therapeutic thought behind seating for stroke patients, according to the guidelines presented here, is based on the importance of body awareness and effective (non-complicated) ADL and mobility over a longer period of time. High rolling resistance (muscles work harder) may increase the tilting of the pelvis backwards. In a short time it causes fatigue and sliding, and a functional sitting position is ruined.

CONCLUSION

Recovery after a stroke includes stimulation of natural responses. The position of the body in space in relation to gravity, in standing as well as in sitting, is important.

Many stroke patients are elderly. They may use a wheelchair temporarily or permanently. Training when seated is an integrated part of the rehabilitation process after stroke.

The position in a wheelchair seat unit directly influences the position of joints and corresponding muscles as well as sense organs responsible for postural corrections. The position of the body in space in relation to gravity influences the quality of the proprioceptive input reaching the brain. The goal is to facilitate daily activities and avoid the consequences seen in long-term seating: pressure sores, contractures and high muscle tone.

Furthermore, the adjustment of the wheelchair propulsion unit, the wheels, can facilitate and stimulate mobility and upper body activity early in the rehabilitation. The purpose is positive physical, mental and social stimulation.

Some of the important points to bear in mind are:

- horizontal or slightly forward sloped – contoured seat
- ischial support – preventing the pelvis from sliding
- sacral support – preventing a backward pelvic tilt
- balance of the trunk – natural thoracic extension
- stimulation of the user to lean forwards
- freedom of motion of the active foot or feet
- low rolling resistance.

32. The health needs of people with stroke: a preliminary study

A. Parry

INTRODUCTION

Strokes continue to be a major cause of disability and institutionalisation among elderly people, taking up just under 16 000 beds in National Health Service hospitals in the UK every day. Consequently, health gain investments in both prevention and rehabilitation are important considerations for purchasers and providers of health care.

North Derbyshire Health Authority is responsible for providing a broad range of services for some 365 000 people in widespread and diverse communities, including areas of great affluence and areas of high unemployment in both its highly industrialised eastern zone and its scenic western and northern rural sectors. Applying the data and ratios from numerous published epidemiological studies (e.g. Bamford et al 1988), approximately 875 new and recurrent strokes can be expected in the district each year, about 30% of sufferers are likely to die within the first 3 weeks and 50–60% will survive for longer than a year.

Wade (1991) has warned that epidemiological studies 'do not help much with planning services because they do not give adequate information on levels of impairment and disability'. We estimate that there are upwards of 1000 people in North Derbyshire at any one time with some residual disability from stroke. 65% will have severe functionally disabling problems and the majority of them and their informal carers will be elderly. If targets for reduction of deaths from stroke by the year 2000 are met, it is reasonable to assume that a significant proportion of the survivors will be disabled and elderly.

The true extent of the burden of stroke on the community is unknown and there is a dearth of information to help planning of services. In response to the British Government's green paper 'The Health of the Nation' which set out national targets to be achieved in the next 15 years, the Health Authority's Department of Research and Information has focused much of its attention on gaining local people's views about existing services and their needs and wishes for development of services. They have influenced development of health strategies, evaluation of services and community initiatives. The small empirical study described in this chapter (Parry et al

1993) focused on the experiences, quality of life and health needs of people with stroke to assist in the development of health strategies. There were three main tasks:

• To prepare a review of the literature on stroke with particular attention to the social and clinical aspects of rehabilitation.

• To provide a qualitative analysis of the range of health needs of people with stroke, to which were added the needs of informal carers.

• To prepare a research proposal for a more comprehensive prospective study of rehabilitation after stroke.

The outcome from the first two tasks has not only provided background information for two applications for research funding but, more importantly, has achieved its main purpose and influenced developments in stroke rehabilitation services.

IMPLICATIONS FOR STROKE REHABILITATION FROM THE LITERATURE

Awareness of the number of deaths and disabilities due to stroke, belief that recovery can be assisted and enhanced, increasing provision of rehabilitation, and consequent escalation in costs have all stimulated research. The physical consequences of stroke are well documented and numerous studies have looked at the effectiveness of ameliorative and restorative interventions in different care settings. Organisation of care and rehabilitation and effective use of resources were major concerns of this study.

In different areas of the UK, 38–60% of patients with stroke are never referred to hospital or for rehabilitation (Dennis 1987) although some of them will have residual deficits. As therapists undertake many activities which are not 'hands-on' treatment of the patient, the relatives of patients who do not have access to rehabilitation do not receive the instruction, counselling and support provided by therapists. Those who are referred may be admitted to general medical wards, units for care of the elderly, intensive stroke units or specialist stroke wards, and they may be transferred from one to another at some stage, when they may or may not be assigned to a specialist stroke team. Brocklehurst et al (1978) noted an apparent paradox: that 17% of stroke patients referred to hospital in the first 2 weeks after stroke could walk unaided but that 33% of those who were not admitted could not stand unaided and 25% could not even turn in bed without assistance. Not surprisingly, they concluded that 'physiotherapy and other forms of therapy are needed by more patients than receive them'.

The quality of many of studies on outcome from rehabilitation is only fair at best, with poorly defined selection criteria and apparent opportunities for biased selection of samples, incomplete data, too much statistical manipulation (sometimes to cover up biased selection) and limited (or selective) interpretation. Despite these flaws and variations in research design and the organisation of rehabilitation, over the last 40 years delayed onset of rehabilitation, i.e. physiotherapy and occupational therapy, has been the most frequently identified variable correlating with poor functional outcome (e.g. Andersen et al 1950, Novack et al 1984). Although poor functional outcome is also said to be correlated with age (e.g. Novack et al 1984), several researchers (e.g. Wade & Langton-Hewer 1987) have found no association and Lind (1982) suggests that outcome appears better in younger patients simply because they are less severely affected by the stroke than older people. Although ability to use the upper limb is essential for functional activities, only Wade (1993) has specifically noted persistence in motor deficits in the upper limb as a significant variable in determining functional outcome.

Recent studies (Young & Forster 1992) suggest that community care and rehabilitation are more cost-effective than hospital care and that outcome is greater and more sustainable; but Acheson (1985) has complained that the term 'community care' is seductive and does not have universal meaning. The need for nursing care is said to be the main reason for admittance to hospital, but this hides a number of social factors and a gender difference – most stroke patients are admitted to hospital because they live alone or because their chief carer cannot manage, and older women, married or single, move into institutionalised care but married men are usually cared for by their wives (Kelly-Hayes et al 1988).

Although relatives are the cornerstone of the British Government's policy of care in the community, apart from Anderson's study (Anderson 1992), the experiences of informal carers have been relatively neglected. It is not clear which aspects of caring cause them most distress: the mood and social behaviour of the patient, or the repetitiveness of daily tasks, or the need for constant watchfulness which restricts their own activities. Access to a 'key person' relieves many of their immediate anxieties and needs (Jones & Vetter 1985).

Brocklehurst and his colleagues (1978) advocated special domiciliary stroke teams that could attend new patients with stroke at short notice to assess needs, deploy resources, instruct the chief carer and prepare the patient for day hospital care at the earliest opportunity. More recently, the York Health Economics Consortium (1992) has suggested that more efficient use of rehabilitation resources would involve 'more combined use of in-patient care, domiciliary services and day care centres'.

ISSUES ARISING FROM THE INTERVIEWS

In depth interviews were conducted in the homes of patients with stroke, four men and four women, who had been referred because they had experience of inpatient and outpatient care in different hospitals within and outside the district. Chief carers and other individuals were present for part or all of the interview in all but two cases. The interviews were tape-recorded and transcribed in full.

The patients were aged between 62 and 77 years and had all been involved in quite complex and changing patterns of care. Three key elements of care were identifiable: self-care, formal care from health and social services and informal care from family, friends and voluntary groups. Most felt that their needs were being met and some were full of praise for health care practitioners and social service workers. Physiotherapists and occupational therapists were singled out for particular commendation. Nurses and doctors were mentioned less frequently, with doctors appearing to be somewhat ephemeral figures in their experiences of care. All respondents but one were dissatisfied with particular aspects of their care or specific episodes of care.

Particular observations which inform health care strategies are:

• Both patients and carers expressed the view that hospital was 'the right place' to be in the early weeks after stroke because carers 'could not have coped' with the situation. The poor health and advanced years of carers and other features of domestic circumstances are clearly of relevance here.

• Contrasting experiences of quality of care came through as a theme. There was evidence that perceived needs were not always being met in hospital during the acute phase when professional attention was concentrated on the patient's medical condition. Transfer from an acute hospital to a community hospital had changed the focus from the condition to the person in most cases, but hospital stay was still subsequently remembered as 'unhappy'.

• Patients need factual information and opportunities to talk about what the stroke means for them now and in the future. A number of respondents gave accounts of trying 'to make sense' of what had happened to them and expressed the need to talk through their experiences with professionals at different stages throughout the aftermath of stroke.

• Patients' preference for, or lack of objection to, time-consuming outpatient visits to therapy departments rather than treatment in their own homes was associated with their need to get out of the house and meet other people socially. Although their carers sometimes attended with them, these visits also gave some spouses a much needed break.

• Both carers and patients raised issues related to the quality and timescale of follow-up rehabilitation. They were convinced that the patient would have benefited from more intensive therapy, particularly physiotherapy but also occupational therapy, and for a longer period.

• In all cases, informal carers made very significant contributions to care of their relatives. They had unmet needs for information and more practical demonstrations of lifting, bathing and assisting or undertaking other activities of daily living. Those who did not live with the patient were involved in complex visiting and support arrangements. Respite care appears to be an important option available to couples and families living with stroke.

CONCLUSIONS

Similar issues related to social and clinical aspects of acute care and rehabilitation were identified from the literature and the interviews. Physiotherapists and occupational therapists appear to play a crucial role as 'key persons' in building up and channelling the motivation of patients with stroke and supporting their carers. This raises questions about the roles of other health care professionals, the coordination of efforts of formal and informal carers, the effects of late commencement of rehabilitation, and the real costs of care in the community.

A mixture of inpatient care, domiciliary services and day care is needed to meet the needs of patients and carers at different times, and therapists and other health care practitioners need to be flexible so that specialist assessment and treatment are available where and when a patient needs them. The structure of the community service in North Derbyshire appears ideally suited to implementation of a service which makes use of different settings, and therapy-led community-based stroke teams will be established in two pilot locations later this year.

As with all research, the study raised more questions than it answered:

• As the 'package of care' is a combination of care-inputs from a range of individuals and agencies, to what extent do patients experience it as integrated and coordinated or disjointed?

• What are the assumptions, policies and practices of family doctors in discussing the alternative options of home and hospital care with patients and their carers immediately after a stroke and in referring patients to hospitals?

• Is there an over-reliance by the statutory services on informal carers? That is, are too many assumptions made about the ability, willingness and capacity of spouses and other family members to take on a substantial caring role?

• Do informal carers, patients and health professionals have conflicting perceptions about what is in the best interests of the patient with stroke?

It is planned to address these and other questions in a more comprehensive prospective study linked with evaluation of the new community stroke teams.

Acknowledgements

This preliminary study was undertaken for North Derbyshire Health Authority by the author and two colleagues in the Health Research Centre at Sheffield Hallam University, Carol Thomas and David Clark, who are sociologists with interests in chronic illness, informal care and the organisation of services in the community. It highlights the benefits of a multidisciplinary approach to health needs assessment. Our mutually beneficial collaboration with Andy Layzell, Director of Research and Information, and Pennie Roberts, Disability Services Manager, both at North Derbyshire Health Authority is continuing.

REFERENCES

Acheson E D 1985 The over-used word community. Health Trends 17: 3
Andersen A L, Hanvik L J, Brown J R 1950 A statistical analysis of rehabilitation in hemiplegia. Geriatrics 5: 214–218
Anderson R 1992 The aftermath of stroke: the experiences of patients and their families. Cambridge University Press, Cambridge
Bamford J, Sandercock P, Dennis M et al 1988 A prospective study of acute cerebrovascular disease in the community: the Oxfordshire community stroke project. 1. Methodology, demography and incident cases of first-ever stroke. Journal of Neurology, Neurosurgery and Psychiatry 51: 1373–1380
Brocklehurst J C, Andrews K, Morris P E, Richards B, Laycock P J 1978 Medical, social and psychological aspects of stroke: final report. University of Manchester, Department of Geriatric Medicine
Dennis M 1987 Incidence of risk factors and outcome. British Journal of Hospital Medicine, March: 194–198
Jones D A, Vetter N J 1985 Formal and informal support received by carers of elderly dependants. British Medical Journal 291: 643–645
Kelly-Hayes M, Wold P A, Kannal W B, Sytkowski P, D'Agostino A, Gresham G E 1988 Factors influencing survival and need for institutionalisation following stroke: the Framingham study. Archives of Physical Medicine and Rehabilitation 69: 416–418
Lind K 1982 A synthesis of studies on stroke rehabilitation. Journal of Chronic Diseases 35: 133–149
Novack T A, Haban G, Graham K, Satterfield W T 1984 Stroke onset and rehabilitation: time lag as a factor in treatment outcome. Archives of Physical Medicine and Rehabilitation 65: 316–319
Parry A, Thomas C, Clark D 1993 The health needs of people with stroke: a preliminary study. Health Research Centre Report No 4, Sheffield Hallam University
Wade D T 1983 Predicting Barthel ADL scores at 6 months after acute stroke. Archives of Physical Medicine and Rehabilitation 64: 24–28
Wade D T 1991 Stroke services: purchasing guidance for District Health Authorities. National Health Service Management Executive, London
Wade D T, Langton-Hewer R 1987 Functional abilities after stroke: measurement, natural history and prognosis. Journal of Neurology, Neurosurgery and Psychiatry 50: 177–182
York Health Economics Consortium 1992 Is rehabilitation cost effective? University of York
Young J B, Forster A 1992 The Bradford community stroke trial: 6 months results. British Medical Journal 304: 1085–1089

33. When the therapist stops and the rest is nursing or less than nursing

D. Christensen

INTRODUCTION

The major focus of this chapter is the following: If the patient's caregiver, whatever his/her educational background, succeeds in providing goal- and method-orientated rehabilitation care for the stroke patient, all other professionals involved in the rehabilitation team will succeed, but if the caregiver does not succeed, then no-one will succeed.

The following topics will be addressed:

- When does the therapist stop?
- What is nursing?
- What is less than nursing?

WHEN DOES THE THERAPIST STOP?

The answer to this question is: Often long before all the rehabilitation objectives have been reached. Many patients with stroke experience the moment the therapist discontinues treatment as the end of everything, as the end of life.

It is therefore extremely important that all those who are involved in the rehabilitation team are very aware of how they imagine and profile themselves as a professional, in relation to other professionals, and in relation to the patients and to their relatives.

Conditions which may be further investigated are:

- Who does actually decide to discontinue treatment?
- Is the decision made formally or informally?

The physician has the formal right, and the power to refer patients and, in some countries, to prescribe and discontinue treatment, be it physiotherapy, occupational therapy or speech therapy. However, when the physician prescribes physiotherapy, for example, what is his/her intention? Does the physiotherapist think in the same way? Do they have the same picture in their minds? Likewise, do they also have the same picture in their minds, when deciding to discontinue treatment?

Therapists do not have the formal right in all countries, but they have the professional power, and perhaps also the informal power, to continue or discontinue treatment. In this way, therapists have the possibility of influencing the physician's decision. Therefore it is important that therapists are exact about the reasons why they choose to discontinue their treatment at a particular time.

Economy, as well as the general attitude towards patients with stroke are factors that influence strongly the decisions that are made. For example, elderly patients with stroke have less possibility of being transferred to a stroke unit than younger patients with stroke. Patients who are to be discharged to nursing homes receive less intensive treatment than those patients who are to return to their own homes. Such attitudes affect all members of the rehabilitation team, including the therapists. Therefore, these factors have to be considered when debating arguments or reasons for discontinuing treatment and discharging the patient.

However, regardless of the arguments, the reality of the situation for the patient with stroke is that, for as long as they live, most patients will need stimulation and rehabilitation care, supervision and guidance, as well as treatment by therapists, in order to encourage normal movement, and to prevent spasticity, pain and unnecessary suffering.

At the time of discharge most patients are facing the fact that daily help and care will be given by a nursing aide or so-called home carer, with no specific training in stroke care.

Therapists are also aware of this fact. Therefore, they want to make sure that the patients can manage at home and will feel secure and safe. Too early in the rehabilitation process therapists feel the need to teach the patients to compensate, or to become able to manage one-handed, e.g. to use a stick in order to keep their balance when walking. However, in doing so, they not only discontinue treatment, but seem also to discontinue the whole rehabilitation process.

The patients may think that nothing more will be done or can be done. Relatives will react in the same way, as will the nurses and the auxiliaries. The rehabilitation process will stop too early, and will not continue as the lifelong process that it really should be.

Therefore, it is extremely important that when therapists discontinue treatment, they make abundantly clear to those taking over:

- that the reasons for discharging the patient at the particular time are valid and are well documented
- that discharge from the hospital does not mean that the rehabilitation objectives have necessarily been reached
- that there are plans for the patients' future care and treatment outside the hospital
- that the plans describe the problems that still have to be worked at, the method to be used, and the time for evaluation and revision of the plans.

The signals sent by therapist to those taking over are highly important, because they pave the way for continuing care, and thereby also for a continuing rehabilitation process.

WHAT IS NURSING?

Nursing care is based on a continuing 24-hour approach. Therefore, nursing care for the stroke patient is as important as therapy, in the long term. It is possible that some therapists do not appreciate this. Some therapists do not set the highest objectives for their patients because they know that nurses are not able or willing to integrate principles of rehabilitation into the daily care programme for the patient. Some of the reasons for this are that:

- the methods which should be used are not communicated openly and clearly by the therapists
- the methods to be used are not accepted by the head nurse, the physician or even by the therapist in charge; therefore everybody can do as they see fit
- nurses do not traditionally accept or respect prescriptions from a therapist, as they do from the physician
- there may be no agreement between the people in charge as to the methods to be used.

However, in some places it seems possible to work together and thereby raise the quality of treatment for the patient with stroke. Where this happens the following may apply:

- Each professional is able to identify his role and responsibilities. This means, that physiotherapists and occupational therapists are giving treatment which belongs solely to their own profession.
- Nurses are doing the nursing, but are so well educated in methods and principles of rehabilitation, that they can integrate the principles of rehabilitation into their nursing care, so that they can participate with confidence in team conferences, and thereby be seen as valuable members of the rehabilitation team.

It must be made clear that therapists may teach others, including nurses, about, for example, their methods, their objectives and what they want to be followed up in the nursing care programme. However, they should not, and cannot, teach nursing care. Therapists should teach principles of treatment and expect nurses to be able to translate those into nursing. It is the responsibility of the nurse in charge to make this happen.

Nurses have to understand that for the patient to be able to benefit from the rehabilitation process, nurses need to carry out the principles of, for example, the Bobath concept, or whichever method or concept has been selected. It is essential for agreement to be reached upon the concepts, principles or methods to be used; only in this way is it possible to build a body of knowledge which is method-based rather than person-based.

Nurses have an obligation to learn about, for example, the Bobath concept themselves, in order to be competent co-workers with therapists. Therapists in turn must understand their obligation to communicate changes in the use of concepts or principles to the nursing staff, in order to be reliable co-workers with nurses.

This may seem to restrict the possibilities that therapists possess to develop methods. However, it is important to understand that the therapist can work as he/she chooses, but that what is communicated to the nursing staff must be within the frame of the principles that are agreed upon, otherwise it is impossible to ensure continuity of treatment and care. The nurse will become confused, and so will the patient. The patient may tend to be too dependent upon the therapist, and may not value time spent in other settings, or with other professionals.

The signals sent to the patients and their relatives should be:

- in whatever setting the patients are treated or cared for, the methods used and the expectations for the patients are the same
- there is a common plan, which refers to the principles used
- it is obvious to all involved that the plan is carried out throughout the day
- that the time spent in the ward is as important as the time spent in therapy.

In this way, the professionals respect the patients and the importance of the learning process, which are the essence of rehabilitation.

WHAT IS LESS THAN NURSING?

'Less than nursing' occurs when the home carers take over which, as mentioned earlier, often takes place in the long term. The home carers may be able to carry out a simple plan and to obey an instruction. They are not able to change plans or prescribe plans, because they have neither the educational background nor the competency to do so. Therefore, therapists have to communicate with the nurse in charge if something has to be corrected or changed.

It is the nurse, not the therapist, who has the responsibility for the quality of the principles and the methods used. The therapist working in home care settings should be aware of the person to whom they should communicate any change in plans, for example. The nurse is legally responsible for the work of the home carer, and is therefore the back-up for the home carer. Many therapists may not be aware of this, which may be one of the reasons why important information from the therapist, about changes in the rehabilitation plan, is not transmitted or transferred to a new plan – simply because the information is communicated at the 'wrong' place or level.

It is important to understand that only those who have formed the plan can change it, and that it is impossible for home carers, as well as other medical personnel, to work systematically and in a goal-orientated manner over time, if new information is not communicated effectively.

The signals sent to the patient and to the relatives should confirm that:

- the methods used in treatment and care are the same, even though the educational background of those carrying out the care may be quite different
- the nurse is responsible for the quality of the nursing care, wherever this takes place
- the nurse is responsible for coordinating the plans between the therapists and the home carer.

When the home carer succeeds in adhering to, for example, the Bobath concept of rehabilitation of the stroke patient, every other nurse and therapist will succeed, too, and the patient's progress will demonstrate this. However, to make this happen is the challenge presented to all those who are involved in the rehabilitation process.

CONCLUSION

In order to ensure quality in the treatment and care of the stroke patient, there has to be:

- agreement on the principles and methods used
- a common plan which reflects the methods used with regard to the specific patient
- a clear understanding of the responsibilities each profession has in relation to each other, and to the patients
- coordination of the rehabilitation treatment and care; this is a matter of leadership.

FURTHER READING

Christensen D 1991 Genoptræning på sygehuse må følges. Op Journal 2: 28–29
Christensen D 1994 Apopleksi i hverdagen. Håndbog for Social- og sundhedshjælpere og andre hjælpere i hjemmet. Munksgaard, København
Daugaard D, Brunn J 1994 Pilotprojekt gav bedre patientbehandling. Danske fysioterapeuter 76(5): 4–5
Muss I 1990 Klinisk sygeplejespecialist i primær sektor? Klinisk Sygepleje 4(1): 2–9
Olsen V, Saksager K, Schmidt M 1993 Udskrivelse fra et apopleksiafsnit. Klinisk Sygepleje 7(1): 14–20
Ryen S 1992 Rehabilitation av store hodeskader. Klinisk Sygepleje 6(4): 15–20

34. Cognitive plasticity and bodily-kinaesthetic intelligence: on neuroplasticity and movement science (abstract)

K. Fredens

Successful treatment of people with brain damage will always be in a permanent mode of change and adaption, in relation to both therapeutic working methods and the patient's sociocultural situation. The challenge of change lies in developing the patient's learning skill and identifying the main barriers to changes, e.g. fear of the unknown, resistance to alteration and a desire to hang onto the familiar.

No-one can cope with situations they do not understand. The patient must become a skilled learner, and must gradually take responsibility for his/her own learning and development in order to gain autonomy. This may not always be easy, and there will be situations where a temporary or permanent compensation due to lack of learning skill may be relevant. However, the skilled learner will develop a sense of fulfilment and confidence to take on problems, and will use more ways of learning and transfer learning more easily from one situation to another.

Learning is not incompatible with training, but a distinction should be drawn between persuasion and conviction. Training is a means of bringing about learning; it has a persuasive power and is focused mostly on the product. Learning is a wider concept; it brings about understanding of the learning process. This is why people do not always have to be trained in order to learn, and why people may learn despite receiving ineffective training.

It is essential, in 'training' patients, to increase the number of ways of learning and to choose appropriately between them. This leads to cognitive plasticity.

Movement science is the art of communicating confidence in and an understanding of the learning ability of one's own bodily-kinaesthetic intelligence.

35. Motor recovery following stroke: towards a disability-orientated assessment of motor dysfunctions

T. Mulder, J. Pauwels, B. Nienhuis

INTRODUCTION

Although most stroke patients suffer from several disabilities which can include hemiparesis, hemianopia, neglect, dysphasia, incontinence and a mix of cognitive, behavioural and emotional dysfunctions, recovery of motor function is still one of the most important goals of rehabilitation. Patients as well as their relatives consider the re-acquisition of their locomotor capacity to be of the utmost importance (Mumma 1986).

However, what is meant when terms such as 'motor recovery' and 'locomotory capacity' are used? What kind of recovery does one have in mind? Increased strength, coordination and control are, indeed, elements of recovery, and conventional motor assessment procedures (e.g. gait labs) focus explicitly on these elements. But although a number of studies indicate that the visual assessment of a patient's gait is inferior to quantitative methods which use gait analysis techniques (Saleh & Murdoch 1985), it is known that these measurements have a limited generalization value for predicting activities of daily living. It is also known that the majority of expensive high-tech facilities are not used as a day-to-day clinical assessment tool (Messenger & Bowker 1987). To solve this problem biomedical engineering has, until now, emphasized the improvement in the technical capacities of the systems.

In this chapter it will be argued that this is the wrong route. It is argued here that for the prediction of functional recovery an assessment approach which differs radically from the conventional one is necessary. Preliminaries for such a novel approach will be discussed here.

MOVEMENT VS SKILL

Movements are the output of a dynamic interaction between muscular forces and peripheral field effects (e.g. gravity, friction, joint reactive forces) and can be described in terms of their pattern, displacement or topology. It is important to note, however, that movement is the means by which an action is realized. The nature of these means, however, is not fixed or stereotyped but is closely related to the context in which the action takes place. Hence, when we rely on the analysis at the movement level we do not learn very much about the action itself. Actions represent the most 'molar' or global level of description and constitute a change in the relationship between the performer and the environment (Gentile 1987). They are organized in terms of major segments (e.g. reaching, lifting, drinking) and each segment in turn is organized in terms of simpler movements. Actions are said to be skilled when their performance has reached a level where they appear to be effortless. In other words, skilled activities are characterized by more or less automatic and smooth performance, more or less independent of cognitive and perceptual control. To prevent misunderstanding, 'automatically' or 'skilled' does not mean without any feedback-dependency or error-monitoring.

There is a conceptual relationship between these terms, and the terms 'impairment' and 'disability' as used in rehabilitation medicine. Impairments are abnormalities or losses of body structures and represent disturbances at the organ level (e.g. loss of muscle strength, decreased range of motion). Disabilities reflect the consequences of impairments in terms of functional performance and activities and thus represent disturbances at the level of the person. One could argue that the analysis of movement refers to the level of impairment, whereas the analysis of skill refers to the level of disability. Against this background a disability can be seen as the final result of the breakdown of skill, characterized by the non-automatic, jerky performance of a sensorimotor task, largely dependent on cognitive and perceptual guidance. Hence, a disability reflects a disturbed functional behaviour as the subject-specific consequence of some disease process. It is important to note that a disability can exist more or less independently of the type of disease; that is to say, different diseases and/or impairments may lead to the same disability, whereas the same disease may result in different disabilities across different subjects.

Since the ultimate goal of rehabilitation is the restoration of skilled behaviour, rehabilitation outcome measurement should focus on this level. However, until now there have been no motor assessment procedures focusing on this disability-orientated level. Most of the available procedures focus on the level of movement impairments.

THE PRINCIPLE OF OUTPUT CONSTANCY

One of the crucial characteristics of human behaviour is its flexibility and adaptability. The behaviour is continuously influenced by multimodal input, i.e. motor behaviour is always the result of an interaction between motor, sensory, and cognitive factors. The relative 'weights' of these factors, however, depend on the complexity of the task, the skilfulness of the performer and the integrity of the motor system. Overlearned tasks such as standing and walking are to a large degree automatized and require minimal cognitive and visual guidance. For example, a healthy adult is perfectly able to maintain a stable, upright position while performing a secondary task such as mental calculation or counting backwards by three or to remain stable with the eyes closed. This is not always possible for a patient with central or peripheral nervous system damage. For example, at the beginning of the rehabilitation process, the balance performance of a lower leg amputee is seriously hindered by the simultaneous performance of a secondary non-motor cognitive task. This dual task interference effect, however, diminishes across time, indicating the reappearance of automaticity (Geurts et al 1991b, Mulder & Geurts 1991).

The same is true for visual guidance. In the beginning, balance performance depends strongly on visual input, whereas across time this dependency decreases. In a series of experiments, it has been shown that a decrease in dual task interference occurs as well as a decrease in visual dependency, reflecting relevant aspects of motor system recovery across time (Geurts & Mulder 1992, Geurts et al 1992). It has also been shown that dual task interference and visual dependency are behavioural aspects which may explain the loss of automaticity so characteristic for patients with traumatic brain injury.

These examples refer to an important property of the motor system which could be termed 'output constancy', and which reflects the tendency of the system to keep the output (action-result) constant by continuously adapting the means to the changing internal and/or external conditions. The system 'selects' the optimal strategies for reaching the environmental goal. When, following a lesion, lower order control strategies are no longer possible, the system shifts to higher order strategies (e.g. visual or cognitive guidance).

This is an important principle because it shows that focusing solely on the output under optimal conditions teaches us nothing about the way the system generates this output. Besides, a significant risk exists that the capacity of the patient will be overestimated. Indeed, in our example the patient could maintain balance and could walk, but the slightest increase in complexity disturbed the performance. The relevance of this point for rehabilitation output measurement may be clarified by the following example: suppose that a patient at the end of a rehabilitation period is able to walk independently. In conventional terms this would probably be seen as the reflection of a successful treatment. However, how successful this therapy is for daily activities also depends on the 'costs' of walking; i.e. when walking is possible only under optimal conditions (e.g. flat floor, no hindrances, no distracting stimuli and no noises), it can be predicted that although the person has the capacity to walk he/she does not have the ability to walk. Indeed, he/she will not be able to walk under normal daily circumstances which are always and in principle characterized by noise, obstacles or distracting stimuli. One could even argue that in this case the rehabilitation process 'delivered' not a successful patient but on the contrary a vulnerable and unsafe patient.

This example stresses the necessity for measuring the performance of patients not only under standard (and often optimal) hospital conditions but under a number of conditions ranging in complexity from very simple to very complex. In other words, assessment procedures should copy as far as possible the requirements of the outside world.

THREE PRINCIPLES OF RECOVERY

Recovery after central nervous system damage may be understood on at least two levels: first, on the level of morphological repair processes and secondly, on the level of the development of novel control strategies. The latter is primarily the domain of physical and occupational therapy and of clinical neuropsychology, and is also the level on which the present chapter focuses.

Until now the mechanisms of central reorganization have been poorly understood and have hardly been studied in the context of rehabilitation medicine. As indicated, motor behaviour should be seen as the result of a continuous interaction between several sources of internal and external input and stored neural rules. From this, it follows that the study of the interaction between input and output patterns may be more important for the understanding of recovery than the analysis of the manifest motor output in isolation.

The majority of clinical research in the field of motor recovery, however, can be characterized by a rather elementary, impairment-orientated approach. Clinical gait studies provide us with ample data on the basic characteristics of pathological gait but they do not deliver much information about the functional or behavioural aspects of recovery. The gap between the laboratory and the everyday world seems to be very large.

The above-mentioned notion of motor control, however, enables us to take a novel standpoint in the assessment debate. Indeed, if motor, sensory and cognitive factors interact permanently in the guidance of behaviour then these factors should be part of any assessment procedure focused on functional recovery.

Three principles of functional reorganization can be distilled from the work performed in recent years in Nijmegen (Geurts et al 1991a, Mulder 1991, 1992, 1993a,b, Mulder & Geurts 1993). It is argued that functional recovery is reflected by:

• a decrease in cognitive regulation
• a decrease in visual dependency
• a restoration of sensorimotor adaptability.

Of course, these principles do not cover the recovery process in toto, since it is well-known that motivational factors and a whole range of neuropsychological factors also play a crucial role in the prediction of the recovery process (Henley et al 1985, Kotila et al 1984). Nevertheless, these principles may form the impetus for the development of novel assessment techniques in the sensorimotor domain.

Decrease in cognitive regulation

In the earlier work on motor learning three stages are outlined:

1. The cognitive stage, in which the learner makes an initial approximation to the skill, based upon background knowledge, observation and instruction.
2. The associative stage in which performance is refined through the elimination of errors.
3. The autonomous stage in which skilled performance is well-established.

During the cognitive stage the performance is slow, jerky, painstaking and under intentional control. Later in practice one may observe a performance which is fast, smooth and not under intentional control (Fitts & Posner 1967).

The first stage of recovery is comparable to a large extent to the cognitive stage in learning, i.e. the patient is very vulnerable to every distraction. To measure whether this vulnerability decreases across time, a dual-task procedure may be employed. This procedure, in fact, is quite simple and can be used without any high-tech facilities: one only has to observe the velocity of a motor task under training (e.g. walking), then a second, non-motor, task is introduced (e.g. counting backwards by three) and the performance of this task is rated, while the patient is sitting. Now one has an impression of the quality of the gait performance, as well as an impression of the ability of the patient to perform the secondary task.

The next step is to combine these tasks (walking while counting backwards) and to measure the effect of the attention-demanding secondary task on the performance of the main task (walking).

If during rehabilitation re-automatization has taken place, it can be predicted that the gait task will be hindered only minimally, or not at all, by the simultaneous performance of a secondary task. However, if at the end of the rehabilitation process the performance of the gait task is still substantially hindered by the performance of a secondary task, this indicates that less re-automatization has taken place.

Decrease in visual dependency

The same logic can be followed for the role of visual information in the control of motor tasks. It has been shown that at the beginning of the rehabilitation process a strong dependency exists on visual input. That is to say, the performance of a task is disproportionally hindered by the withdrawal of visual input (eyes closed), which is probably a reflection of the fact that the lesion affected the redundancy of sensory input. The post-lesion input specifications are no longer known to neural networks. As long as novel and stable input–output relations do not exist the system cannot depend on the somatosensory input and is forced to switch to a bypass strategy (visual guidance). The duration of this bypass strategy is an indication, albeit indirect, of the capacity of the system to employ somatosensory input, a capacity which is crucial for normal and skilled behaviour.

A restoration of sensorimotor adaptability

Normal behaviour is characterized by a large amount of flexibility, i.e. the skilled performer is able to avoid obstacles in a fluent and smooth way, and even if they appear in a sudden and unpredictable manner, they form no real problem for the performer. In patients, however, the capacity to anticipate or react to obstacles is markedly reduced, leading to a slow and unstable gait. It is argued here that restoration of sensorimotor adaptability is an important ingredient of recovery and therefore has to be measured.

Preliminaries for a disability-orientated task set for balance and gait

The above discussion leads to the design of a task set which differs substantially from the conventional clinical movement analysis procedures. Figure 35.1 demonstrates the ingredients for a balance assessment task, whereas Figure 35.2 shows the ingredients for a gait assessment task set.

I **Basic measurements:** quiet upright standing under optimal conditions.
Aim: determination of reference values.

II **Perceptual manipulations:** quiet upright standing under impoverished illumination conditions (dark glasses, milky white glasses).
Aim: determination of visual dependency.

III **Cognitive manipulations:** quiet upright standing while performing a concurrent cognitive task (mental calculation).
Aim: determination of cognitive dependency.

IV **Motor manipulations:** quiet upright standing while waiting for a disturbance. Type and moment of perturbation is known (anticipation). Type and moment of perturbation is not known (reaction).
Aim: determination of the capability of the system to implement future disturbances into a motor programme under construction and to determine the capability of the system to react adequately to sudden environmental changes.

Fig. 35.1 Design of disability-orientated motor tasks for the assessment of balance.

I   Basic measurements: flat level walking, optimal conditions.
Aim: determination of reference values.

II   Perceptual manipulations: walking under impoverished illumination conditions. Walking with 'impaired' peripheral vision. Walking with 'impaired' central vision.
Aim: determination of visual dependency.

III Cognitive manipulations: walking under conditions of loud noise (traffic noise). Walking while performing a concurrent task (auditory Stroop task).
Aim: determination of cognitive dependency.

IV   Motor manipulations: walking at a certain (firm) speed while approaching a clearly visible hindrance (a walkway/escalator). The subject has to step on the walkway without losing speed (anticipation). Walking at a certain (firm) speed towards a hindrance which has to be taken. At unpredictable moments the hindrance shifts from the left to the right or vice versa (reaction).
Aim: determination of the capability of the system to anticipate future but expected disturbances and to react adequately to sudden and unexpected changes in the environment.

FIg. 35.2   Design of disability-orientated motor tasks for the assessment of locomotion.

CONCLUSION

The suggested task sets reflect all the theoretical aspects discussed in this chapter. These task sets enable clinicians to gain insight, not only into the visible end result of a task, but also into the processes leading to this end result. It is argued here that shifts in these control processes across time give an objective indication of recovery. It is further argued that these aspects of recovery have more relevance for the prediction of activities of daily living than the conventional biomechanical parameters. Indeed, if at the end of a treatment programme a patient still shows a strong cognitive and/or visual dependency as well as an impaired ability to negotiate obstacles it will be clear that this patient is at risk under normal environmental circumstances. Assessment procedures used currently do not deliver this information since they focus primarily on output parameters acquired under optimal conditions.

At present only a prototype version of the task sets exists and the generalization value of the collected data has to be established in order to answer the question of whether this approach has real additional value for rehabilitation research. Therefore, patients who perform poorly at the end of rehabilitation should be monitored across time to test whether they really are at risk in terms of, for example, safety, dependency and skillfulness, compared to patients who performed well at the end of rehabilitation. Besides, more research is also needed to determine the dependent variables most sensitive for recovery. Hence, there is still a long way to go before a disability-orientated motor assessment task is ready, and only the first few steps have been described in this chapter.

REFERENCES

Fitts P M, Posner M I 1967 Human performance. Brooks/Cole, Belmont
Gentile A M 1987 Skill acquisition: action movement and neuromotor processes. In: Carr J H, Shepherd R B, Gordon J, Gentile A M, Held J M (eds) Foundations for physical therapy in rehabilitation. Aspen, Rockville, ch 3, pp 93–154
Geurts A C H, Mulder T 1992 Reorganization of postural control following lower limb amputation. Physiotherapy Theory and Practice 8: 145–157
Geurts A C H, Mulder T, Rijken R A J, Nienhuis B 1991a From the analysis of movements to the analysis of skills: bridging the gap between laboratory and clinic. Journal of Rehabilitation Sciences 4: 9–12
Geurts A C H, Mulder T, Nienhuis B, Rijken R A J 1991b Dual task assessment of reorganization of postural control in persons with lower limb amputation. Archives of Physical Medicine and Rehabilitation 72: 1059–1064
Geurts A C H, Mulder T, Nienhuis B, Rijken R A J 1992 Postural reorganization following lower limb amputation: possible motor and sensory determinants of recovery. Scandinavian Journal of Rehabilitation Medicine 24: 83–90
Henley S, Petit S, Todd-Pokropek A, Tupper A 1985 Who goes home? Predictive factors in stroke recovery. Journal of Neurology, Neurosurgery and Psychiatry 48: 1–6
Kotila M, Waltimo O, Niemi M L, Laaksonen R, Lempinen M 1984 The profile of recovery from stroke and factors influencing outcome. Stroke 15: 1039–1044
Messenger N, Bowker P 1987 The role of gait analysis in clinical medicine: a survey of UK centres. Engineering in Medicine 16: 221–227
Mulder T 1991 A process-oriented model of motor behavior: towards a theory based rehabilitation approach. Physical Therapy 71: 157–164
Mulder T 1992 Current ideas on motor control and learning: implications for therapy. In: Illis L (ed) Spinal cord dysfunction, vol. II, Intervention and treatment, Oxford University Press, Oxford, ch 11, pp 187–209
Mulder T 1993a Current topics in motor control: implications for rehabilitation. In: Greenwood R J, Barnes M P, McMillan T M, Ward C D (eds) Neurological rehabilitation. Churchill Livingstone, Edinburgh, ch 11, pp 125–133
Mulder T 1993b The learning machine: ideas about adaptation and learning following nervous system damage. In: Doorenbosch C A M, Out L, Commissaris D A C M, Oudejans R R D, Wimmers R H, Roszek B, Stins J F (eds) Learning motor skills: proceedings of the third symposium of the graduate institute of human movement. Free University Press, Amsterdam, ch 2, pp 29–47
Mulder T, Geurts A C H 1991 The assessment of motor dysfunctions: preliminaries to a disability-oriented approach. Human Movement Sciences 10: 565–574
Mulder T, Geurts A C H 1993 Recovery of motor skill following nervous system disorder: a behavioral approach. Baillière's Clinical Neurology 2: 1–13
Mumma C M 1986 Perceived losses following stroke. Rehabilitation Nursing 11: 19–24
Saleh M, Murdoch G 1985 In defence of gait analysis. Journal of Bone and Joint Surgery 67B: 237–241

36. Management and organization of community care in stroke rehabilitation

E. Viel

INTRODUCTION

Patient education and family autonomy in the face of adversity are touted today as solutions to offset increases in the cost of health services. In the field of rehabilitation, this philosophy has been practised for years. Physiotherapists, collectively, are guilty of not broadcasting an ability which is theirs by tradition. Today, the nursing profession speaks of community-based rehabilitation programmes and, instead of asking for advice, propagates the notion that it has invented the process.

This chapter deals with concrete examples culled from the author's own experience. No doubt many colleagues can add to the registry of successful experiments in the linkage of services.

An overview of past achievements

The Rehabilitation Institute of Oregon (RIO) model

In the early 1960s, when working in Oregon, the author coordinated a 'linked system' of referral. The rehabilitation facility had an understanding with acute care hospitals which referred patients with cerebrovascular accidents (CVA) automatically. As soon as the patient was transferred to RIO, in the case of a young person, he/she was 'linked' with the Department of Vocational Rehabilitation. Shortly before leaving Oregon in 1967 the author became a member of the Professional Advisory Committee to the Home Health Agency, adding the last link – a strategy for the early return home.

The Tokyo Toritsu model

In the early 1970s, the author worked for the Metropolitan Government of Tokyo. There was a need for care of patients with CVA at home, so in collaboration with a Japanese therapist a pamphlet was produced to teach families how to manage a hemiplegic person who lives on the floor, as Japanese families do (Iwasaki 1974). A 'linkage' experiment was conducted between hospitals, the Metropolitan Social Services, and the School of Physical Therapy. The brochure is still in use today.

The Deggendorf model

In Europe, a tradition of long-term treatment of patients with CVA made it impossible for many years to reach the same level of efficiency, until the laws of economics made therapists change under duress.

Leaping forward from the 1960s to the 1990s, a concrete example of linkage is presented by the Deggendorf model (Birnberger 1993). In this Bavarian community, the general hospital and the rehabilitation facilities work jointly to ensure that the patient returns home as soon as possible, and that the home environment is satisfactory.

The AGEFIPH model

In the area of France where the author is now located, the Graduate School of Physical Therapy has signed an agreement with the health insurance authorities. An ergonomic assessment of the workplace is carried out for those younger patients with CVA who are able to return to employment. The linkage of services regroups general hospitals, a rehabilitation centre, and the Ergonomics department of the Graduate School, which provides the expertise of its students and teachers.

ASSESSING THE QUALITY OF CARE: FIVE PRIORITIES

When a quality care programme is designed, the consultant must bear in mind that the client (i.e. the person who is cared for) does not choose the product, and usually (where there is health insurance) does not pay for it. Yet, the patient and his family do create a 'virtual client' who must be treated with consideration and must end up satisfied with the service.

The specific points to assess are as follows (not necessarily in this order):

- ethical considerations (and informed consent)
- the burden/deficit score assessed from different viewpoints
- quality as seen by the patient and his family
- case manager or coordinator?
- evaluation techniques.

The thorny question of ethics

In setting up a community-based rehabilitation service, including instructional courses for the families and education of the patient, one of the obvious moves was to create an electronic mail service (e-mail) accessible by linked computers. This system would make use of the communication highways as they came gradually into operation. The family could ask questions without the necessity of travelling several miles to meet a professional, and the answer would be on-screen the next day.

A positive aspect was the fact that the younger members of the family would gain status and become involved in the care of one of the older family members. It can be postulated that a 14-year-old boy will be better able to handle the e-mail than his mother. Drawing generations together around a computer will be a desired outcome of the operation.

The next obvious step is the screening of information that can be passed on to the patient; this is, quite obviously, the task of the case manager. This person must, therefore, be trained in the latest concepts of ethics for rehabilitation specialists who are not doctors of medicine.

Respect for the patient's expectations becomes obvious when the solutions envisaged for their life after discharge are discussed with patient and family. The necessary 'informed consent' requested by rules of ethics with regard to research programmes as well as medical or surgical procedures is sought. It is good policy to obtain informed consent when planning a home care programme. The patient's cooperation is required, and there is no better way to secure it.

The burden/deficit score – scored by whom?

Keeping in mind that the impairment is based on damage suffered, that disability means a cluster of symptoms and that a handicap is the residual amount of insurmountable damage, it becomes essential to establish a deficit score and an importance score, to detect which former activities the patient can abandon without regrets, and which will create a feeling of deep loss.

To simplify this, let it be stated that the objective 'burden' must be divided into the burden for the patient and the burden for the family: loss of mobility can weigh more heavily on family members than on a person who is of a passive nature. The subjective burden can be similarly divided, since an eventual return to work is dependent on the educational level and the perception that patients have of their disability.

The subjective burden for the family can be overcome, in most cases, by commonsense and practical advice. This subjective burden, a whole array of hurdles which are made more daunting because of the unknown aspects of the situation, will dissipate when proper assistance is offered, hence the idea of an e-mail system which lets the families express their concern. Putting it into words lessens the burden, and some of the obstacles will vanish during the intra-family debate which precedes the translation of a problem for the keyboard.

In order to score the burden, work and leisure have to be reviewed. The scorer can also take advantage of the opportunity to assess the general attitude of the patient and his family.

After several weeks or months, the relatives of a surviving patient with CVA will realize the size of the handicap (which was denied at first) and the amount of work which is required of them (the burden). Patient education and family education will become effective only when the interested parties are ready to listen; this will occur at different times with different people. Just as it does no good to browbeat a child who cannot yet tie his shoelaces, it does not help to try to speed up the relatives' understanding of their future burden.

Patient and family education must concentrate on a picture of remaining abilities (clearly listed), and not on the sum of the patient's organic lesions. One of the most useful tools for assessing these remaining abilities is the functional independence measurement (FIM), which provides a standardized scorecard and leaves no stone unturned.

There are three stages to disability assessment:

1. Related: what the patient tells the therapist about their impairment.
2. Observed: things that the therapist knows that the patient cannot do alone.
3. Measured: how fast? how often? how much? All the measuring equipment may not be available because some of it is expensive, but a comprehensive rehabilitation programme cannot overlook the importance of measurement.

Quality as assessed by the patient and their family

Speaking with the patient and their family often yields surprising dividends. Some people readily give up activities which seem important to the therapists, and conversely, they will fight tooth and nail to regain abilities which the staff tends to rate in second or third place. It is the patient's life; they are the best judges of their own priorities.

It is the responsibility of the case manager, or of the coordinator of services, to record:

• Quality of results as seen by the medical profession.
• Quality of results as measured by rehabilitation professionals; therapists have seen many a patient with head trauma classified as 'excellent result' (medically-speaking) who turns out to be a disaster in terms of social integration.
• Quality of result as defined by the patient.
• Quality of result as defined by the family.

The last two are the 'independent observer evaluation' that is sought. The team cannot self-evaluate; there is need for an assessment of quality seen through the eye of 'the consumer'.

Identity of the client

This leads on to the essential question: who is the client? Is it the health insurance company which pays the cost? Is it the doctor who referred the patient? Is it the patient? Or is it the patient's family?

The client is all four persons combined into one. In those countries where health insurance is available on a voluntary basis, and where it is provided by the State, the individual patient is not a real client, because he/she does not choose and does not pay for the services.

The health insurance company is not a traditional client, because it pays for something which is not of its choosing, and something that it will not use. As an example, an individual does not mind paying a little extra for a personal automobile, but will only buy the basic model when it is a company car.

The referring physician must be satisfied, but he or she is likely to assess the result at least in part through the patient's eyes. Professionals operate in a poorly-defined environment, and therefore are bound to use ill-defined logic.

It must be remembered that quality of life is a 'pay on delivery' item. As long as it has not been delivered, the client will not be satisfied. Change must be consensual, and the goals and losses must be clearly spelled out. Every time a difficulty is encountered one must ask:

- What is the obstacle?
- What is the cause?
- Is there an instrument to help overcome that hurdle?

Quality issues (including quality of life) can be addressed by total quality management (TQM) techniques (Shiba 1992), beginning with the three steps given above.

To assess the quality of life, therapists must:

- take into consideration the subjective burden as well as the objective burden
- evaluate the optimism/helplessness of that particular patient and their family
- evaluate the patient's level of self-esteem.

Satisfaction with the outcome of rehabilitation will depend on the evaluation of the results obtained so far and the expression of expectations for future improvement. Constant monitoring is necessary, to ascertain that the patient does not habour unreasonable expectations which cannot be met and which will be used as an excuse for not performing. Some people are willing to become aware of inevitable deficits, others are not.

In every case, the patient and their family will need to restructure their environment, which is why the intervention of a case manager or a coordinator of services is essential; he or she is the person who can 'tie up the loose ends', by examining every aspect of the problem.

Case manager or coordinator?

A decision must be made concerning the qualification of the person who will be in charge. If the option of a case manager is taken the designated

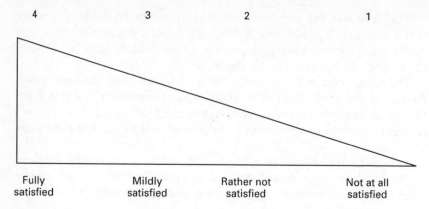

Fig. 36.1 The Osgood scale of satisfaction: a simple type of metrics easily applicable to the evaluation of results in rehabilitation.

specialist varies according to the type of patient. If the option is for a coordinator, the same person handles every patient file.

In every case, the 'manager' will have to act as arbitrator and defuse the minefield of personal and professional interests; each profession thinks its contribution is paramount, and presents requests for large chunks of the client's time. Reason must prevail, and apportionment of time will tax the coordinator's diplomatic abilities to the full. The coordinator must harness their professional efforts towards the best possible result in rehabilitation, in medical and social terms.

It must be assumed that the patients act in their own best self-interest. Making life difficult for them by complicating procedures must be avoided. That should be the burden of the coordinator.

Evaluation techniques

This is where most rehabilitation programmes are weakest. The functional independence measurement (FIM) has already been mentioned. The problem-oriented medical record (POMR) is also useful. Speech therapists and vocational counsellors are generally well equipped with a battery of tests. It remains for the physiotherapists to develop and use specific charts which concentrate on the benefits derived from physiotherapy (Fig. 36.1).

These records must be client-orientated, not written for the internal satisfaction of the staff. All measurements must be carried out with the patient and their family as co-graders of the outcome (Fig. 36.2), and report-writing must be clear and concise to satisfy the 'client'.

With regard to measurements, the use of the seven steps in total quality management (TQM) (Shiba 1992) is advocated, for the reason that the outcome is evaluated every step of the way. To sum up, in the words of an

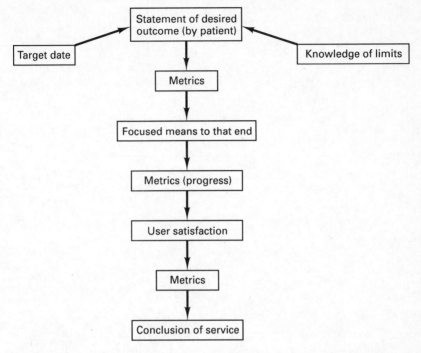

Fig. 36.2 The TQM approach to systemic assessment of a community-based rehabilitation programme for the individual client.

expert in quality management (Mizuno 1988): 'If one is equipped only with a hammer, every single problem is a nail'.

CONCLUSION

The linkage of facilities is the essence of comprehensive rehabilitation programmes. The author proposes that physiotherapists must make a concerted effort to publicize their expertise relevant to the present-day preoccupation with community-based rehabilitation services.

REFERENCES

Birnberger K F 1993 Ein umfassendes regionales Versogungssystem in der Neurorehabilitation. Proceedings of the symposium 'Neurorehabilitation: Eine perspective für die Zukunft'. Deggendorf 13–15 May, unpublished
Iwasaki T 1974 The patient returns home: a handling vademecum. Social Services, Tokyo Metropolitan Government
Mizuno S 1988 Management for quality improvement. Productivity Press, Cambridge (Mass)
Shiba S 1992 Les outils du management de la qualité. Mouvement Français pour la Qualité, Paris

37. Cross-country skiing and the Bobath concept

M. Gerber

INTRODUCTION

One of the problems that limits the quality of life of a stroke patient is undoubtedly a lack of endurance. In the early phase an appropriate retraining programme with the aim of increasing the level of endurance, and adapted to the stage of recovery, is to be recommended.

Being involved in a sport such as cross-country skiing, which has been adapted to the Bobath concept, is a motivating alternative to more traditional therapy, as long as certain requirements have previously been met. A training programme will be offered to the patient when they have reached a sufficient level of recovery (i.e. stable cardiovascular system, and enough concentration and muscle tone to achieve the task) to permit such sports activities as, for example, swimming, 'work out' on machines, walking or cross-country skiing.

THERAPEUTIC ASPECTS

The therapeutic aspects of cross-country skiing adapted for hemiparetic patients are multiple: rhythmical mobilization of the trunk including flexion, extension and rotation, in posterior, anterior and lateral directions, improvement of the 'passive' swing phase in gait, coordination, endurance and lastly the psychological aspect of improved well-being.

Preparation

Indoor preparation with a skateboard or roller-skis enables the patient to become used to the kinetics of skiing. It is important to note that when using a skateboard, the healthy foot should be raised to the same level as the hemiparetic foot to avoid a lateral flexion of the hemiparetic side.

The patient practises upward and downward movements, which he/she will have ample opportunity to use when on skis.

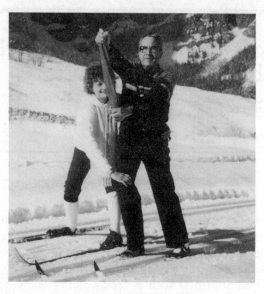

Fig. 37.1 The patient walks slowly on the ski track. The therapist facilitates the weight bearing of his right paretic lower limb and the external rotation of his hip. His arm activity influences positively the elongation of right paretic trunk and allows better hip control.

Techniques

Three techniques will be favoured on the well-prepared ski track: slow walking, sliding and alternate paces (Fig. 37.1). While slow walking on skis, the optimal unipodal weight bearing on the paretic foot enables the other leg to advance. It will be combined with exercises for the trunk and upper limbs. In a sliding walk, during the stance phase, the ski slides forwards and the weight is transferred to the other leg. Finally, the alternate pace, which represents the patient's optimal goal is tackled (Fig. 37.2). As a precaution, an anti-supination Bobath bandage is applied to the shoe worn on the paretic foot.

All three techniques are accomplished without ski sticks, as these could present a danger of injury to the thorax and abdomen. During treatment, the therapist facilitates movement from the paretic side.

Intervention and evaluation

The therapist intervenes by carefully preparing the stance phase and during the swing phase by stabilising the trunk or, if necessary, by realigning the paretic foot. The most significant therapeutic aspect is the improvement of the swing phase in gait, a probable consequence of the proprioceptive information of the patient integrating the notion of passivity of the swing phase experienced during this specific treatment.

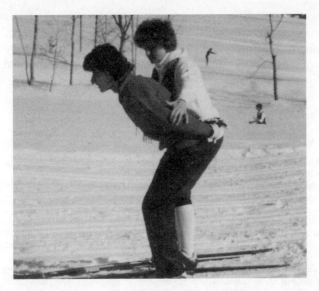

Fig. 37.2 Patient at an advanced level: preparation for sliding down a slope. The sliding is possible due to the symmetrical weight distribution on both legs. The arm position allows balance to be controlled by the trunk and not by the upper limbs.

If the patient wishes to improve his/her endurance, a 20–30 minute session three times a week (e.g. Tuesdays, Thursdays and Saturdays) will be advised as an ideal goal; this will correspond to a medium-intensity programme, with a heart rate of approximately 170 minus half the patient's age.

A monitoring of the heartbeat during therapy will be a valuable help in evaluating the patient's reaction and in comparing the results with the subjective evaluation of muscle tonicity.

Empirical experience has shown that a lapse of time of about 2 hours after finishing the sports activity allows a judicious evaluation of the intensity of the effort expended by the patient. A feeling of well-being without great fatigue should be felt.

Psychological benefits

The psychological aspect is unquestionable, whether the aim is an improvement in endurance or in gait. The mere act of coming out of the protective isolation of the therapy room can transform the anguish of the winter season into pleasure.

CONCLUSION

Many patients wish to be able to participate in a family sports activity, however limited their participation may be. This is particularly appreciated where small children are concerned.

The success of this therapy depends on the notion of pleasure which should be constantly present.

The Bobath concept, with its holistic approach, lends itself very easily to this type of adaptation. With the example of cross-country skiing it is possible to improve a patient's gait and endurance while respecting the principles of the concept.

FURTHER READING

Davies P 1986 Steps to follow. Springer Verlag, Berlin

Ducommun A M 1978 Skions malgré tout. Delta SA, Vevey

Gerber M 1987 Skilanglauf adaptiert nach dem Bobath-Konzept für Hemiplegiker/Ski de fond adapté selon le concept Bobath pour les hémiplégiques. Swiss Journal of Physiotherapie 5: 8–16

Gerber M 1990 Variations de la fréquence cardiaque chez l'hémiplégique adulte lors d'un traitement-type d'après le concept Bobath. Annales de kinésithérapie 17: 421–432

Gerber M 1992 Ski-langlaufen voor patiënten met een hemiplegie, aangepast aan het Bobath (NDT)-concept. Dutch Studiegroep voor NDT/Bobath 4: 33–39

Gerber M, Vaney C 1994 Verlust selektiver Rumpfaktivität und deren Auswirkungen bei Erwachsenen mit Hemiparese. Krankengymnastik 3: 328–341 P Flaum, Munchen

Imhof U 1985 Langlauf als Therapie. Skilanglauf 1: 18–20

Villiger B, Egger K, Lerch R, Probst HP, Schneider W, Spring H, Tritschler T 1991 R. Gym 3. Ausdauer Thieme, Stuttgart, New York

38. Aerobics with hemiplegic patients: results of physical aerobic fitness training in stroke rehabilitation

G. Rasmussen

INTRODUCTION

The Centre for Rehabilitation of Brain Injury, at the University of Copenhagen, is a private institution and opened in 1985. The treatment fee is usually paid in full by public authorities. The centre admits post-acute adult patients in groups of approximately 10–15 twice a year. Patients attend the centre for 4 days a week, 6 hours per day for a little over 4 months. The types of diagnoses referred to the centre are 30% strokes, 50% cranial trauma and 20% infections, tumours, etc.

The age criterion is 16–50 years, and the treatment programme typically starts 1–4 years post-injury. The neuropsychological programme is Luria inspired and holistic in orientation. It includes, besides physical training, other elements such as cognitive training, group psychotherapy and speech therapy where required. Patients are called 'students'. This reflects an attitude which supports the person with brain injury in leaving the patient role and taking responsibility for their own education and training. The physiotherapists do not 'treat' in this stage of the rehabilitation but act as consultants and teachers.

Physical training takes place several times a week and serves more than one function. In part it helps to restore the often much neglected physical condition of the clients who, in many cases, have been physically inactive since their injury. In addition, since the training is planned to follow precisely established and structured routines it supplements the cognitive training, and since it is a group activity, it furthermore promotes social interaction between the students.

LURIA

The interdisciplinary treatment approach at the Centre has been inspired by the Russian neuropsychologist and medical doctor A.R. Luria. His views on motor recovery are described in the chapter entitled 'Restoration of motor function after brain injury' in his book *Restoration of function after brain injury* (Luria 1968).

Luria suggested early implementation of compensatory strategies for motor deficits following injuries at lower cortical levels of integration such as pareses and disorders of tone and coordination. As opposed to lesions at lower cortical levels of integration, lesions at higher cortical levels permit reorganization strategies. The examiner should first try to establish the psychological nature of apraxia, and then find the defective link primarily responsible for disintegration of the motor act. Only then can the examiner try to correct this deficit by introducing the disturbed function into a new and intact system. This method of intersystemic reorganization is the main method of correction of the deficits in these cases. Luria also stated that it is more important to find out and analyze the intact functional systems than to list the deficits.

Since the early days of the Centre for Rehabilitation of Brain Injury, physical rehabilitation in the programme has developed from an initially more traditional neurological treatment approach. The term 'physiotherapy' in the programme has changed to *physical training and education*. Education about their own dysfunctions and deficits affords the students an opportunity to improve their physical condition. The integration, into physiotherapy, of awareness of cognitive deficits such as memory, learning and concentration problems, has produced treatment principles called *cognitive physiotherapy*.

Two other facts have been essential for the development of new treatment principles. The first of these is the nature of the persistent physical deficits most commonly seen in patients referred to the Centre. The main physical problems proved to be a very poor physical condition and lack of endurance. Spasticity may be a great physical problem, but it is also a psychological one.

The second essential fact is that the Centre is located in a university environment rather than a hospital setting. This has turned out to be important. The students use the same public transport, buy lunch in the same canteen, and sometimes even buy sweatshirts with the insignia of the 'University of Copenhagen' just as any other student attending the university might do. These circumstances increase their self-confidence. The students start and end their training programme following the semesters of the university.

However, the university buildings do not have suitable facilities for physical training and the fitness club of a nearby large hotel is therefore used (where students mingle freely with hotel guests and former students). Some activities, including aerobics, volleyball and a dance session do take place on the premises of the university. The wide open area in which the university is located also gives the opportunity for jogging.

FITNESS STUDY OF STUDENTS WITH A STROKE

Subjects

For the last 5 years (1989–1994), 42 people with stroke were followed with special regard to their physical fitness and outcome before and after completing a highly structured aerobic fitness training programme.

Among the students with stroke, 80% had haemorrhage and 20% an infarct. 50% were men and 50% were women. 79% of the cases had a right-sided hemiparesis, 14% had a left-sided hemiparesis and 2% had hemiparesis in both sides. Only 5% had no sign of paresis. 38% had severe aphasia. The average age of the students at the time of stroke was 36 years (s.d. 9 years). The students started the programme on average 2.1 years (s.d. 1.8 years) after the onset of their stroke. It was, therefore, mainly quite young people with a lesion in the left hemisphere who were admitted to the programme. However, the Centre also offers a training programme for smaller groups of older people with a stroke, and the training results do not differ very much from the outcome of the younger group.

Physical and cognitive dysfunctions

Prior to this period (1989–1994) all students were subjected to a neurological and physiotherapeutic examination and all physical and neurological data were recorded. This was not very motivating to the students because the end of the programme saw a reiteration of the same deficits. The data were more diagnostic than a measure of improvement. Furthermore reports from both the students and their relatives indicated that the physical deficits played a far less important role at this stage of the rehabilitation period than psychosocial dysfunctions.

The main physical deficits which were observed apart from the very poor physical condition were: epileptic seizure, decreased respiratory capacity, paresis, impaired balance and ambulation, slow psychomotor speed, liability, tiredness and arterial hypertension.

The main cognitive deficits which have proved to be the greatest problems when planning a physical training programme are: poor attention and concentration, distractability, poor memory and learning, aphasia, apraxia, neglect, reduced sense of time, sequencing confusion, lack of initiative, perseveration, change of personality and lack of motivation.

Methods

The physical examination

At present the most important tools in the physical examination are fitness indices derived from three different tests:

- the Åstrand bicycle test,
- the Harvard step test
- the Cooper walking or running distance test.

The advantages of these tests are that they are easy and quick to perform in a modified form. Moreover, the patients become motivated to continue physical training. It is easy to measure an improvement within a short time (e.g. over a period of 3–4 weeks). Because the students are in such a poor physical condition at the start, even a moderate investment in physical training quickly shows results, which also promotes increased self-confidence. The tests are repeated at the end of the programme and at 1 and 3 years post-programme. At the end of a programme the students will receive a diploma illustrating the results of the physical training (Fig. 38.1).

The Åstrand bicycle test comprises a Swedish ergometer bicycle (Monark), a pulse-rater around the chest of the 'respiratory' type VAS (visual analogue scale), Borg's subjective exertion scale, and the scoring system recommended by the Danish Heart Association (Åstrand 1970). By means of this system, it is possible to calculate the average fitness level of the student and to show it as a figure. The test takes approximately 6 minutes, which is the time it takes for the pulse to reach a steady state at a certain resistance.

People with a severe spastic hemiparetic side may have difficulty maintaining the constant speed of 60 revolutions per minute which is necessary in order to obtain a heart rate of at least 120 beats per minute, from which the result may be calculated. Sometimes it is impossible to carry out the test at the beginning of the programme, but usually it is possible at the end of the physical programme of 16 weeks.

The Harvard step test involves stepping up onto a 50 cm high footstool, at a rate of 30 times per minute for 5 consecutive minutes. Thereafter, over a period of 5 consecutive minutes, measurements are taken of the pulse rate decline. The readings are inserted in a formula, and the resulting figure is another indication of physical fitness and endurance. Most hemiparetic persons will have difficulty maintaining the speed of 30 steps per minute. The goal in this testing is therefore to do as many steps as possible during the 5 minutes and thus to endure a physical exercise for this period of time.

The Cooper walking and running distance test comprises two tasks. The first task is to cover a 1 200 m outdoor distance running or walking as quickly as possible. The students have to concentrate for perhaps up to 15 or 30 minutes despite noise and visual distraction from the very busy passing traffic. The second task is performed on a treadmill in a fitness centre. The students are asked to run and/or walk as many metres as they can within 12 minutes. From these results, an index is obtained that shows the level of physical condition and possibly how much the cognitive deficits affect their physical performance.

The physical training programme

At the Centre there are three main physical activities:

- leading the morning gymnastic exercises; a sequence of 10 exercises have to be learned and performed
- work-out in a fitness centre once a week
- aerobics or wateraerobics once a week.

Furthermore trying out potential sport and leisure activities is also regarded as very important and this is therefore often incorporated in the intensive training programme.

In addition, there are some supplementary activities where these are required:

- transport programme
- ball games: volleyball, badminton, squash
- dancing: folkdance, les lanciers (a French minuet), flamenco
- tai chi (Chinese slow movements, shadow boxing)
- making a home aerobics programme on a videocassette or audiocassette with the individual student's favourite rhythmic music.

Most of the physical training is performed in groups, with due consideration given to the students' various cognitive deficits. However, individual physical training does take place. Typically, this can include supervising the student in his or her own home, an exercise programme, applying for and employing personal aids, education and support in diet maintenance, or even teaching the patients to ride a bike or drive a car again in their local environment. Treatments such as manipulation, ultrasound, shortwave, laser or manual active/passive exercises are no longer applied. Relaxation therapy and massage have been attempted but with little or no success. This type of 'therapy' tends to lower the general level of concentration and alertness to the detriment of the cognitive training. What most patients need is stimulation and support to minimize the initiation difficulties and the general psychomotor slowing which are so often seen as sequelae of stroke.

Structure of work-out training

The training in the fitness centre or following an aerobic class is structured in the same way as an ordinary aerobic class. It serves the purpose of teaching the students to endure a longer period of increased heart rate. The structure is as follows:

- 10 minutes of warming-up exercises
- 20 minutes of aerobics, where the heart rate can be up to 60% of the maximum heart rate

- 10–12 minutes for cooling-down exercises
- 10 minutes for strengthening and endurance exercises
- 5 minutes or more for stretching out.

Spasticity may increase for the first 2 or 3 minutes, which is the same time it takes to achieve a steady heart rate. It seems that the spasticity decreases for a longer time period after a work-out session. The students feel generally more relaxed and comfortable.

The normal movement pattern is stimulated in ways other than the Bobath concept. At the fitness centre once or twice a week, the students have to fill out their own chart during their training. Here, the aim of the physical training is not only improvement of strength, endurance and fitness but also body awareness, social behaviour, memory, concentration, and general awareness.

The bicycle test. After the bicycle warm-up, the students measure their own pulse, calorie output, resistance, revolutions per minute, and duration of the warm-up. They have to remember four figures on a display before they stop pedalling because the display disappears as soon as they stop.

The treadmill. To start and read the display of the treadmill is another cognitive challenge. At the end of a day's work-out the results have to be plotted on a chart, which shows the progressive points of calorie output and the amount lifted in kilos. The plotting of the chart is very motivating to the students, giving them an incentive to undertake more physical training.

Besides improving physical condition, the treadmill is also suitable for training balance and stride. It is the general impression and experience among the students that the spasticity does not increase by performing strengthening exercises on the apparatus; in fact, the contrary is true. For the first 2 or 3 minutes an increase of spasticity may be seen, but this is also the case for the pulse rate. During the first 2 minutes the body adjusts to the increased demand of exercising. The pulse rate will increase to a steady state and the level of spasticity will decrease again.

Water aerobics is another alternative which is very popular and effective regarding training of balance, strength and endurance. In the swimming pool, typically two or three people within any group learn to swim again. The physical training described here, with its focus upon cardiovascular circulation, tends to stimulate the students to use the normal movement pattern and is yet another alternative to a motor relearning programme.

Other physical activities offered are badminton, table-tennis, billiards, jogging, and sailing, in order to enable students to try out sporting and leisure activities with potential for future activity or to rekindle an old interest. Many sport and leisure activities provide a setting where movement patterns are enhanced far more functionally than is possible in a traditional physical training programme. Thus coordination can be integrated while sailing, arm movement can be trained during flamenco dancing, balance can be achieved through tai chi.

Transport training. Two or three students per group require tansport training. They are often afraid to travel by bus, train, car or bicycle because of:

• a tendency to epileptic seizures
• sudden increases of spasticity
• orientation and memory problems
• a sense of uneasiness in public places.

Results

An example of the physical training results of a 34-year-old woman with a severe right-sided hemiparesis is illustrated in Figure 38.1. She improved the bicycle test by 48%, the step test by 87% and the walking/running test by 6%. It is quite remarkable how great the improvement can be in some cases, but it is due to the fact that the students are in such a poor condition at the start of the programme, with a very low oxidative capacity and level of endurance. It should be noted that traditional physiotherapy for patients with stroke in hospital and outpatient settings has not emphasized cardiovascular treatment (although this is done with heart disease patients). Therefore, even a moderate investment in physical training quickly shows results, which is very encouraging to the students and the therapists.

Figure 38.2 summarizes the results of 32 persons with a stroke who were tested pre- and post-programme in the Åstrand bicycle test. The black blocks illustrate the ranges from the 25th to the 75th percentiles. The white lines are the median values. There is a significant improvement from pre- to post-programme (Wilcoxon matched-pair test p = 0.001). The Harvard step test and the Cooper's walking or running test also show significant improvement (p < 0.01).

Conclusions

During the last 8 years, the physiotherapeutic treatment at the Centre for Rehabilitation of Brain Injury has changed from being traditionally neurologically-oriented to being more functional and pedagogically cognitive. It has been inspired by Luria, whose ideas constitute the basis of the retraining principles used by all the members of the interdisciplinary team.

The physiotherapists do not provide 'treatment' but rather physical training, consultation, and education. The physical training takes place in normal surroundings, and has demonstrated a greater degree of transfer effect than has been possible to achieve in an institutional environment. The results presented here show that the effect of fitness training for stroke patients can be measured and that progress is easily achieved during the 4-month period of training. The very fact of being able to carry through the

DIPLOMA

FOR

S.G.

PHYSICAL TEST RESULTS

Name:	START	FINISH
Åstrand Bicycle Test	31	46
Harvard Step Test	42	78,67
Cooper's Walking/Running Test (1270 m)	8,30 min	7,56 min
Cooper's Treadmill (12 min.)		1530 m

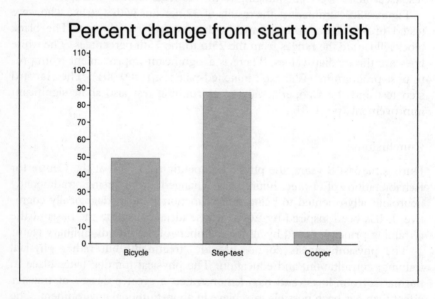

Fig. 38.1   Centre for Rehabilitation of Brain Injury diploma

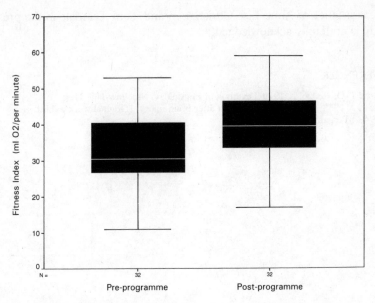

Fig. 38.2 Åstrand bicycle test.

tests themselves is motivating to the students, and encourages them to continue the physical training.

Sport and leisure activities also play an important role when planning the rehabilitation programme, as the students with a stroke can very seldom return to their former job.

SUMMARY

In future, physiotherapists will need to integrate the cognitive, psychological and social deficits into their physical rehabilitation programme. To make spasticity disappear permanently is not a realistic objective. However, the physiotherapist derives more satisfaction from the challenge of offering a greater repertoire than from vainly targeting spasticity.

There are many directions for the physiotherapists to take in stroke rehabilitation, and physical aerobic fitness training is only one option. This training can be of great physical benefit, since the cardiovascular system is generally affected in people who suffer a stroke. Furthermore it can also meet the special cognitive and perceptive deficits that are encountered in a person with a stroke. It is important to see progress, to feel successful and to focus not on the deficits but on the remaining resources, as Luria pointed out many years ago.

Acknowledgements

The assistance of Anne-Lise Christensen and Tom Teasdale in the present study is gratefully acknowledged.

REFERENCES

Åstrand P-O, Rodahl K 1970 Textbook of physiology. McGraw-Hill, New York
Luria L A 1968 Restoration of function after brain injury. (Original work published in 1948.) Pergamon, New York

39. Volleyball, music and balance, archery and riding with stroke patients

K. Malmström,   S. Johansson,   M. Sallnäs

INTRODUCTION

The intention of this chapter is to present neuropsychology and to show its importance for physiotherapists working within stroke rehabilitation. Also presented are four different activities which demonstrate neuropsychological theory and which can be suitable for patients with stroke. The authors believe that the activities are quite untraditional in stroke rehabilitation.

NEUROPSYCHOLOGY

Neuropsychology is the study of how different functions of the brain interact and to what behaviours the interactions lead. There are many different schools of thought. One example is Alexander Luria, who developed a neuropsychological theory in Russia during and after the Second World War (Luria 1980).

The functional system

An important concept in neuropsychology is the *functional system*. In every activity of man, many parts of the brain are activated. All these parts together can be called a functional system for a special activity. When carrying out a motor performance many parts of the brain are activated. This can be verified by different measurements of regional cerebral blood flow. The motor cortex cannot be isolated from the rest of the brain, as the brain always functions as a whole.

To have a sound understanding of the brain one has to know what takes place in different parts of it and how they interact in, for example, motor performance. One needs to know the difference between the right and the left hemispheres and how they interact. The specific function of each lobe and deeper structures such as the basal ganglia have to be understood. Examples are:

• How and where the sensory information from each receptor is analysed and stored, and how and where information is put together.

• How motor performance is executed and which parts of the motor- and pre-motor cortex as well as deeper structures are activated.

Neuropsychological theory will help with this.

Well-localized brain damage may interfere with many different motor behaviours. The patient does not need to have a paretic limb to fail in a goal-oriented motor activity. Any missing link in the functional system will interfere with motor performance. Some examples are:

• Does the patient have enough energy?
• Is the patient missing the idea of the movement?
• Can all sensory information be analysed and put together?

If any of these links is missing, the 'motor output' will be affected.

The motor relearning programme

Through neuropsychology one may obtain an explanation for the behaviour of a patient with stroke. When a structured neuropsychological analysis is made, the patient's resources and deficits will be discovered. The resources are very important because they have to be used in the motor relearning programme. Neuropsychological theory helps the therapist to find the main problem of the patient with stroke and what to focus on during rehabilitation. It also tells the therapist what to demand from each patient with stroke. In practical terms, this means adjusting treatment to each individual patient with stroke depending on his/her special problems and resources.

An example of this is to ask the question: 'Can exactly the same treatment be used for a patient with hemiparesis and apraxia or neglect?' The answer is that it cannot. The patients have different main problems. For the 'neglect patients' half of their body and half of the world does not exist in their own mind, while the patient with apraxia often has difficulties in performing a motor activity on demand. The solutions must be different. Before commencing any motor relearning programme for the patient with neglect one has to make the patient try to integrate the whole of their body and the whole world into their own mind, perhaps through logic if they have that resource. To ask a patient with apraxia to perform a motor activity only leads to frustration. Instead one has to use other techniques such as manual guiding or different automatic reactions at the outset.

Neuropsychological theory is essential for the whole team working with patients with stroke. It helps to build up efficient rehabilitation where everyone has a common language and where everyone uses the patient's resources to attain the best function. It also lessens frustration if success is not achieved, and helps the team to find new ways within the rehabilitation programme.

In the presentation of four activities more examples will be given of how neuropsychological thinking is used in treatment.

VOLLEYBALL WITH BALLOON

An ordinary indoor badminton net and a large balloon are used. There are two teams with approximately six members in each; the patients can sit or stand. There are two leaders, one for each team. The duration of the game is 30 minutes. The balloon has to be passed three times within the team before it is passed over to the other side. The reasons for this are to activate as many team members as possible, to use cognitive function in planning and cooperation and to use more spatial relationships between the patients, the balloon and the net.

What is achieved?

A number of functions are required for successful participation:

• One goal for the activity is balance and, for some patients, motor activity of the paretic arm.

• The concentration is intense and the awareness is on the balloon all the time. Therefore, it is a good exercise for patients lacking awareness, but it is necessary that the patient knows the reason for participating.

• The patient has to use spatial relationships – coordination of the eyes with the hand in relation to the environment. The balloon is a sensitive instrument which gives direct feedback relating to the force used by the arm and the direction of the movement.

• Cognitive functions that have to be used are, e.g. planning, concentration and decision-making. For example, the patient has to decide if it is their turn to hit the balloon over the net or if it should be passed to any of the others in the team.

• Alertness is stimulated by many stimuli such as movements of the balloon, the other team members and the leaders. The leader is especially important because he/she has to be the 'driving force' of the team. The leader has to continually activate, stimulate, correct and motivate the team members.

There are different reasons for the patient's participation in this activity. It is important that the leaders and the patient are aware of these reasons. There are often many laughs and most patients do enjoy this activity. It can be a useful way of increasing motivation for treatment.

MUSIC AND BALANCE

This activity is used in the treatment of patients with stroke who are able to work in standing and walking, sometimes with personal support from their own physiotherpaist. The group consists of one leader and 10–15 participants with various dysfunctions. The programme lasts for approximately 30 minutes, usually with a short break at halftime, when participants can sit down and have something to drink. The music which is used is chosen so that different tempos, rhythms and characters may be experienced.

In this treatment the group itself is used as an instrument. Many functions are required to interact with other people. The individual has to concentrate on their own body, and try to find the right rhythm and the right movements in a continuously changing environment. The music itself can stimulate the patient to start to move. Everyone has memories of movements which can be activated when listening to and 'feeling' the right kind of music.

What is achieved?

Stimulation is achieved in a variety of forms:

• Alertness is stimulated through a massive sensory input (especially from the music).

• Training of balance where there is a change in the centre of gravity in relation to different tempos and rhythms is occurring continuously.

• Motor relearning is emphasized by the music.

• Cognitive functions that have to be used are, e.g. concentration and planning. The individual has to concentrate on the leader's commands and his/her own movements and has to plan continuously, e.g. what they are and where they are supposed to lead.

• Perceptual functions are needed. Here, spatial relationships between oneself and other people and the room are used. The individual also has to be able to walk in the right direction at the right time.

• Being together with other people gives the patients social stimulation. This, together with the music, can give them courage and joy in movement.

ARCHERY

Archery is an individual treatment which uses ordinary bow, arrows and target. The distance is approximately 10 metres. The patient can sit or stand. The treatment includes preparing for the activity (e.g. putting on a forearm shield, moving into the correct position) as well as shooting, inspecting/evaluating the result, removing the arrows from the target and returning to the starting point.

What is achieved?

The following functions are required:

• Motor function and coordination of both arms as well as maintaining balance.

• Cognitive functions such as concentration and planning. For example, the patient has to use different motor performances in a continuous series to achieve a result. Direct feedback from the motor activity is gained from the arrow at the target. If it is successful the patient has to replicate it. If not, a different strategy has to be found for the next attempt. The concentration has to be intense.

• Perceptual functions such as awareness and spatial relationships. Placing the patient in a special position requires crossing the eyes over the midline to see the target. Of course the patient then needs to know the purpose of the activity. The patient needs to use many sensory inputs to make a spatial analysis of all the information in order to orientate the body in relation to the target, to put the arrow on the string and to pull the string against the chin. If any input is missing the physiotherapist has to try to help the patient to compensate with other sensory components.

For many patients, archery is a new experience. Therefore a comparison cannot be made with performance before the stroke.

The ability to hit the target can give the patient satisfaction and pleasure for many days afterwards.

THERAPEUTIC RIDING

Erstagårdskliniken in Sweden has used therapeutic riding in the treatment of patients with stroke for approximately 10 years. At a nearby riding school there are horses which are well-trained for this purpose. Every week, four patients with various dysfunctions go to the riding school, together with four helpers (physiotherapists and occupational therapists), all of whom are familiar with horses.

At the riding school the patients participate, as much as they can, in the preparation of the horses. Ordinary saddles, mostly without stirrups, are used; sometimes a sheepskin is used. A large handle is fixed to the front of the saddle or is put directly on the sheepskin. The reins are shortened if the rider rides with one hand ('cowboy style').

Each patient's ride lasts approximately 30 minutes. An individual programme is worked out; the patient is taught to ride and one of the major goals is to become an 'independent' rider.

The horse is a sensitive instrument which responds immediately to the rider's behaviour. It responds to the rider's way of moving his/her legs and arms as well as to the way they shift their body weight. The horse responds to the way the rider gives commands, with or without words.

What is achieved?

The following functions are called upon:

• Balance and coordination. The whole body is involved. The horse responds distinctly and directly to the rider's signals. All the time the rider has to maintain balance when sitting on a moving horse and during that time he/she also has to shift their body weight in order to make the horse do what is required! For example, if the riders move their weight to the left (intentionally or unintentionally) the horse will turn to the left. Together with weight shifting, the rider also has to use the reins to make the horse go where he/she wants it to go – the whole body must be coordinated.

• Cognitive functions such as concentration and planning. The rider has to listen to the instructions from the instructor, give the right instructions to the horse and respond in the right way to the horse's behaviour. The rider is asked to ride the horse through cones in serpentines and then halt. To do this he/she has to plan their strategy in advance. The rider has to start the horse, make the horse keep on walking, give the right signals for turning and then make the horse halt. All these components have to be performed with exact timing. Afterwards the patient has to ask the questions: 'Did I achieve the goal? How was my motor performance?'

• Perceptual functions. Relationships between horse and rider, and also between horse, rider and the environment must be considered. For example, to reinforce spatial relationships the rider can ride through serpentines or circles. The rider needs to control and be aware of all parts of the body when communicating with the horse, e.g. if a rider with neglect to the left is asked to ride in a circle to the left, he/she must be aware of the left side of the body and the amount of space required to ensure a successful performance.

• Communication. For riders with aphasia riding can be a source of satisfaction because of the possibility of 'speaking' with the horse without words.

For many patients, horseback riding is a new, exciting experience. To learn something new, in a situation where most aspects of daily living remind the patients of their disability, can give a new dimension to their lives.

CONCLUSION

Physiotherapists at Erstagårdskliniken have had help from members of many other professions, especially the occupational therapists, speech pathologists and the neuropsychologist, in understanding and learning the meaning of neuropsychological theory and how it affects motor relearning. It has been a long process, but theory can now be transferred into practice. A long-standing assumption has been that physiotherapists work only with motor function but, like all other professions, they do in fact work with the whole brain, including cognition, as well as perception.

It is hoped that this chapter has given some new ideas as well as stimulation for further development in physiotherapy for the patient with stroke.

REFERENCES

Luria A R 1980 Higher cortical functions in man, 2nd edn. Basic Books, New York

FURTHER READING

Eriksson H 1988 Neuropsykologi vid demenser och avgränsade hjärnskador. Norstedts
    Förlag AB, Stockholm
Luria A R 1973 The working brain. Penguin, London

Appendix 1: Poster abstracts

Different types of feedforward in the hemiparetic's early motor reeducation
St. Baykouchev[*], *J. Paralingov*[†]
[*] Neurological Clinic Medical University, 15A V. Aprilov str, 4000 Plovdiv, Bulgaria.
[†] Hospital for Pulmonary Patients, 4000 Plovdiv, Bulgaria.

The rehabilitation of gait in stroke patients with multichannel functional electrical stimulation
U. Bogataj PhD[*], *N. Gros*, RP[†], *M. Kljajić* PhD[*], *R. Aćimović* MD[†],
M. Malezič BSc[*]
[*] J. Stefan Institute, Jamova 39, SI-61111 Ljubljana, Slovenia. [†] Institute of Republic of Slovenia for Rehabilitation, Linhartova 51, SI-61000 Ljubljana, Slovenia.

Correction of drop foot using a common peroneal stimulator surface electrodes and a pressure sensitive foot switch: a pilot study
J. H. Burridge MCSP, *P. N. Taylor* MSc, *S. A. Hagan* BSc, *I. D.* Swain PhD
Department of Medical Physics and Biomedical Engineering, Glanville Centre, Salisbury District Hospital, Salisbury, Wiltshire, SP2 8BJ, UK.

From the humoral medicine of Hippocrates, to a 20th century humoral therapy, the manual lymphatic drainage ad modum Vodder
V. Cool
Physiotherapist, Center MLD Vodder, 66300 Llauro (PYR.-OR.) France.

Forced use technique to improve chronic motor deficit after stroke to overcome the effect of learned non-use
N. Eckstein PT Cert Neurological PT
Yair Ben Yair Day Center for Long Term Rehabilitation, Dubnov St. 14, Holon 58808, Israel.

An attempt in rehabilitation of post-stroke lower extremity amputees
D. Ganchev, E. Dimitrova
Department of Kinesitherapy, National Sports Academy, Sofia, Bulgaria.

313

Effect of intense physiotherapy using the Bobath concept on the capacity of stroke patients for symmetrical walking

J. Goldman-Reznik, B. Stillman
The University of Melbourne School of Physiotherapy, Victoria Australia.

Indicator of physical progress following stroke

P. M. Hodgson, C. Watkins, L. Juby
Stroke Unit, Nottingham City Hospital (NHS) Trust, Hucknall Road, Nottingham, UK.

Rehabilitation at home after stroke – an exploratory pilot study on design and contents

M. Holm*, L. Widén Holmqvist†
* Department of Physical Therapy, † Division of Neurology, Department of Clinical Neuroscience and Family Medicine, Karolinska Institute, Huddinge Hospital, S–141 86 Huddinge, Sweden.

Neurogenic hand and finger oedema in hemiplegic patients treated with manual lymph drainage

P. Hutzschenreuter, H. Brümmer, G. T. Werner*
Department of Experimental Surgery II, University of Ulm (Germany) and Hospital of Physical Medicine*, Munich-Bogenhausen (Germany).

The organisation of outpatient rehabilitation in Lithuania (Klaipeda)

V. Janusonis, R. Miciuniene, R. Radziuviene
Klaipéda City hospital, Liepojos str. 15, Klaipéda, Lithuania.

Facing the challenge of spasticity

M. Johnstone, A. Thorp
Derriford House, Linton Bank Drive, West Linton, Peeblesshire, UK. Johnstone Teaching Centre, care of Dr Selz, Bürgerspital Solothurn, Solothurn, CH-4500, Switzerland.

An evaluation of rehabilitation services for stroke patients in hospital

L. C. Juby, N. B Lincoln, P. Berman
Stroke Research Unit, Nottingham City Hospital (NHS) Trust, Nottingham, UK.

Correlation of perceptual performance and activities of daily living in stroke patients

H. Kayihan PhD PT Assoc Professor, M. Uyanik PT, A. Ergun PT, T. Akcay PT, G. Hazar PT
School of Physiotherapy and Rehabilitation Center, Ankara, Turkey.

The motor relearning programme in a stroke unit: a comparative study of stroke patients

S. Knútsdóttir, E. Hafsteinsdóttir
Physiotherapists, Department of Rehabilitation and Neurology, Borgarspítalinn, 108 Reykjavík, Iceland.

Predicting disability after stroke: a critical literature review

Drs. G. Kwakkel
Physical Therapist, Movement Scientist Dept. Physiotherapy, Free University, Amsterdam.

Use of the 'gaitway' system for the assessment of anomalies of gait in patients following stroke and other conditions affecting the pattern of locomotion

H. T. Law PhD
Department of Orthopaedic Surgery, University of Edinburgh Teviot Place, Edinburgh, UK

Effect of different models of multidisciplinary teamwork on length of stay of patients on a stroke unit

P. Laidler MCSP, W. Wilson PhD MA DipCST
Hillside Cottage, Station Road, Wickham Bishops, Essex, UK.

Educational programme for stroke patients

H. Lund*, L. Lauesen[†]
* Physiotherapist, [†] Occupational Therapist,
Voksenskolen, Albertslund, Liljens Kvarter 2, 2620 Albertslund, Denmark.

BBH'S fysioterapeutiske apopleksiscore (BFA-score)

H. Lund, A. Krogh Møller, K. Brandt Nielsen, A. Castberg
Physiotherapists, Bispebjerg Hospital, Bispebjerg Bakke 23, 2400 København NV.

Intensified multidisciplinary individual training in groups of patients diagnosed as suffering from apoplexia cerebri

H. Lund*, L. Lauesen[†], B. Greby*, I. Schmidt Hansen[†]
* Physiotherapists, [†] Occupational Therapists, Bispebjerg Hospital,
Bispebjerg Bakke 23, 2400 København NV, Denmark.

Video based pendulum test: procedure and normal response

J. M. McMeeken, B.C. Stillman
School of Physiotherapy, The University of Melbourne, Australia.

Physiotherapy at Erstagårdskliniken, Stockholm

P.T. Kenth Malmström, P.T. Helena Sallnäs
Ersta sjukhus Erstagårdskliniken Hästhagsvägen 9 S-131 33 nacka, Sweden.

Comparison of Brunnstrom and Todd–Davies methods in early rehabilitation of hemiplegic patients

* A.S. Otman, * N. Kose, [†] U. Cavlak
* Hacettepe University, School of Physical Therapy and Rehabilitation, Ankara, Turkey.
[†] Dokuz Eylül University, School of Physical Therapy and Rehabilitation, Izmir, Turkey.

The effect of Bobath concept treatment on the upper extremity of the hemiplegic person

E. Panturin Z. Dvir
School of Physiotherepy, Faculty of Medicine, Tel Aviv University, Israel.

Preliminary study – the reciprocal effect of prone knee bending and straight leg raising in the hemiplegic person
E. Panturin
School of Physiotherapy, School of Medicine, Tel Aviv University, Israel.

Outcome assessment of gross function and qualitative parameters in the recovery of motor function after stroke
G. Preishuber, C. Asteiner, M. - L. Seisenbacher
Rehabilitationszentrum Großgmain - Salzburg, A-5084 Großgmain, Austria.

Physical fitness and aerobics in stroke rehabilitation
G. Rasmussen
Centre for Rehabilitation of Brain Injury, University of Copenhagen, Denmark.

Sailing – also for stroke patients
G. Rasmussen
Centre for Rehabilitation of Brain Injury, University of Copenhagen, Denmark.

Hemiplegic gait – analysis of temporal – distance measurements obtained from ink footprints
M. C. Riley MCSP
Johannesburg Hospital, Private Bag X39, Johannesburg, South Africa.

Concept organizing rehabilitation and care for neurological disabled patients in Germany
W. Schupp
Dep. f. Neurology/Neuropsychology, Fachklinik Enzensberg, Hopfen am See/Füssen, Germany.

Physiotherapy in stroke patients on a neurophysiological basis within a multiprofessional interdisciplinary rehabilitation team
W. Schupp, W. Münz, R. Pfundstein
Dep. f. Neurology and Dep. f. Physiotherapy, Fachklinik Enzensberg, Hopfen am See/ Füssen, Germany.

Sitting balance in elderly people and CVA patients measured by a force-stool system
B. Smits-Engelsman, L. Schomaker
Nijmegen Institute for Cognition and Information, P.O. Box 9104, N 6500 HE, The Netherlands.

Characterization of the pusher syndrome in 143 stroke patients
L. Stukalin, R. Alter, T. Teplytsky, R. Cohen
Stroke Rehabilitation Unit, Beth Rivka Geriatric Medical Center, Petach Tikva, Israel.

Self-reported functional and psychosocial outcome and physiotherapy after stroke: 1 year follow-up study

L. Suhonen MSc PT, O. Joki PT, S. Leisti MD, E. Mälkiä PhD PT, J. Savolainen MD
Department of Physiatrics, Kymenlaakso Central Hospital, FIN-48210 Kotka, Finland.

A model for analysing gait of the stroke patient

A. B. Svendsen, I. Sørensen, R. Larsen, J. Severinsen, G. Madsen
Physiotherapists, Dept. of Rheumatology, Copenhagen County Hospital/University of Copenhagen.

The Development of physiotherapy for patients with neglect

P. Taskinen
Senior Physiotherapist, Master of Health Science, Pirkanmaan Erikoiskuntoutus, Vellamonkatu 11, 33500 Tampere, Finland.

A Clinical method for measuring functional capacity after a stroke

Talvitie. Ulla, Turunen Ulla, T. Ritva, U. Nina, A. Sirpa, S. Sanna
University of Jyväskylä, Department of Health Sciences, P.O. Box 35, FIN-40351 Jyväskylä, Finland.

The spasticity reduction splint as an adjunct to physiotherapy

F. Uygur, K. Armutlu, N. Bek, G. Sener, S. Aksu
Physical Therapy Rehabilitation School-Hacettepe University, Ankara, Turkey.

A stroke protocol for physiotherapy in primary health care

D. van Ravensberg, J. Halfens, R. Oostendorp
National Institute for Research and Postgraduate Education in Physical Therapy/ SWSF, P.O. Box 1161, 3800 BD Amersfoort, The Netherlands.

Orthokinetic therapy for clients with stroke

A. Warden-Flood, [†]R. Burns, [*]R.A. Frick, M.H. Sharpe
School of Physiotherapy, [*] School of Mathematics, University of South Australia, North Terrace, Adelaide, South Australia, 5000. [†] Department of Neurology, Finders Medical Centre, Australia.

Evaluation of a package of domiciliary rehabilitation after discharge from hospital

C. Watson MCSP[*], A.G. Rudd PhD[†], C. Wolfe Phd[‡]
[*] Senior Physiotherapist, Community Stroke Team, St. Thomas' Hospital, London, UK. [†] Consultant Physician, Stroke Unit, St. Thomas' Hospital, London, UK. [‡] Senior Lecturer, Public Health Medicine, St. Thomas' Hospital, London, UK.

Our experience on modifying some PNF techniques in movement recovery of stroke patients

V. Zelev[*], *L. Venova*[†]

[*] Institute of Emergency Medical Care Pirogov, Sofia, Bulgaria. [†] Department of Kinesitherapy, National Sports Academy, Sofia, Bulgaria

Appendix 2: Video abstracts

Effect of intense physiotherapy using the Bobath concept on the capacity of stroke patients for symmetrical walking

J. Goldman-Reznik, B. Stillman
The University of Melbourne School of Physiotherapy, Victoria Australia.

Use of the 'gaitway' system for the assessment of anomalies of gait in patients following stroke and other conditions affecting the pattern of locomotion

H.T. Law Phd
Department of Orthopaedic Surgery, University of Edinburgh Teviot Place, Edinburgh, UK.

Physiotherapy and the City Hospital

A.L. Rold Sørensen, A.W. Brown, K. Eriksen
Physiotherapists at the City Hospital in conjunction with Video Medie Centret, Copenhagen Physiotherapy Department, Kommunehospitalet, Øster Farimagsgade 5, 1399 Copenhagen, Denmark.

Apoplexia – Bobath – working postures

M. Telling, D. Kløvgaard, M. Carlsen, V. Nielsen.
Department of Neurology, Hvidovre Hospital, Kettegård Alle 30, Hvidovre, Denmark.

The rehabilitation of an acute stroke patient in the stroke unit

V. Väyrynen, M. Karinen, T. Aura
OULU University Central Hospital, Department of Physical Medicine and Rehabilitation, Kajaanintie 50, 90220 Oulu, Finland.

Stroke management simplified

M. Wilson, J. Harcourt-Wood, C. Sharratt
Leipoldt House, 59 Mile End Road, Dieprivier, 7800, South Africa.

Appendix 3: Workshops

Lymph drainage in the treatment of stroke
V. Cool
Ecole de Drainage Lymphatique
66300 Llauro, Pyrénées-Orientales, France.

Bobath treatment: a clinical demonstration
O. Gjelsvik
Haukeland Sykehus, N-5021 Norge, Norway.

Functional electrical stimulation
L. Harreby J. Nielsen
Hovedgaden 21 A, DK-3460 Birkerød, Denmark.

PNF in the treatment of upper limb dysfunction
K. Hartmann
Schosterweg 3a, D-48155 Münster, Germany.

Discussion of indicators for good physiotherapy practice in stroke management
B. Ireland
Lemchesvej 24, DK-2900 Hellerup, Denmark.

Facing the challenge of spasticity
M. Johnstone
Derriford House, Linton Bank Drive, West Linton, Peeblesshire, UK.

Perception as a key to motor performances
K. Nielsen
Konrad Adenauerstr 21, D-8876 Jettingen, Germany.

Adverse neural tension
E. Panturin
112/3 Derech Bet Lechem, Jerusalem 93630, Israel.

The trunk in hemiplegia
E. Panturin
112/3 Derech Bet Lechem, Jerusalem 93630, Israel.

Author index

Subject index